Clinical
Impulse-Control
Disorders

MW00984448

Clinical Manual of Impulse-Control Disorders

Edited by

Eric Hollander, M.D.

Dan J. Stein, M.D., Ph.D.

Copyright © 2006 American Psychiatric Publishing, Inc.
ALL RIGHTS RESERVED
Manufactured in the United States of America on acid-free paper
10   09   08   07   06   5   4   3   2   1
First Edition
Typeset in Adobe's AGaramond and Formata.

American Psychiatric Publishing, Inc.
1000 Wilson Boulevard
Arlington, VA 22209-3901
www.appi.org

Library of Congress Cataloging-in-Publication Data
Clinical manual of impulse-control disorders / edited by Eric Hollander, Dan J. Stein.—
1st ed.
     p. ; cm.
    Includes bibliographical references and index.
    ISBN 1-58562-136-6 (pbk. : alk. paper)
    1. Impulse control disorders.
    [DNLM: 1. Impulse Control Disorders. WM 190 C6413 2005] I. Hollander, Eric, 1957–   II. Stein, Dan J.

    RC569.5.I46C56 2005
    616.85'84—dc22
                                   2005008195

British Library Cataloguing in Publication Data
A CIP record is available from the British Library.

Contents

7 Trichotillomania 149

Martin E. Franklin, Ph.D.
David F. Tolin, Ph.D.
Gretchen J. Diefenbach, Ph.D.

8 Kleptomania 175

Jon E. Grant, J.D., M.D.

Contributors

Jean Adès, M.D.
Professor of Psychiatry, Louis Mourier Hospital, Colombes, France

Andrea Allen, Ph.D.
Assistant Professor, Department of Psychiatry, The Mount Sinai School of Medicine, New York, New York

Bryann R. Baker, B.A.
Clinical Research Coordinator, Department of Psychiatry, The Mount Sinai School of Medicine, New York, New York

Donald W. Black, M.D.
Professor, Department of Psychiatry, University of Iowa Roy J. and Lucille A. Carver College of Medicine, Iowa City, Iowa

Emil F. Coccaro, M.D.
Professor, Department of Psychiatry, The University of Chicago, Chicago, Illinois

Melany Danehy, M.D.
Clinical Neuroscience and Psychopharmacology Research Unit, Department of Psychiatry, The University of Chicago, Chicago, Illinois

Gretchen J. Diefenbach, Ph.D.
Staff Psychologist, Anxiety Disorders Center, The Institute of Living/Hartford Hospital, University of Connecticut School of Medicine, Hartford, Connecticut

Stephen J. Donovan, M.D.
Assistant Professor of Clinical Psychiatry, College of Physicians and Surgeons, Columbia University; Research Psychiatrist, New York State Psychiatric Institute, New York, New York

Martin E. Franklin, Ph.D.
Associate Professor of Psychiatry and Director, Center for the Treatment and
Study of Anxiety, Department of Psychiatry, University of Pennsylvania
School of Medicine, Philadelphia, Pennsylvania

Toby D. Goldsmith, M.D.
Assistant Professor, Department of Psychiatry, University of Florida College
of Medicine, Gainesville, Florida

Jon E. Grant, J.D., M.D.
Assistant Professor, Department of Psychiatry and Human Behavior, Brown
Medical School and Butler Hospital, Providence, Rhode Island

Brian Harvey, Ph.D.
Professor of Pharmacology, School of Pharmacy, University of the Northwest,
Potchefstroom, South Africa

Eric Hollander, M.D.
Professor of Psychiatry and Director of Compulsive, Impulsive, and Anxiety
Disorders Program, Department of Psychiatry, The Mount Sinai School of
Medicine, New York, New York

Jessica Kahn
Intern, Department of Psychiatry, The Mount Sinai School of Medicine,
New York, New York

Renu Kotwal, M.D.
Assistant Professor of Clinical Psychiatry, Division of Psychopharmacology
Research, Department of Psychiatry, University of Cincinnati College of
Medicine, Cincinnati, Ohio

Michel Lejoyeux, M.D., Ph.D.
Professor of Psychiatry, Bichat-Claude Bernard Hospital, Paris, France

Susan L. McElroy, M.D.
Professor of Psychiatry and Neuroscience, Division of Psychopharmacology Research, University of Cincinnati College of Medicine, Cincinnati, Ohio

Mary McLoughlin, Ph.D.
Doctor in Psychology, Bichat-Claude Bernard Hospital, Paris, France

Stefano Pallanti, M.D., Ph.D.
Visiting Professor, Department of Psychiatry, The Mount Sinai School of Medicine, New York; Professor of Psychiatry, University of the Studies of Florence, Florence, Italy

Nicolò Baldini Rossi, M.D., Ph.D.
Research Fellow, Department of Psychiatry, The Mount Sinai School of Medicine, New York; Research Fellow, Department of Psychiatry, Neurobiology, Pharmacology, and Biotechnology, University of Pisa, Pisa, Italy

Soraya Seedat, M.B., Ch.B., F.R.C.Psych.
Associate Professor of Psychiatry, University of Stellenbosch, Cape Town, South Africa

Nathan A. Shapira, M.D., Ph.D.
Assistant Professor, Department of Psychiatry, University of Florida College of Medicine, Gainesville, Florida

Daphne Simeon, M.D.
Associate Professor, Department of Psychiatry, Mount Sinai School of Medicine, New York, New York

Dan J. Stein, M.D., Ph.D.
Professor and Chair, Department of Psychiatry, University of Cape Town, Cape Town, South Africa

David F. Tolin, Ph.D.
Director, Anxiety Disorders Center, The Institute of Living/Hartford Hospital; Assistant Professor of Psychiatry, University of Connecticut School of Medicine, Hartford, Connecticut

Preface

The impulse-control disorders (ICDs) have burst onto the scene in psychiatry, as well as in popular culture, in recent years. In psychiatry, this may be due to an ascertainment bias, because clinicians and researchers are doing a better job screening for and diagnosing these conditions and new types of ICDs have been proposed. The media is also intrigued by what they view as bad behavior, especially among celebrities in the public eye. However, changes in our society and technological developments may also have contributed to the importance of ICDs. Moral issues have been of prime concern in recent presidential elections in the United States. Changes in the nuclear and extended family, examples of impulse dyscontrol in the popular media, and the development of the Internet may have all contributed to increases in impulsive behavior.

This clinical manual provides cutting-edge, concise, and practical information about the ICDs for use by researchers, clinicians, family members, and individuals with these disorders. Hollander and colleagues (Chapter 1) describe the conceptualization and classification of the ICDs, including the phenomenology, assessment, and classification of impulsivity as a core symptom domain that cuts across and drives the ICDs. Cognitive aspects and dimensional approaches to impulsivity, comparison with compulsivity, and assessment tools are described. The impact of comorbidity on course of illness and treatment response are also highlighted.

Coccaro and Danehy (Chapter 2) highlight the one ICD characterized by impulsive aggression, intermittent explosive disorder (IED). They describe how the nosology of IED-R (revised) was developed for research studies, how the disorder is frequently overlooked, and how it is frequently comorbid with bipolar, other impulse-control, and Cluster B personality disorders. Genetic contributions, biological correlates, and functional neurocircuitry of the disorder are described. Finally, psychosocial and pharmacological treatments of value are described.

Donovan (Chapter 3) describes childhood conduct disorder and the antisocial spectrum. Conduct disorder and oppositional defiant disorder, which are examples of the disruptive behavior disorders of childhood, are common, frequently comorbid with attention-deficit/hyperactivity disorder, expressed as antisocial behavior that violates social norms, and mediated by affective or impulsive aggression. Various underlying mechanisms may contribute to aggression, and this helps inform the assessment and treatment of such behavior.

Simeon (Chapter 4) describes self-injurious behaviors (SIBs), which currently do not fit neatly into the DSM classification system. Four major categories of SIB have been proposed, including stereotypic, major, compulsive, and impulsive. The relationship of SIB to impulsive aggression and childhood trauma is described. Of interest, the pharmacological and psychosocial treatment of SIB differs based on the category of SIB.

Allen and Hollander (Chapter 5) highlight sexual compulsions, which have been conceptualized as addictive, impulsive, or compulsive disorders. They may be proposed for DSM-V as impulsive/compulsive sexual behavior disorder, but are currently referred to as nonparaphilic sexual addictions and may or may not occur with paraphilias. More work is needed in developing effective pharmacological and psychosocial treatments for this increasingly recognized problem with serious public health implications.

McElroy and Kotwal (Chapter 6) describe the history of binge eating as a symptom and discuss whether it should be considered as an ICD distinct from other eating, compulsive, and affective disorders. The prevalence of binge eating is influenced by how broadly it is defined, but it is associated with serious medical complications and psychopathology. It is clearly a highly familial disorder, and a number of successful strategies are emerging to reduce binge eating and its complications.

Franklin and colleagues (Chapter 7) describe trichotillomania, an ICD characterized by hair pulling that results in hair loss. The functional impairment of this disorder may be out of proportion to the hair loss, and it may be related to phenomena such as obsessive-compulsive disorder (OCD), skin picking, and nail biting. A hair-pulling cycle may be triggered by internal or contextual cues and may be reinforced by various sensations. Randomized controlled trials have been conducted, but more effective treatments are needed.

Grant (Chapter 8) highlights kleptomania, or the failure to resist impulses to steal, associated with arousal, remorse, and functional impairment. The disorder may be heterogeneous; shares features with mood, anxiety, ICD, and addictive disorders; and has had limited study to date. Early evidence suggests that opioid antagonists, selective serotonin reuptake inhibitors (SSRIs), mood stabilizers, and behavioral treatments may be effective.

Black (Chapter 9) describes compulsive shopping, or poorly controlled shopping urges leading to functional impairment, which is more common in females and has only recently been studied. Psychiatric comorbidity is the rule rather than the exception with this disorder. Self-help, financial counseling, psychodynamic, marital, and behavioral treatments have been examined, and trials with SSRIs have been mixed, perhaps owing to the high placebo response rate.

Lejoyeux and colleagues (Chapter 10) highlight pyromania, or impulsive behavior leading to motiveless arson. Pyromania must be differentiated from arson, and pyromania frequently occurs with depression or alcohol dependence. Psychodynamic aspects of pyromania as well as the disorder's relationship to impulsivity, sensation seeking, and the OCD spectrum are described. Few who repetitively set fires are caught, and few of the set fires are committed by people with pyromania, but the consequences are important.

Pallanti and colleagues (Chapter 11) describe pathological gambling as maladaptive and suggest that the disorder is rapidly growing in association with the growth of legalized gambling and Internet gambling, especially among the young. It shares many features of addictive disorders and may thus be considered a behavioral addiction. It may also be frequently comorbid with attention-deficit/hyperactivity disorder (ADHD), the broader bipolar spectrum, and OCD. Genetic contributions and the functional neurocircuitry of the disorder are being elucidated. Psychosocial treatments include self-help (Gamblers Anonymous) and behavioral and psychodynamic treatments. Medication treatments have been adapted from treatments of OCD (SSRIs), bipolar disorder (mood stabilizers), ADHD (dopaminergic agents), and addictive disorders (opiate antagonists) with some real successes.

Finally, Goldsmith and Shapira (Chapter 12) describe problematic Internet use, or Internet addiction, which can range from excessive seeking of medical information to dangerous sexual behaviors facilitated by the Internet. Treatment studies are still in their infancy.

Stein and colleagues (Chapter 13) describe themes for treatment that run throughout the ICDs. These are complex conditions, and currently no U.S. Food and Drug Administration–approved medication or standardized cognitive-behavioral therapy manual exists for the ICDs. Correct diagnosis is the first step, and assessment of comorbidity is essential for choosing the correct treatment approach. Antidepressants, mood stabilizers, antipsychotics, stimulants, and opioid antagonists may have a role in the management of impulsivity, and flexible and eclectic psychotherapies also seem reasonable. These patients represent a real challenge to clinicians, and emerging research from cognitive-affective neuroscience models may yield new treatments for impulsivity.

Eric Hollander, M.D.
Dan J. Stein, M.D., Ph.D.

Conceptualizing and Assessing Impulse-Control Disorders

Eric Hollander, M.D.
Bryann R. Baker, B.A.
Jessica Kahn
Dan J. Stein, M.D., Ph.D.

This chapter provides an overview of the conceptualization and assessment of impulse-control disorders (ICDs). In addition, to fully understand the ICDs, it is also helpful to describe the nature of impulsivity as a core symptom domain that contributes to these disorders.

This work was supported in part by the National Institute on Drug Abuse (grant 5 RO1 DA10234–03) and the Paula and Bill Oppenheim Foundation.

Conceptualization and Classification of the Impulse-Control Disorders

ICDs are of increasing importance to clinicians and researchers as the consequences of impulsivity and ICDs affect society to an ever greater degree. Of interest, changes in society and new technological developments may partially account for a rise in these ICDs. With the development of the Internet and its unlimited access to sex, gambling, shopping, and stock trading, there has been a subsequent rise in impulsive behavior and even new forms of impulsive behavior, such as Internet addiction. With the rise in legalized gambling in the United States (48 states have legalized gambling) and increased access to casinos and Internet gambling, pathological gambling is increasingly common. Additionally, the amount of retail sales lost to shoplifting is on the rise and in 2002 totaled 10 billion U.S. dollars (Hollinger and Davis 2003). Clinicians now see more patients in their practice presenting with ICDs and even newer forms of ICDs and therefore need to know how to classify them appropriately.

Whereas ICDs were once conceptualized as either addictive or compulsive behaviors, they are now classified within the DSM-IV-TR (American Psychiatric Association 2000) ICD category. These include intermittent explosive disorder (failure to resist aggressive impulses), kleptomania (failure to resist urges to steal items), pyromania (failure to resist urges to set fires), pathological gambling (failure to resist urges to gamble), and trichotillomania (failure to resist urges to pull one's hair) (Table 1–1). However, behaviors characteristic of these disorders may be notable in individuals as symptoms of another mental disorder. If the symptoms progress to such a point that they occur in distinct, frequent episodes and begin to interfere with the person's normal functioning, they may then be classified as a distinct ICD.

There are also a number of other disorders that are not included as a distinct category but are categorized as ICDs not otherwise specified in DSM-IV-TR. These include sexual compulsions, compulsive shopping, skin picking, and Internet addiction. One proposal for the research agenda leading up to DSM-V is to include these emerging disorders as new and unique ICDs rather than lumping them together as ICDs not otherwise specified. These disorders are unique in that they share features of both impulsivity and compulsivity and might be labeled as ICDs. Patients afflicted with these disorders engage in the behavior to increase arousal. However, there is a compulsive

Table 1–1. DSM-IV-TR impulse-control disorders

Impulse-control disorders not elsewhere classified
Intermittent explosive disorder
Kleptomania
Pyromania
Pathological gambling
Trichotillomania

Impulse-control disorders not otherwise specified
Impulsive-compulsive sexual disorder
Impulsive-compulsive self-injurious disorder
Impulsive-compulsive Internet usage disorder
Impulsive-compulsive buying disorder

Other disorders with impulsivity
Childhood conduct disorders
Binge eating disorder
Bulimia nervosa
Paraphilias
    Exhibitionism
    Fetishism
    Frotteurism
    Pedophilia
    Sexual masochism
    Sexual sadism
    Transvestic fetishism
    Voyeurism
    Paraphilia not otherwise specified
Bipolar disorder
Attention-deficit/hyperactivity disorder
Substance use disorders
Cluster B personality disorders
Neurological disorder with disinhibition

Source. American Psychiatric Association 2000.

component in which the patient continues to engage in the behavior to decrease dysphoria. An area of discussion for DSM-V may include whether these disorders should be recognized as distinct ICDs.

In DSM-IV-TR, ICDs are characterized by five stages of symptomatic behavior (Table 1–2). First is the increased sense of tension or arousal, followed by the failure to resist the urge to act. Third, there is a heightened sense of arousal. Once the act has been completed, there is a sense of relief from the urge. Finally, the patient experiences guilt and remorse at having committed the act.

Table 1–2. Core features of impulse-control disorders

Essential features	Failure to resist an impulse, drive, or temptation to perform an act that is harmful to the person or to others
Before the act	The individual feels an increasing sense of tension or arousal
At the time of committing the act	The individual experiences pleasure, gratification, or relief
After the act	The individual experiences a sense of relief from the urge
The individual may or may not feel regret, self-reproach, or guilt

Source. American Psychiatric Association 2000.

Impulsivity

To properly conceptualize ICDs, it is helpful to understand the role of impulsivity within them. Impulsivity is a defining characteristic of many psychiatric illnesses, even those not classified as ICDs, including Cluster B personality disorders such as borderline and antisocial personality disorder, neurological disorders characterized by disinhibited behavior, attention-deficit/hyperactivity disorder (ADHD), substance and alcohol abuse, conduct disorder, binge eating, bulimia, and paraphilias. It is important for clinicians to recognize that individuals who are prone to impulsivity and ICDs are often afflicted with a cluster of related conditions including sexual compulsions, substance use disorders, and posttraumatic stress disorder and to screen for comorbid conditions such as bipolar spectrum disorders and ADHD that contribute to impulsivity (Figure 1–1).

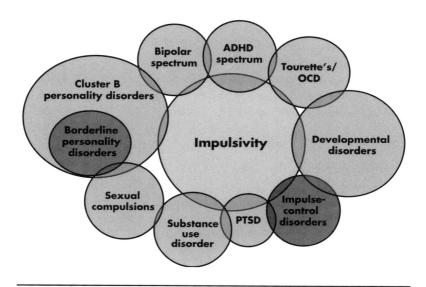

Figure 1–1. Impulsive disorder spectrum.
ADHD = attention-deficit/hyperactivity disorder; OCD = obsessive-compulsive disorder; PTSD = posttraumatic stress disorder.
Source. Hollander E: "Treating Impulsivity in Impulse Control and Personality Disorders." Paper presented at the 156th annual meeting of the American Psychiatric Association, San Francisco, CA, May 2003.

Impulsivity research has been conducted both in disorders characterized by impulsivity, such as borderline personality disorder, antisocial personality disorder, and conduct disorder, and in traditional ICDs such as intermittent explosive disorder. As such, the basic tenets of impulsivity can be applied both to the ICDs and to other related psychiatric conditions.

Impulsivity—the failure to resist an impulse, drive, or temptation that is potentially harmful to oneself or others—is both a common clinical problem and a core feature of human behavior. An impulse is rash and lacks deliberation. It may be sudden and ephemeral, or a steady rise in tension may reach a climax in an explosive expression of the impulse, which may result in careless actions without regard for self or others. Impulsivity is evidenced behaviorally as carelessness, an underestimated sense of harm, extroversion, impatience, including the inability to delay gratification, and a tendency toward risk taking, pleasure, and sensation seeking (Hollander et al. 2002). What makes an impulse pathological is an inability to resist it and its expression. The nature of impulsivity as a core symptom domain within the ICDs allows it to be distinguished as either a symptom or a distinct disorder, much in the same way as anxiety or depression.

Cognitive Aspects of Impulsivity

Three major cognitive components play a role in modulating impulsivity. The first is the *inability to delay gratification.* Individuals with disorders involving impulsivity make decisions with the goal of attaining an immediate reward, regardless of how small the reward or what the likely long-term negative consequences of the decision are. The second cognitive component is *distractibility,* or the inability to maintain sustained attention on a particular task. Finally, impulsivity is characterized cognitively by *disinhibition,* or the inability to restrain behavior in a manner that would be expected based on cultural norms and constraints.

Dimensional Approaches to Impulsivity

Impulsivity can also be approached from a dimensional standpoint as occurring along a spectrum of compulsivity and impulsivity (Figure 1–2). On one end of the spectrum are compulsive individuals, who are highly risk aversive; they perceive their environment as risky and threatening, and they carry out ritualistic behaviors to neutralize the threat and reduce their anxiety. On the opposite end of the spectrum are impulsive individuals, who tend to underestimate the degree of harm in the environment and therefore repeatedly engage in high-risk behaviors, after which they fail to learn from their errors in judgment. In the middle are individuals with conditions such as Tourette's syndrome, trichotillomania, and autism, which have features of both compulsively driven behaviors to reduce anxiety and impulsive behaviors associated with arousal, pleasure, or gratification. It is not unusual for both components to be present in the same individual, either simultaneously or at different times in the course of the same illness.

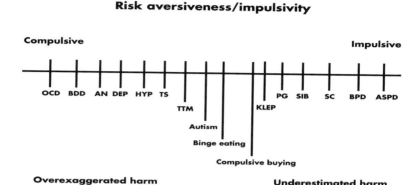

Figure 1–2. A dimensional approach to impulsivity and compulsivity. AN = anorexia nervosa; ASPD = antisocial personality disorder; BDD = body dysmorphic disorder; BPD = borderline personality disorder; DEP = depersonalization disorder; HYP=hypochondriasis; KLEP=kleptomania; OCD=obsessive-compulsive disorder; PG = pathological gambling; SC = sexual compulsions; SIB = self-injurious behavior; TS=Tourette's syndrome; TTM=trichotillomania. *Source.* Hollander E, Rosen J: "Impulsivity." *Journal of Psychopharmacology* 14 (suppl 1):S39–S44, 2000.

Contrast With Compulsivity

The driving force behind the behavior is what distinguishes compulsivity from impulsivity. Whereas the former is driven by an effort to reduce anxiety, the latter is driven by an effort to obtain arousal and gratification. However, individuals at both ends of the spectrum have in common the inability to refrain from repetitive behaviors (Hollander et al. 2000b; Stein et al. 1993). In addition to this difference in motivation or drive between ICDs and obsessive-compulsive disorder (OCD), *impulsive* disorders are usually perceived to be ego-syntonic, whereas *compulsive* disorders tend to be more ego-dystonic. Instead of being the dimensional opposite of OCDs, ICDs possibly represent a different phenomenological manifestation of a group of disorders sharing the feature of decreased capacity to extinguish motor responses to affective states. In fact, ICDs retain similarities to obsessive-compulsive and related disorders, which are characterized by engagement in repetitive behaviors, often in response to obsessions that are associated with anxiety. Although ICDs begin in response to an urge to engage in an action that is pleasurable, over time some behavior may become compulsively driven in an attempt to reduce anxiety and discomfort.

Impulsive Aggression

In several disorders, such as intermittent explosive disorder, impulsivity is linked to aggression. *Impulsive aggression* is defined as deliberate, nonpremeditated aggressive acts, either of a verbal or physical nature, that are directed at another person, object, or the self and intended to cause harm (Coccaro 1998; Moeller et al. 2001). Impulsive aggressive behaviors are associated with morbidity and mortality, leading to profound impairment in social, vocational, and family functioning. Also, impulsive aggressive behaviors are often at the root of violent crimes such as rape, murder and assault, and accidents (Hollander et al. 2002). Patients with Cluster B personality disorders such as antisocial personality disorder may present with both premeditated aggression and impulsive aggression, and these individuals are frequently seen in forensic settings and in the legal system. Also, impulsivity and aggression have been directly linked to suicide (Busch et al. 2003; Fawcett et al. 1987; Hall et al. 1999). It has been asserted that a motivation for suicide may not be solely despair, but an urgent and uninhibited impulse to act on self-directed anger (Hollander et al. 2002).

Not all impulsive acts are aggressive, but impulsivity and aggression can coincide in the same action. For example, self-mutilation is usually an impulse to act aggressively toward the self. By cutting oneself with no premeditation, both impulsivity and self-aggression intersect within a singular behavior. When behavior is simultaneously impulsive and aggressive, it is referred to as impulsive aggression.

Conduct Disorder

One disorder that exemplifies the link between impulsivity and aggression is conduct disorder. Symptoms of conduct disorder usually manifest in early childhood or adolescence and include aggressive actions that cause physical harm to others, damage to property, deceitfulness, theft, and serious violations of rules. Other hallmarks of conduct disorder are risk taking and impulsive behavior, such as early onset of sexual behavior, drinking, smoking, drug use, and reckless behavior. A person afflicted with conduct disorder may display aggressive features, but it takes an impulsive nature to carry out the reckless actions associated with conduct disorder. It is the combination of aggression and impulsivity that causes the person to act out on his or her aggression in an impulsive manner. Additionally, conduct disorder is often a childhood precursor for the development of adult ICDs.

However, impulsivity and aggression are not constantly synonymous. For example, pathological gamblers are impulsive but not necessarily aggressive. Similarly, a premeditated murder is aggressive but not necessarily impulsive. Although these traits or symptoms can be expressed in the same action, not all impulsive actions are aggressive nor vice versa.

Comorbidity Influences Treatment

In patients with an ICD, comorbid disorders are often present, including bipolar spectrum disorders, substance abuse, OCD, anxiety disorders, ADHD, and depressive disorders (Hollander et al. 2000a; Pallanti et al. 2002) (Figure 1–3). When treating ICDs, it is crucial for clinicians to identify the comorbid disorders precisely because they have an important impact on the treatment of ICDs. For example, in pathological gambling, one pharmacological approach that has been investigated is the use of selective serotonin reuptake inhibitors (SSRIs; Hollander et al. 1998, 2000b). However, not all pathological gamblers respond to SSRIs. Based on previous findings suggesting a connection between impulsivity and bipolarity (including a comorbidity rate of about 30% between the two), our group undertook a single-blind study in which patients were treated with either lithium or valproate (Pallanti et al. 2002). Fifty-two percent of the lithium-treated pathological gambling patients and 57.9% of the valproate-treated pathological gambling patients responded to treatment (Pallanti et al. 2002). In a subsequent placebo-controlled trial of sustained-release lithium in 40 patients who met criteria for both pathological gambling and the broader bipolar spectrum (including bipolar II disorder, hypomania, mixed states, rapid cycling, or cyclothymia), lithium was significantly superior to placebo in reducing both impulsive gambling and mania scores (Hollander et al. 2005). It remains unclear whether improvement in impulsivity reduces affective instability, or improvement in affective instability results in decreased impulsivity. Thus, it is essential for the clinician to identify comorbid disorders and choose the treatment accordingly.

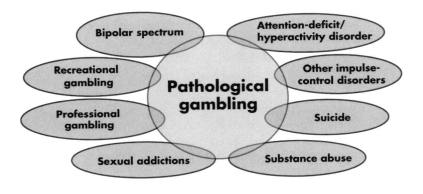

Figure 1–3.   Pathological gambling: presentation and comorbidity.
Source.   Hollander E: "Treating Impulsivity in Impulse Control and Personality Disorders." Paper presented at the 156th annual meeting of the American Psychiatric Association, San Francisco, CA, May 2003.

Impact of Gender

The ICDs, and more specifically impulsivity, are manifested in different ways across the genders. Prevalence rates within all of the ICDs have not been thoroughly researched; however, pathological gambling, pyromania, sexual compulsions, and intermittent explosive disorder appear to be more prevalent in males, whereas kleptomania, trichotillomania, compulsive shopping, self-injurious behavior, and binge eating disorder seem to be more prevalent in females (Table 1–3). In these disorders, outwardly directed and aggressive impulsive behaviors are more common in men, whereas inwardly directed, nonaggressive, impulsive behaviors predominate in women. These gender differences could conceivably be the result of genetic factors, hormonal differences (i.e., testosterone), or differences in the modulation of serotonin and other peptides such as vasopressin (Coccaro et al. 1998) but may also derive from sociocultural factors.

Table 1–3.   Gender predominance in the impulse-control disorders

Male	Female
Pathological gambling	Kleptomania
Intermittent explosive behavior	Trichotillomania
Pyromania	Self-injurious behavior
Sexual compulsions	Compulsive buying
	Binge eating

Impulse-Control Disorders and Cluster B Personality Disorders

It was previously thought that ICDs and personality disorders (such as borderline personality disorder) were mutually exclusive (DSM-IV; American Psychiatric Association 1994). However, it is now clear that impulsive aggression as a symptom domain within Cluster B personality disorders may progress to the point where it is considered a separate ICD (i.e., intermittent explosive disorder). This has been clarified in DSM-IV-TR; patients may be diagnosed with both a personality disorder and an ICD, and this is frequently the case. For example, patients with borderline personality disorder might also meet criteria for kleptomania, trichotillomania, self-injurious behavior, or binge eating disorder.

Biological Basis of Impulsivity That Informs the Conceptualization of Impulse-Control Disorders

The following is a brief summary of the biological basis of impulsivity that helps to inform the conceptualization of the ICDs. However, a lengthy description of the neurobiology of impulsivity and the ICDs is beyond the scope of this chapter and is elucidated in greater detail in subsequent chapters. Several neurotransmitters are implicated in the manifestation of impulsivity. Extensive evidence in animals and humans suggests that a deficiency of central serotonin (5-hydroxytryptamine [5-HT]) is associated with greater impulsivity (Brown et al. 1989; Higley and Linnoila 1997; Linnoila et al. 1983). Also, populations with high levels of impulsivity, such as bullfighters (Carrasco et al. 1999) and bulimic patients (Carrasco et al. 2000), present with lower levels of platelet monoamine oxidase. Additionally other neurotransmitters, such as γ-aminobutyric acid (GABA), norepinephrine, and dopamine, have been linked to modulation of impulsivity and aggression (Oquendo and Mann 2000).

Lesion studies also help to identify a neuroanatomic basis of impulsivity (Hollander and Evers 2001). In rats, lesions in the nucleus accumbens, orbitofrontal cortex, and basolateral amygdala are associated with impulsive choice on delayed reward tasks (Cardinal 2001; Mobini et al. 2002; Winstanley et al. 2004). Frontal lobe lesions in humans are correlated with impulsive behavior on cognitive risk-taking tasks (Miller 1992). Specifically, patients with lesions in the region of the ventromedial prefrontal cortex perform more impulsively in delayed reinforcement tasks (Bechara et al. 1994, 2000). Patients with lesions of the orbitofrontal cortex are more impulsive on self-report measures and cognitive-behavioral measures than patients with lesions in the prefrontal cortex and normal control subjects (Berlin et al. 2004). Of interest, there may be a different motivational salience that alters the functional neurocircuitry for each disorder. For example, pathological gamblers may activate the neurocircuitry of goal-directed behavior in response to monetary stimuli, whereas binge eaters do so in response to food and sexually compulsive patients in response to sexual stimuli.

Genetic Basis of Impulse-Control Disorders That Inform Conceptualization

Some studies support strong genetic contributions to the ICDs. In pathological gamblers, 20% have a first-degree relative who is also a pathological gambler (Lesieur 1988). Twin pair studies have found a common genetic vulnerability for both pathological gambling and alcohol dependence (Eisen et al. 1998, 2001; Slutske et al. 2001). Studies support an association between a major mood disorder and alcohol and substance abuse in first-degree relatives of individuals with kleptomania and pathological gambling (Linden et al. 1986; Ramirez et al. 1983). Associations between anxiety disorders in the families of individuals with kleptomania and violent behavior and ADHD in families of individuals with intermittent explosive disorder have also been reported (McElroy et al. 1991).

Assessment of Impulsivity and the Impulse-Control Disorders

Differentiating Symptoms From a Disorder

Many patients present with symptoms of ICDs such as gambling or self-injurious behavior, and it is important to establish whether they are symptoms of another disorder or a distinct ICD. For example, not all gambling is pathological, and it is clinically important to differentiate the pathological gambler from the recreational or professional gambler. The latter are capable of accurately calculating risks or odds, are able to control the impulse to gamble, and have no functional impairment as a consequence of gambling. Pathological gamblers, by contrast, allow gambling to severely interfere with their daily lives. They may lose their spouses and social networks, their jobs, and their savings to gambling. They may be forced to declare bankruptcy or may turn to embezzlement to obtain money for gambling. The distress produced by these secondary complications may cause such patients to gamble at a higher frequency, resulting in a downward spiral into financial, vocational, and social ruin (Hollander et al. 2000a). Additionally, biological factors may distinguish pathological from nonpathological gambling populations.

Assessment Measures

Currently, measures available to assess ICDs are limited. Most of the commonly used measures, such as the Barratt Impulsiveness Scale Version 11 (BIS-11) and the Overt Aggression Scale–Modified (OAS-M) evaluate the symptoms of impulsivity or aggression. Other scales, such as the South Oaks Gambling Screen and the Psychiatric Institute Trichotillomania Scale, are used to screen for the presence of the disorder. Self-report assessments such as the Buss-Durkee Hostility Inventory (BDHI), the Hostility and Direction of Hostility Questionnaire (HDHQ), and the Spielberger State-Trait Anger Expression Inventory (STAEI) evaluate impulsive aggression. Of note, existing scales initially developed for OCD, such as the Yale-Brown Obsessive-Compulsive Scale (Y-BOCS), have been modified to measure the severity of specific ICDs. These variations of the original test are administered in the same manner and use items pertaining specifically to the given behavior. Four such modifications of the Y-BOCS have been created for pathological gambling, compulsive shopping, binge eating, and sexual compulsions. Laboratory measures of impulsivity are beyond the scope of this chapter and are not described here.

The BIS-11 measures impulsivity in terms of three domains: motor impulsiveness, nonplanning impulsiveness, and attentional impulsiveness. By evaluating a patient's severity in each of the three domains, the scale is able to provide a description of impulsivity in mentally healthy individuals. It is a clinician-rated scale that should take 10–15 minutes to complete the 30 items. When tested with undergraduates, the mean score averaged 63.8 ± 0.2 but in male prison inmates it averaged 76.3 ± 11.9 (Patton et al. 1995). The BIS-11 is among the more commonly used measures of impulsivity. This is due to a number of factors. It is a simple scale to administer and it is widely known. However, at extreme levels its sensitivity decreases, and the items on the test are aimed at a more middle-class population.

The OAS-M is a clinician-rated, semistructured interview that measures the severity and frequency of aggressive behavior (Coccaro et al. 1991). The OAS-M measures current levels of aggression through four subscales: verbal assault, assault against objects, assault against self, assault against others. The scale has high interrater reliability (Endicott et al. 2002). The OAS-M is often used to measure impulsive aggression.

Self-report assessments include the BDHI, the HDHQ, and the STAEI. As their names imply, all three are used to measure a patient's impulsive aggression through a variety of items and questions.

The BDHI contains 75 true/false items broken up into eight subscales that measure hostility, aggression, and danger. The primary goal of the scale is to determine the various components of hostility, both as an overall characteristic and as a complex trait, in a subject. Although this measure is the best known and oldest hostility scale, there are still no established norms, so interpretation of individual scores is difficult. The true/false format of the scale decreases sensitivity, and at extreme levels sensitivity is further reduced. It has also been noted that the test focuses on feelings of aggression, which aggressive individuals are apt to misrepresent, and neglects severe aggression entirely. However, its high test-retest reliability allows it to be an effective tool in medical research.

A much longer scale for aggression is the Anger, Irritability and Assault Questionnaire (AIAQ). Like the BDHI, it is a self-report. The 210 items are rated on a scale of one to four and each question is rated on three time frames (past week, past month, my adulthood). There are five subscales from which the scores are computed. In addition, the scale has no standardized norms and takes about 50 minutes for the newer version to be completed. Validity testing has shown the AIAQ to be a useful tool in determining impulsive aggression, and its efficacy has been shown in both clinical and research purposes.

It is true that measuring impulsivity is difficult, especially due to large discrepancies between a self-report and an observer report. Impulsivity is not socially acceptable; therefore patients tend to answer questions untruthfully. In addition, an individual may not appear or act as impulsively in an interview as he or she does at home or in public. Some patients may even act more antagonistically in the interview as a result of the stresses inherent in the nature of the interview. Thus, an accurate concept of the severity of the patient's disorder is most clearly obtained with a combination of both types of scales.

Conclusion

ICDs are a growing concern to society. ICDs by definition follow a similar pattern of mounting tension before the act, pleasurable feelings and relief from tension while committing the act, and a sense of guilt and remorse after committing the act. DSM-IV-TR specifically describes five ICDs, although in DSM-V four new ICD diagnoses may be added as data regarding epidemiology, classification, neurobiology, and treatment of specific ICDs not otherwise specified are reported. Much progress has been made in our understanding of the ICDs, but more research is clearly needed to fully characterize the underlying phenomenology, classification, and assessment of these growing problems.

References

American Psychiatric Association: Diagnostic and Statistical Manual of Mental Disorders, 4th Edition. Washington, DC, American Psychiatric Association, 1994

American Psychiatric Association: Diagnostic and Statistical Manual of Mental Disorders, 4th Edition, Text Revision. Washington, DC, American Psychiatric Association, 2000

Bechara A, Damasio AR, Damasio H, et al: Insensitivity to future consequences following damage to human prefrontal cortex. Cognition 50:7–15, 1994

Bechara A, Tranel D, Damasio H: Characterization of the decision-making deficit of patients with ventromedial prefrontal cortex lesions. Brain 123:2189–2202, 2000

Berlin HA, Rolls ET, Kischka U: Impulsivity, time perception, emotion and reinforcement sensitivity in patients with orbitofrontal cortex lesions. Brain 127:1108–1126, 2004

Brown CS, Kent TA, Bryant SG, et al: Blood platelet uptake of serotonin in episodic aggression. Psychiatry Res 27:5–12, 1989

Busch KA, Fawcett J, Jacobs DG: Clinical correlates of inpatient suicide. J Clin Psychiatry 64:14–19, 2003

Cardinal RN: Impulsive choice induced in rats by lesions of the nucleus accumbens core. Science 292:2499–2501, 2001

Carrasco JL, Saiz-Ruiz J, Diaz-Marsa M, et al: Low platelet monoamine oxidase activity in sensation-seeking bullfighters. CNS Spectr 4:21–24, 1999

Carrasco JL, Diaz-Marsa M, Hollander E, et al: Decreased platelet monoamine oxidase activity in female bulimia nervosa. Eur Neuropsychopharmacol 10:113–117, 2000

Coccaro EF: Impulsive aggression: a behavior in search of clinical definition. Harv Rev Psychiatry 5:336–339, 1998

Coccaro EF, Harvey PD, Kupsaw-Lawrence E, et al: Development of neuropharmacologically based behavioral assessments of impulsive aggressive behavior. J Neuropsychiatry Clin Neurosci 3:S44–S51, 1991

Coccaro EF, Kavoussi RJ, Hauger RL, et al: Cerebrospinal fluid vasopressin levels: correlates with aggression serotonin function in personality-disordered subjects. Arch Gen Psychiatry 55:708–714, 1998

Eisen SA, Lin N, Lyons MJ, et al: Familial influences on gambling behavior: an analysis of 3359 twin pairs. Addiction 93:1375–1384, 1998

Eisen SA, Slutske WS, Lyons MJ, et al: The genetics of pathological gambling. Semin Clin Neuropsychiatry 6:195–204, 2001

Endicott J, Tracy K, Burt D, et al: A novel approach to assess inter-rater reliability in the use of the Over Aggression Scale-Modified. Psychiatry Res 112:153–159, 2002

Fawcett J, Scheftner W, Clark D, et al: Clinical predictors of suicide in patients with major affective disorders: a controlled prospective study. Am J Psychiatry 144:35–40, 1987

Hall RCW, Platt DE, Hall RCW: Suicide risk assessment: a review of risk factors for suicide in 100 patients who made severe suicide attempts. Psychosomatics 40:18–27, 1999

Higley JD, Linnoila M: Low central nervous system serotonergic activity is traitlike and correlates with impulsive behavior: a nonhuman primate model investigating genetic and environmental influences on neurotransmission. Ann N Y Acad Sci 836:39–56, 1997

Hollander E: Impulsive and compulsive disorders, in Neuropsychopharmacology: The Fifth Generation in Progress. Edited by Davis K, Charney D, Coyle J, et al. New York, American College of Neuropsychopharmacology, 2002, pp 1591–1757

Hollander E, Evers M: New developments in impulsivity. Lancet 358:949–950, 2001

Hollander E, DeCaria CM, Mari E, et al: Short-term single-blind fluvoxamine treatment of pathological gambling. Am J Psychiatry 155:1781–1783, 1998

Hollander E, Buchalter AJ, DeCaria CM: Pathological gambling. Psychiatr Clin North Am 23:629–642, 2000a

Hollander E, DeCaria CM, Finkell JN, et al: A randomized double-blind fluvoxamine/placebo crossover trial in pathological gambling. Biol Psychiatry 47:813–817, 2000b

Hollander E, Posner N, Cherkasky S: Neuropsychiatric aspects of impulse-control disorders, in American Psychiatric Press Textbook of Neuropsychiatry. Edited by Yudofsky SC, Hales RE. Washington, DC, American Psychiatric Publishing, 2002, pp 579–596

Hollander E, Pallanti S, Baldini-Rossi N, et al: Sustained release lithium/placebo treatment response in bipolar spectrum pathological gamblers. Am J Psychiatry 162:137–145

Hollinger RC, Davis JL: 2002 national retail security survey: final report. Available at: http://web.soc.ufl.edu/SRP/finalreport_2002.pdf. Accessed October 1, 2003

Lesieur HR: The female pathological gambler, in Gambling Research: Proceedings of the Seventh International Conference on Gambling and Risk Taking. Edited by Eadington WR. Reno, NV, Bureau of Business & Economic Research, University of Nevada, 1988

Linden RD, Pope HG Jr, Jonas JM: Pathological gambling and major affective disorder: preliminary findings. J Clin Psychiatry 47:201–203, 1986

Linnoila M, Virkkunen M, Scheinin M, et al: Low cerebrospinal fluid 5-hydroxyindoleacetic acid concentration differentiates impulsive from non-impulsive violent behavior. Life Sci 33:2609–2614, 1983

McElroy SL, Hudson JI, Pope HG, et al: Kleptomania: clinical characteristics and associated psychopathology. Psychol Med 21:93–108, 1991

Miller LA: Impulsivity, risk-taking, and the ability to synthesize fragmented information after frontal lobectomy. Neuropsychologia 30:69–79, 1992

Mobini S, Body S, Ho MY, et al: Effects of lesions of the orbitofrontal cortex on sensitivity to delayed and probabilistic reinforcement. Psychopharmacology 160:290–298, 2002

Moeller FG, Barratt ES, Dougherty DM, et al: Psychiatric aspects of impulsivity. Am J Psychiatry 158:1783–1793, 2001

Oquendo MA, Mann JJ: The biology of impulsivity and suicidality. Psychiatr Clin North Am 23:11–25, 2000

Pallanti S, Quercioli L, Sood E, et al: Lithium and valproate treatment of pathological gambling: a randomized single-blind study. J Clin Psychiatry 63:559–564, 2002

Patton JH, Stanford MS, Barratt ES: Factor structure of the Barratt impulsiveness scale. J Clin Psychol 51:768–774, 1995

Ramirez LF, McCormick RA, Russo AM, et al: Patterns of substance abuse in pathological gamblers undergoing treatment. Addict Behav 8:425–428, 1983

Slutske WS, Eisen S, Xian H, et al: A twin study of the relationship between pathological gambling and antisocial personality disorder. J Abnorm Psychol 110:297–308, 2001

Stein DJ, Hollander E, Liebowitz MR: Neurobiology of impulsivity and the impulse control disorders. J Neuropsychiatry Clin Neurosci 5:9–17, 1993

Winstanley CA, Theobald DE, Cardinal RN, et al: Contrasting roles of basolateral amygdala and orbitofrontal cortex in impulsive choice. J Neurosci 24:4718–4722, 2004

2

Intermittent Explosive Disorder

Emil F. Coccaro, M.D.
Melany Danehy, M.D.

Intermittent explosive disorder (IED) is a DSM diagnosis that has come into use to describe the pathology of people with impulsive aggression. Surprisingly, many clinicians and researchers rarely consider the diagnosis of IED, although impulsive aggressive behavior is relatively common. In community surveys, 12%–25% of men and women in the United States reported engaging in physical fights as adults, a frequent manifestation of impulsive aggression (Robins and Regier 1991). Impulsive aggressive behavior usually is pathological and causes substantial psychosocial distress/dysfunction (Mattes 1990; McElroy et al. 1998). Being on the receiving end of impulsive aggressive behavior can lead to similar behavior in a child who grows up in this environment (Huesmann et al. 1984). A description of the development of IED diagnostic criteria and information about the epidemiology, genetics, neurobiology, and treatment of impulsive aggression are included in this chapter.

19

Nosology

DSM-I Through DSM-III-R

Prior descriptions of impulsive aggressive behavior fell under the labels of Type A personality, passive-aggressive personality (aggressive type), or explosive personality. Until most recently, little research was done using categorical expressions of impulsive aggression due to difficulties with the DSM criteria. This section describes the process by which the current research criteria for IED were developed.

"Intermittent explosive disorder" was named for the first time in DSM-III (American Psychiatric Association 1980). However, these criteria were not specific enough to make the diagnosis in more than a handful of subjects. The IED diagnostic criteria were revised for DSM-III-R (American Psychiatric Association 1987), but they proved to be overly restrictive. IED could only be diagnosed by DSM-III-R in 20% of violent male volunteers with clinically impulsive aggressive pathology, due in no small part to the exclusion of generalized impulsive aggressive behavior in between aggressive outbursts (Felthous et al. 1991).

Research Criteria for Intermittent Explosive Disorder– Revised

To use an IED diagnosis in research studies, research criteria were created. The research criteria for IED–revised (IED-R) described five criteria for IED, emphasizing the severity, impulsive nature, frequency, and pathology of the impulsive aggressive behavior. Less severe impulsive aggressive behavior (i.e., verbal aggression or aggression toward property) was included because these forms of aggression had been shown to respond to treatment (Coccaro and Kavoussi 1997; Salzman et al. 1995). The criteria also specified that *impulsive,* not *premeditated* aggression would be required for this diagnosis. Prior research had shown psychosocial, biological, and treatment response findings specific to only impulsive and not premeditated aggression. A minimal frequency of aggressive acts was required to increase the reliability of the IED diagnosis and exclude those without severe symptoms. Finally, to distinguish the IED diagnosis as pathological, the criteria required the presence of subjective distress and/or social or occupational dysfunction.

The new IED-R criteria also included inclusion/exclusion changes. The past exclusion of subjects with borderline personality disorder (BPD) and antisocial personality disorder (ASPD) had seemed reasonable at the time of the publication of DSM-III. Individuals with BPD are diagnosed in part by their impulsivity and frequent expressions of anger, and those with ASPD are often irritable and aggressive. Impulsive aggression, however, is not present in all BPD/ASPD subjects. Moreover, familial, twin, biological, and treatment response data suggest that impulsive aggressive behavior, although present in many BPD/ASPD subjects, has specific clinical relevance separately from the remaining diagnostic features of these personality disorders (Barratt et al. 1997; Coccaro et al. 1989; Cowdry and Gardner 1988; Linehan et al. 1994; Moss et al. 1990; Sheard et al. 1976; Silverman et al. 1991; Torgerson 1984).

Other mental illnesses with impulsive aggressive outbursts include bipolar disorder, major depression, substance abuse, and mental retardation; these, among others, should be excluded from an IED diagnosis. Although most impulsive aggressive behaviors occurring in patients with these disorders can be explained by the primary diagnosis, aggressive outbursts occurring in the context of major depression (Fava et al. 1993) may be particularly difficult to distinguish from IED. However, irritability and aggressive outbursts occurring only during an episode of major depression are most likely due to the depression, and thus comorbid IED should not be diagnosed unless there is evidence that impulsive aggressive behavior occurs in the absence of major depressive episodes.

Application of Intermittent Explosive Disorder—Revised Criteria

A study of DSM-III-R IED versus IED-R criteria was first published in 1998 with 188 subjects with personality disorder, nearly half of whom were seeking treatment for impulsive aggressive behavior (Coccaro et al. 1998b). A very low 2% of subjects met DSM-III-R IED criteria (10% would have met DSM-IV [American Psychiatric Association 1994] criteria). In contrast, 40.4% met IED-R criteria. The subjects diagnosed by either set of criteria had many characteristics that differentiated them from non-IED subjects, including elevated aggression and impulsivity scores. IED subjects had lower Global Assessment of Functioning scores compared with non-IED subjects even when age, race, gender, and other relevant variables were accounted for. Current and past mood disorders, as well as alcohol and substance dependence, were more frequently found in those with IED but did not affect these findings. Subjects with IED were more likely to have BPD, although most (62%) did not have either BPD or ASPD. Moreover, aggression and impulsivity scores were still elevated when the comorbidity of these disorders was accounted for, indicating that features of the IED subjects were not due to BPD/ASPD.

IED-R and DSM-IV Criteria: Defining Integrated Research Criteria for Intermittent Explosive Disorder

Although DSM-IV made some changes to the IED criteria, it still did not provide criteria useful for research. The "aggressive acts" of criterion A did not give specific definitions for its terms or a number of acts or time frame during which the acts had to occur. Apparently, no official guidelines for these items had been determined or considered by the DSM-IV subcommittee.

Clinically, subjects with impairment from IED may fit a variety of descriptions. Example of descriptions include 1) subjects with frequent, small-scale, nonassaultive/nondestructive explosive episodes associated with distress and/or impairment (IED-R); 2) subjects with relatively infrequent but severely assaultive/destructive episodes in addition to frequent small-scale, less severely assaultive/destructive episodes (both IED-R and DSM-IV IED); and 3) subjects with relatively infrequent but severely assaultive/destructive episodes (DSM-IV IED). Using research criteria for IED-R and DSM-IV IED in the same subjects used in the original IED-R series, 69% of subjects met both IED-R and DSM-IV IED diagnoses, 20% met criteria for only DSM-IV IED, and 11% met criteria for only IED-R. Analyses done to compare subject groups found no differences in aggression and impulsivity levels and a significant difference between the total IED group and non-IED subjects. Because the two criteria sets did not differentiate groups with different aggression and impulsivity levels, and each alone leaves a number of subjects undiagnosed, integrated research criteria (IED-IR) were created to allow subjects from any or both of these groups to be identified.

Epidemiology

DSM-IV-TR (American Psychiatric Association 2000) describes IED as "apparently rare." However, clinical interview or survey data give a different picture. A number of studies have looked at clinical populations, and one community survey has been done to determine the prevalence of IED. Numbers range between 1.1% and 6.3%. The evaluation of studies is complicated by the variety of defining criteria used, from DSM-III to current research criteria and IED-IR. Initially, Monopolis and Lions (1983) reported that only 1.1% of hospitalized patients met DSM-III criteria for IED. More recently, Zimmerman et al. (1998) used the Structured Clinical Interview for DSM-IV (SCID) to study current or lifetime IED in 411 outpatient psychiatric subjects at Rhode Island Hospital. They reported a rate of 3.8% for current IED and 6.2% for lifetime IED by DSM-IV criteria. A recent reanalysis of a much larger sample from the same population revealed similar rates of IED (Coccaro et al., in press). Moreover, data from a pilot community sample study revealed a community rate of lifetime IED by DSM-IV-TR criteria at 4.0% and by IED-IR criteria at 5.1% (Coccaro et al. 2004). Considering the rates found in these more recent studies, IED could be as common as other major psychiatric disorders such as schizophrenia or bipolar illness.

Clinical Features

The age of onset and course of IED distinguish the disorder as separate from its comorbid diagnoses. A mean age at onset of 16 years and an average duration of about 20 years has been described for IED (McElroy et al. 1998). Preliminary data from the Rhode Island Hospital Study (Coccaro et al., in press) confirm these findings and indicate that onset of IED by DSM-IV-TR is seen by the end of the first decade in 31%, by the end of the second decade in 44%, by the end of the third decade in 19%, and by the end of the fourth decade in only 6%. IED comes on rapidly, without a prodromal period. Aggressive episodes typically last less than 30 minutes and involve one or a combination of the following: verbal assault, destruction of property, or physical assault. If any provocation is identifiable, it is from a known person and is seemingly minor in nature (Felthous et al. 1991; Mattes 1990; McElroy et al. 1998). As discussed earlier, many IED subjects who have severely aggressive/destructive episodes frequently have minor aggressive episodes in the interim. Substantial distress, social, occupational, legal, or financial impairments typically result from these episodes. Data on gender differences in IED are limited, but most published data suggest that males outnumber females in this regard. More recent, unpublished data from the Rhode Island Hospital Study (Coccaro et al., in press), however, suggest that the male:female ratio is closer to 1:1.

Comorbidity With Axis I and II Disorders

Subjects with IED most frequently have other Axis I and II disorders. The most frequent Axis I diagnoses comorbid with IED lifetime include mood, anxiety, substance, eating, and other impulse-control disorders ranging in frequency from 7% to 89% (Coccaro et al. 1998b; McElroy et al. 1998). Such Axis I comorbidity rates raise the question of whether IED constitutes a separate disorder. However, recent data finding earlier onset of IED compared with all disorders, except for phobic-type anxiety disorders, suggest that IED is not secondary to these other disorders (Coccaro et al., in press). That noted, the possible comorbidity with bipolar disorder and other impulse-control disorders deserves more detailed consideration.

Bipolar Disorder

McElroy et al. (1998) reported that the aggressive episodes observed in their subjects resembled "microdysphoric" manic episodes. Symptoms in common with both manic and IED episodes included irritability (79%–92%), increased energy (83%–96%), racing thoughts (62%–67%), anxiety (21%–42%), and depressed (dysphoric) mood (17%–33%). However, this finding may not be surprising, because 56% of the subjects in question had a comorbid bipolar diagnosis of some type (bipolar I, 33%; bipolar II, 11%; bipolar not otherwise specified or cyclothymia, 11%). Two other studies suggest a much lower rate of comorbid bipolar illness, with rates of 11% (bipolar I, 5%; bipolar II, 5%; bipolar not otherwise specified, 1%) noted in the Rhode Island Hospital Study (Coccaro et al., in press) and only 10% (bipolar II only) noted by Gavlovski et al. (2002). Regardless, clinicians should fully evaluate for bipolar disorder prior to determining treatment for IED, because mood stabilizers, rather than selective serotonin reuptake inhibitors (SSRIs), would be the first-line treatment for IED comorbid with bipolar disorder.

Other Impulse-Control Disorders

McElroy et al. (1998) reported that up to 44% of their IED subjects had another impulse-control–type disorder such as compulsive buying (37%) or kleptomania (19%). In the Coccaro et al. (1998b) study, however, few IED subjects had a comorbid impulse-control disorder, and only 5% of IED subjects had another impulse-control disorder in the Rhode Island Hospital Study (Coccaro et al., in press).

Borderline and Antisocial Personality Disorders

The rate of BPD and/or ASPD in IED subjects has been reported at 38% (Coccaro et al. 1998b). However, rates of IED in subjects with BPD have been noted at 78% and in subjects with ASPD at 58% (Coccaro et al. 1998b). A review of unpublished data from the author's (E.H. Hollander 2005) research program suggests that these rates are lower among subjects not seeking treatment and are lowest in the community (23% for BPD and/or ASPD; Coccaro et al. 2002). Regardless, BPD and ASPD subjects with a comorbid diagnosis of IED do appear to have higher scores for aggression and lower scores for general psychosocial function than do BPD/ASPD subjects without IED (Coccaro et al., in press).

Pathogenesis

Familial and Genetic Correlates

Family and Twin Studies

Clinical observation and family history data suggest that IED is familial. Violent behavior or a history of violent behavior in probands correlates with violent behavior in first-degree relatives (Bach-Y-Rita et al. 1971; Maletsky 1973). Familial aggregation of temper outbursts and IED has been reported in psychiatric patients with "temper problems" (Mattes and Fink 1987), and McElroy et al. (1998) reported that nearly a third of first-degree relatives of IED probands had IED. A recent blinded, controlled, family history study using IED-IR criteria (Coccaro 1999) found a morbid risk of IED of 26% in relatives of IED-IR probands compared with 8% among the relatives of control probands, a significant difference. Although twin studies have confirmed the hypothesis that both impulsivity (Seroczynski et al. 1999) and aggression (Coccaro et al. 1997a) are under substantial genetic influence, there are no twin studies of IED itself. Genetic influence for these two traits ranges from 28% to 47%, with nonshared environmental influences making up the lion's share of the remaining variance.

Molecular Genetic Studies

Studies of particular genes in aggressive populations have used the candidate gene approach. Candidate genes are those genes for proteins with a suspected, or proven, biological association to a disorder (e.g., serotonin [5-HT] receptors in aggression). The polymorphism HTR1B/G861C and short tandem repeat locus D6S284 are part of the gene for the 5-HT$_{1B}$ receptor for serotonin. These genetic sites were examined in 350 Finnish sibling pairs and in 305 Southwestern American Indian sibling pairs, both with a high rate of alcoholism. The diagnoses of ASPD and IED were used to examine the traits of impulsivity and aggression. The rate of IED in relatives of ASPD probands was 15%, and the relatives of healthy control subjects had neither IED nor ASPD. Lappalainen et al. (1998) were able to discover that the gene predisposing to ASPD alcoholism resides close to the HTR1B version of the coding sequence. They concluded that impulsivity and aggression might be influenced, in part, by 5-HT$_{1B}$ receptors. Other candidate genes include the genes for tryptophan hydroxylase and monoamine oxidase A. Manuck et al. (1999, 2000) revealed an association of the traits of aggression, impulsivity, and serotonin activity (tested by *d,l-Fen* challenge) with variations in both the tryptophan hydroxylase and monoamine oxidase A genes in community samples.

Biological Correlates

Serotonin

Serotonin and other centrally acting neurotransmitters are the most studied biological factors in aggression. Measures examining central (as well as peripheral) serotonin function correlate inversely with life history, questionnaire, and laboratory measures of aggression. This relationship has been demonstrated by cerebrospinal fluid 5-hydroxyindoleacetic acid (G.L. Brown et al. 1979; Linnoila et al. 1983; Virkkunen et al. 1994), physiological responses to serotonin agonist probes (Coccaro et al. 1989, 1997b; Dolan et al. 2001; Manuck et al. 1998; Moss et al. 1990; O'Keane et al. 1992), and platelet measures of serotonin activity (Birmaher et al. 1990; C.S. Brown et al. 1989; Coccaro et al. 1996; Stoff et al. 1987). The type of aggression associated with reduced central serotonin function appears to be *impulsive,* as opposed to *nonimpulsive,* aggression (Linnoila et al. 1983; Virkkunen et al. 1994). These findings suggest that impulsive aggressive behavior can be distinguished biologically from nonimpulsive aggression.

Other Neurotransmitter Systems:
Dopamine, Norepinephrine, Vasopressin,
and Brain-Derived Neurotrophic Factor

There is also emerging evidence to support the role of other nonserotonergic brain systems and modulators in impulsive aggression. These findings suggest a facilitating role for dopamine (Depue et al. 1994), norepinephrine (Coccaro et al. 1991), vasopressin (Coccaro et al. 1998a), brain-derived neurotrophic factor (BDNF; Lyons et al. 1991), opiates (Post et al. 1984), and testosterone (Archer 1991; Virkkunen et al. 1994) and an inhibitory interaction between neuronal nitric oxide synthase and testosterone in rodents (Kriegsfeld et al. 1997). The relationship of catecholamines and vasopressin to aggression and serotonin is noteworthy. The inverse relationship between aggression and serotonin is not observed when catecholamine system function is impaired. Among depressed subjects, who typically demonstrate diminished norepinephrine system function, the relationship between serotonin and aggression is not found (Coccaro et al. 1989; Wetzler et al. 1991). In the case of central vasopressin and aggression, serotonin appears to be inversely related to both central vasopressin and to aggression in both animal (Ferris and Delville 1994) and human subjects (Coccaro et al. 1998a). In human subjects, the relationship between central vasopressin and aggression is present even after the relationship with serotonin is taken into account. In animal studies, both central vasopressin activity and aggression can be suppressed by treatment with SSRI agents (Ferris and Delville 1994). In other animal studies, SSRI agents were able to suppress the overaggressiveness of mice deficient in BDNF (BDNF± mice), revealing a role for BDNF in both aggressiveness and serotonin regulation (Lyons et al. 1991).

Imaging and Brain Localization

The availability of modern imaging devices, especially functional imaging, allows for examination of the neurocircuitry of emotion and behavior. Although many localization and functional studies have been done in the depressed population, few studies have looked at impulsive aggression or IED. Soloff et al. (2000) used fluorodeoxyglucose positron emission tomography (FDG-PET) and serotonin stimulation to compare brain activity of BPD patients with that of normal control subjects. Prior to stimulation, the control group had greater uptake in all regions examined. However, the BPD patients had decreased uptake in the medial and orbital regions of the right prefrontal cortex, areas associated with impulsive aggression. Similarly, in the context of FDG-PET, Siever et al. (1999) found blunted glucose utilization responses to serotonin stimulation in the orbitofrontal cortex of IED subjects with BPD. More recently, New et al. (2002) reported a similar finding in the anterior cingulate after stimulation with the direct serotonin agonist *m*-chlorophenylpiperazine.

Parsey et al. (2002) used PET with a 5-HT$_{1A}$ antagonist to examine the relationship between serotonin receptor binding and lifetime aggression. Looking at the dorsal raphe, anterior cingulate cortex, cingulate body, hippocampus, amygdala, medial prefrontal cortex, and orbital prefrontal cortex, all areas except the cingulate and hippocampus demonstrated association with lower serotonin binding and aggression. The study was done in healthy volunteers. Best et al. (2002) provided support for a possible dysfunctional frontal circuit using neuropsychological testing performance in subjects with impulsive aggression. Further work in this area of emotion regulation, and new attention to the abnormalities in information processing, will likely reveal more specifics of functional brain abnormalities in individuals with impulsive aggression.

Treatment

There are few studies in which subjects with IED have been the focus of treatment. A number of studies in which the treatment of impulsive aggression in related subjects has been examined are reviewed in the following sections.

Psychotherapy

Anger treatment studies focus on treatment of anger as a component of other psychiatric illnesses. It is true that anger can largely contribute to the dysfunction caused by a disorder, particularly in adolescents or children; in patients with substance abuse, posttraumatic stress disorder, depression, and domestic violence; and in forensic and mentally impaired populations. In these cases, therapy for anger and aggression focuses on cognitive-behavioral group therapy. In a few rare cases, anger is addressed as the primary or only problem, and a limited number of treatments have been described. "Imaginational exposure therapy," used frequently in anxiety disorders, was studied by Grodnitzky and Tafrate (2000) in a noncontrolled pilot study of anger treatment. Subjects habituated to anger-provoking scenarios, and the treatment was felt to be useful. Studies on driving anger provide the only controlled studies of anger treatment in a population without other psychopathology. Deffenbacher et al. (2000) reported on an initial controlled trial comparing two treatments versus an assessment-only control condition in a self-identified, high–driving anger population of college-student volunteers who received research credit for participation. Group treatment conditions consisted of pure relaxation training compared with relaxation training combined with cognitive therapy and an assessment-only control. Neither treatment condition demonstrated improvement on general trait anger, but both active treatments improved driving anger. The same researchers repeated these interventions in a different population using drivers with higher anger levels than in the first study (Deffenbacher et al. 2002). This time, both treatments lowered trait anger. The second study gave some attention to the generalization of skill use to other sources of anger. Overall, because relaxation training with cognitive therapy provided little gain over pure relaxation training, relaxation training in itself may be an adequate treatment for driving anger.

Other versions of cognitive-behavioral therapy, such as Marsha Linehan's dialectical behavior therapy, have been studied in BPD patients. A study in 26 BPD subjects showed improvement in anger, social adjustment, and global functioning compared with a treatment-as-usual condition (Linehan et al. 1994). In addition, studies of dialectical behavior therapy have been done in subjects with many diagnoses, and improvement in impulsivity and anger scores has been shown. No double-blind, placebo-controlled studies on IED subjects in therapy have been published, but studies of therapy in IED subjects are ongoing.

Pharmacotherapy

A number of medications in different classes have been used to treat impulsive aggression, from tricyclic antidepressants to benzodiazepines, mood stabilizers, and neuroleptics. Most recently, studies of the pharmacotherapy of aggression have turned to SSRIs and mood stabilizers as first-line treatments.

Fluoxetine and other SSRIs have been studied in IED patients and impulsive aggressive subjects. In our published fluoxetine treatment trial of subjects meeting IED-IR criteria, impulsive aggressive behavior did respond to fluoxetine (Coccaro and Kavoussi 1997). The past use of non-serotonin-specific antidepressants in impulsive aggression had little benefit and many side effects in treatment studies. Soloff et al. (1986a) looked at amitriptyline in a group of inpatients with BPD and schizotypal personality disorder. Although affective symptoms improved during the 5-week study in some patients, there was a set of patients with worsening of impulsivity and aggression. This worsening could have been due to the noradrenergic effects of tricyclic antidepressants (Links et al. 1990). Accordingly, the use of the new dual-action antidepressants in these patients should be approached with caution.

Monoamine oxidase inhibitors such as tranylcypromine and phenelzine have also been studied in impulsively aggressive subjects. Soloff et al. (1993) examined the response of BPD patients to treatment with phenelzine versus haloperidol. Compared with placebo and haloperidol, phenelzine produced a moderate reduction in anger and hostility in this double-blind comparison. However, a 16-week continuation phase revealed that the subjects had experienced only minor benefits in depression and irritability, and the subjects remained substantially impaired after the treatment phase (Cornelius et al. 1993; Soloff et al. 1993). Cowdry and Gardner's (1988) study of tranylcypromine, trifluoperazine, alprazolam, and carbamazepine in patients with treatment-resistant BPD (all of whom had a substantial history of impulsive aggressive outbursts) revealed little benefit for tranylcypromine. This double-blind, placebo-controlled crossover study was also of interest due to the results from the other medications. Cowdry and Gardner (1988) revealed a worsening of behavior among subjects given alprazolam. Episodes of serious dyscontrol increased in frequency among those subjects with a history of similar episodes and BPD. The authors theorized that the benzodiazepine treatment might have released the subjects' control or inhibition of these episodes. Treatment of such patients with benzodiazepines should only be instituted under close watch and after considering the other options.

Mood stabilizers have also been used to treat aggression. Initially, controlled trials examined lithium and its affects on mood and impulsive aggression in two different populations, BPD outpatients and chronically aggressive prisoners. Links et al. (1990) compared lithium with desipramine and placebo. Objective ratings of anger and suicidality improved the most on lithium; however, the subjects and their clinicians did not report any improvement in mood. Sheard et al. (1976) found an improvement using lithium versus placebo in chronically aggressive prisoners. However, again, only objective findings supported this; subjectively, no improvement was reported. Barratt et al. (1997) also reported a reduction in aggression with diphenylhydantoin treatment in impulsively aggressive prison inmates.

The other mood stabilizers studied for impulsive aggression have been carbamazepine and divalproex. Referring back to the Cowdry and Gardner (1988) study, carbamazepine did lessen episodes of impulsive aggression in BPD subjects. However, 18% of these subjects noticed a worsening in their mood, which improved once carbamazepine was stopped. Recently, Kavoussi and Coccaro (1998) and Hollander et al. (2003) reported an antiaggressive effect of divalproex sodium in IED subjects with a Cluster B personality disorders. Divalproex reduced overt aggression scores to a greater degree than did placebo, especially by the third month of treatment. Surprisingly, IED subjects without a Cluster B personality disorder responded equally well to divalproex and placebo. Reasons for an absence of a differential antiaggressive effect of divalproex in this population is unknown at this time. Given the relative adverse event profiles for SSRIs versus mood stabilizers, it is likely that clinical treatment of IED patients should start with SSRIs unless the subject is extremely aggressive or has a history of a bipolar disorder, in which case treatment with a mood stabilizer would be more appropriate.

The neuroleptics haloperidol, trifluoperazine, and depot flupenthixol have all been studied in BPD populations. In Cowdry and Gardner's (1988) study, subjects showed significant improvement in depression and anxiety objective ratings with trifluoperazine; however, subjective ratings did not support this finding. Trifluoperazine was seen as less useful than tranylcypromine (a monoamine oxidase inhibitor) and carbamazepine in improving behavior and affect among the subjects. Soloff et al. (1986b, 1989) examined haloperidol versus amitriptyline in hospitalized BPD patients with or without schizotypal personality disorder. These subjects improved on hostility and global function measurements, but considerable depression remained. Soloff afterward described haloperidol as a nonspecific tranquilizer in BPD patients. A 6-month study of depot flupenthixol by Montgomery and Montgomery (1982) found decreased suicidal and parasuicidal behavior in the treatment group compared with the placebo group among individuals with a history of such behaviors.

Atypical antipsychotics provide a new class of possible treatments for impulsive aggressive behavior. Few studies in this area are controlled trials. Zanarini and Frankenburg (2001) compared olanzapine with placebo in outpatients with BPD. The treatment improved anger, hostility, and other symptoms, but not depression. The patients remained quite ill.

Conclusion

As a diagnostic entity, IED has been poorly characterized over the years. However, the behavioral phenomenon underlying IED (i.e., impulsive aggression) has been well studied for more than two decades, and research in this area has led to important insights into the biology and treatment of the core behaviors in IED. Given the emerging evidence suggesting several treatment options that may effectively reduce impulsive aggressive behavior, IED should now be systematically investigated so that patients with this disorder can be offered potentially efficacious treatments (psychopharmacological and/or cognitive-behavioral treatments) and can be identified for further research in this area.

References

American Psychiatric Association: Diagnostic and Statistical Manual of Mental Disorders, 3rd Edition. Washington, DC, American Psychiatric Association, 1980

American Psychiatric Association: Diagnostic and Statistical Manual of Mental Disorders, 3rd Edition, Revised. Washington, DC, American Psychiatric Association, 1987

American Psychiatric Association: Diagnostic and Statistical Manual of Mental Disorders, 4th Edition. Washington, DC, American Psychiatric Association, 1994

American Psychiatric Association: Diagnostic and Statistical Manual of Mental Disorders, 4th Edition, Text Revision. Washington, DC, American Psychiatric Association, 2000

Archer J: The influence of testosterone on human aggression. Br J Psychol 82:1–28, 1991

Bach-Y-Rita G, Lion JR, Climent CF, et al: Episodic dyscontrol: a study of 130 violent patients. Am J Psychiatry 127:1473–1478, 1971

Barratt ES, Stanford MS, Felthous AR, et al: The effects of diphenylhydantoin on impulsive and premeditated aggression: a controlled study. J Clin Psychopharmacol 17:341–349, 1997

Best M, Williams JM, Coccaro EF: Evidence for a dysfunctional prefrontal circuit in patients with an impulsive aggressive disorder. Proc Natl Acad Sci U S A 99:8448–8453, 2002

Birmaher B, Stanley M, Greenhill L, et al: Platelet imipramine binding in children and adolescents with impulsive behavior. J Am Acad Child Adolesc Psychiatry 29:914–918, 1990

Brown CS, Kent TA, Bryant SG, et al: Blood platelet uptake of serotonin in episodic aggression. Psychiatry Res 27:5–12, 1989

Brown GL, Goodwin FK, Ballenger JC, et al: Aggression in humans correlates with cerebrospinal fluid amine metabolites. Psychiatry Res 1:131–139, 1979

Coccaro EF: Family history study of intermittent explosive disorder. Paper presented at the 152nd annual meeting of the American Psychiatric Association, Washington, DC, May 1999

Coccaro EF, Kavoussi RJ: Fluoxetine and impulsive aggressive behavior in personality disordered subjects. Arch Gen Psychiatry 54:1081–1088, 1997

Coccaro EF, Siever LJ, Klar HM, et al: Serotonergic studies in affective and personality disorder: correlates with suicidal and impulsive aggressive behavior. Arch Gen Psychiatry 46:587–599, 1989

Coccaro EF, Lawrence T, Trestman R, et al: Growth hormone responses to intravenous clonidine challenge correlate with behavioral irritability in psychiatric patients and healthy volunteers. Psychiatry Res 39:129–139, 1991

Coccaro EF, Kavoussi RJ, Sheline YI, et al: Impulsive aggression in personality disorder correlates with tritiated paroxetine binding in the platelet. Arch Gen Psychiatry 53:531–536, 1996

Coccaro EF, Bergeman CS, Kavoussi RJ, et al: Heritability of aggression and irritability: a twin study of the Buss-Durkee Aggression Scales in adult male subjects. Biol Psychiatry 41:273–284, 1997a

Coccaro EF, Kavoussi RJ, Hauger RL: Serotonin function and anti-aggressive responses to fluoxetine: a pilot study. Biol Psychiatry 42:546–552, 1997b

Coccaro EF, Kavoussi RJ, Hauger RL, et al: Cerebrospinal fluid vasopressin: correlates with aggression and serotonin function in personality disordered subjects. Arch Gen Psychiatry 55:708–714, 1998a

Coccaro EF, Kavoussi RJ, Berman ME, et al: Intermittent explosive disorder-revised: development, reliability and validity of research criteria. Compr Psychiatry 39:368–376, 1998b

Coccaro EF, Schmidt CA, Samuels JF, et al: Lifetime and 1-month prevalence rates of intermittent explosive disorder in a community sample. J Clin Psychiatry 65:820–824, 2004

Coccaro EF, Posternak MA, Zimmerman M: Prevalence and features of intermittent explosive disorder in a clinical setting. J Clin Psychiatry (in press)

Cornelius JR, Soloff P, Perel JM, et al: Continuation pharmacotherapy of borderline personality disorder with haloperidol and phenelzine. Arch Gen Psychiatry 150:1843–1848, 1993

Cowdry RW, Gardner DL: Pharmacotherapy of borderline personality disorder: alprazolam, carbamazepine, trifluoperazine, and tranylcypromine. Arch Gen Psychiatry 45:111–119, 1988

Deffenbacher JL, Lynch RS, Oetting ER, et al: Characteristics and treatment of high-anger drivers. J Couns Psychol 47:5–17, 2000

Deffenbacher JL, Filetti LB, Lynch RS, et al: Cognitive-behavioral treatment of high anger drivers. Behav Res Ther 40:895–910, 2002

DePue RA, Luciana M, Arbisi P, et al: Dopamine and the structure of personality: relation of agonist-induced dopamine activity to positive emotionality. J Pers Soc Psychol 67:485–498, 1994

Dolan M, Anderson IM, Deakin JF: Relationship between 5-HT function and impulsivity and aggression in males offenders with personality disorders. Br J Psychiatry 178:352–359, 2001

Fava M, Rosenbaum JF, Pava JA, et al: Anger attacks in unipolar depression, part 1: clinical correlates and response to fluoxetine treatment. Am J Psychiatry 150:1158–1163, 1993

Felthous AR, Bryant G, Wingerter CB, et al: The diagnosis of intermittent explosive disorder in violent men. Bull Am Acad Psychiatry Law 19:71–79, 1991

Ferris CF, Delville Y: Vasopressin and serotonin interactions in the control of agonistic behavior. Psychoneuroendocrinology 19:593–601, 1994

Grodnitzky GR, Tafrate RC: Imaginal exposure for anger reduction in adult outpatients: a pilot study. J Behav Ther Exp Psychiatry 31:259–279, 2000

Hollander E, Tracy KA, Swann AC, et al: Divalproex in the treatment of impulsive aggression: efficacy in cluster B personality disorders. Neuropsychopharmacology 28:1186–1197, 2003

Huesmann LR, Leonard E, Lefkowitz M, et al: Stability of aggression over time and generations. Dev Psychopathol 20:1120–1134, 1984

Kavoussi RK, Coccaro EF: Divalproex sodium for impulsive aggressive behavior in patients with personality disorder. J Clin Psychiatry 59:676–680, 1998

Kriegsfeld LJ, Dawson TM, Dawson VL, et al: Aggressive behavior in male mice lacking the gene for neuronal nitric oxide synthase requires testosterone. Brain Res 769:66–70, 1997

Lappalainen J, Long JC, Eggert M, et al: Linkage of antisocial alcoholism to the serotonin 5-HT1B receptor gene in 2 populations. Arch Gen Psychiatry 55:989–994, 1998

Linehan MM, Tutek DA, Heard HL, et al: Interpersonal outcome of cognitive behavioral treatment for chronically suicidal borderline patients. Am J Psychiatry 151:1771–1776, 1994

Links PS, Steiner M, Boiago I, et al: Lithium therapy for borderline patients: preliminary findings. J Personal Disord 4:173–181,1990

Linnoila M, Virkkunen M, Scheinin M, et al: Low cerebrospinal fluid 5-hydroxyindoleacetic acid concentration differentiates impulsive from non-impulsive violent behavior. Life Sci 33:2609–2614, 1983

Lyons WE, Mamounas LA, Ricaurte GA: Brain-derived neurotrophic factor-deficient mice develop aggressiveness and hyperphagia in conjunction with brain serotonergic abnormalities. Proc Natl Acad Sci U S A 96:15239–15244, 1991

Maletsky BM: The episodic dyscontrol syndrome. Dis Nerv Syst 36:178–185, 1973

Manuck SB, Flory JD, McCaffery JM, et al: Aggression, impulsivity, and central nervous system serotonergic responsivity in a nonpatient sample. Neuropsychopharmacology 19:287–299, 1998

Manuck SB, Flory JD, Ferrell RE, et al: Aggression and anger-related traits associated with a polymorphism of the tryptophan hydroxylase gene. Biol Psychiatry 45:603–614, 1999

Manuck SB, Flory JD, Ferrell RE, et al: A regulatory polymorphism of the monoamine oxidase-A gene may be associated with variability in aggression, impulsivity, and central nervous system serotonergic responsivity. Psychiatry Res 95:9–23, 2000

Mattes JA: Comparative effectiveness of carbamazepine and propranolol for rage outbursts. J Neuropsychiatry Clin Neurosci 2:159–164, 1990

Mattes JA, Fink M: A family study of patients with temper outbursts. J Psychiatr Res 21:249–255, 1987

McElroy SL, Soutullo CA, Beckman DA, et al: DSM-IV intermittent explosive disorder: a report of 27 cases. J Clin Psychiatry 59:203–210, 1998

Monopolis S, Lion JR: Problems in the diagnosis of intermittent explosive disorder. Am J Psychiatry 140:1200–1202, 1983

Montgomery SA, Montgomery D: Pharmacological prevention of suicidal behavior. J Affect Disord 4:291–298, 1982

Moss HB, Yao JK, Panzak GL: Serotonergic responsivity and behavioral dimensions in antisocial personality disorder with substance abuse. Biol Psychiatry 28:325–338, 1990

New AS, Hazlett EA, Buchsbaum MS: Blunted prefrontal cortical [18]fluorodeoxyglucose positron emission tomography response to meta-chlorophenylpiperazine in impulsive aggression. Arch Gen Psychiatry 59:621–629, 2002

O'Keane V, Moloney E, O'Neill H: Blunted prolactin responses to *d*-fenfluramine in sociopathy: evidence of subsensitivity of central serotonergic function. Br J Psychiatry 160:643–646, 1992

Parsey RV, Oquendo MA, Simpson NR, et al: Effects of sex, age, and aggressive traits in man on brain serotonin 5-HT$_{1A}$ receptor binding potential measured by PET using [C-11]WAY-100635. Brain Res 954:173–182, 2002

Post RM, Pickar D, Ballenger JC, et al: Endogenous opiates in cerebrospinal fluid: relationship to mood and anxiety, in Neurobiology of Mood Disorders. Edited by Post RM, Ballenger JC. Baltimore, MD, Williams & Wilkins, 1984, pp 356–368

Robins LN, Regier DA: Psychiatric Disorders in America. New York, Free Press, 1991

Salzman C, Wolfson AN, Schatzberg A, et al: Effect of fluoxetine on anger in symptomatic volunteers with borderline personality disorder. J Clin Psychopharmacol 15:23–29, 1995

Seroczynski AD, Bergeman CS, Coccaro EF: Etiology of the impulsivity/aggression relationship: genes or environment? Psychiatry Res 86:41–57, 1999

Sheard M, Manini J, Bridges C, et al: The effect of lithium on impulsive aggressive behavior in man. Am J Psychiatry 133:1409–1413, 1976

Siever LJ, Buchsbaum MS, New AS, et al: *d,l*-Fenfluramine response in impulsive personality disorder assessed with [18F]fluorodeoxyglucose positron emission tomography. Neuropsychopharmacology 20:413–423, 1999

Silverman JM, Pinkham L, Horvath TB, et al: Affective and impulsive personality disorder traits in the relatives of patients with borderline personality disorder. Am J Psychiatry 148:1378–1385, 1991

Soloff PH, George A, Nathan RS, et al: Paradoxical effects of amitriptyline in borderline patients. Am J Psychiatry 143:1603–1605, 1986a

Soloff PH, George A, Nathan RS, et al: Progress in pharmacotherapy of borderline disorders. Arch Gen Psychiatry 43:691–697, 1986b

Soloff PH, George A, Nathan RS, et al: Amitriptyline versus haloperidol in borderlines: final outcomes and predictors of response. J Clin Psychopharmacol 9:238–246, 1989

Soloff PH, Cornelius J, Anselm G, et al: Efficacy of phenelzine and haloperidol in borderline personality disorder. Arch Gen Psychiatry 50:377–385, 1993

Soloff PH, Meltzer CC, Greer PJ, et al: A fenfluramine-activated FDG-PET study of borderline personality disorder. Biol Psychiatry 47:540–547, 2000

Stoff DM, Pollock L, Vitiello B: Reduction of (3H)-imipramine binding sites on platelets of conduct disordered children. Neuropsychopharmacology 1:55–62, 1987

Torgerson S: Genetic and nosological aspects of schizotypal and borderline personality disorder. Arch Gen Psychiatry 41:546–554, 1984

Virkkunen M, Rawlings R, Tokola R, et al: CSF biochemistries, glucose metabolism, and diurnal activity rhythms in alcoholic, violent offenders, fire setters, and healthy volunteers. Arch Gen Psychiatry 51:20–27, 1994

Wetzler S, Kahn RS, Asnis GM, et al: Serotonin receptor sensitivity and aggression. Psychiatry Res 37:271–279, 1991

Zanarini MC, Frankenburg FR: Olanzapine treatment of female borderline personality disorder patients: a double-blind, placebo-controlled pilot study. J Clin Psychiatry 62:849–854, 2001

Zimmerman M, Mattia J, Younken S, et al: The prevalence of DSM-IV impulse control disorders in psychiatric outpatients (NR265), in 1998 New Research Program and Abstracts, American Psychiatric Association 151st Annual Meeting, Toronto, Ontario, May 30–June 4, 1998. Washington, DC, American Psychiatric Association, 1998

3

Childhood Conduct Disorder and the Antisocial Spectrum

Stephen J. Donovan, M.D.

Conduct disorder (CD) is the most serious of three disruptive behavior disorders of childhood and adolescence. The others are oppositional defiant disorder (ODD) and disruptive behavior disorder not otherwise specified (American Psychiatric Association 2000). The term *disruptive behavior disorder* is used in this chapter to refer to all three disorders. They are characterized by persistent antisocial spectrum behaviors (Table 3–1) and affect between 5% and 10% of the child and adolescent populations in industrialized countries (Loeber et al. 2000). Combined with attention-deficit/hyperactivity disorder (ADHD), they account for more than 50% of clinic referrals (Waschbusch 2002). There are many reviews of the disruptive behavior disorder literature (Dishion et al. 1995b; Earls and Mezzacappa 2002; Loeber et al. 2000). Most summarize the history of the construct, the vast epidemiologic literature, and some of the psychotherapeutic treatment theories, but they devote little space to psychopharmacology, despite the fact that pharmacological treatment of children with these disorders is very common (Pappadopulos et al. 2003; Schur et al. 2003). Although treatment guidelines for disruptive behavior disorders have been proposed, there is no theory-driven approach to the pediatric psychopharmacology of antisocial spectrum problems. Physicians therefore empirically treat target symptoms and comorbidities, and this remains the pharmacological standard of care (Kutcher et al. 2004). The most common target symptom is aggression (Bassarath 2003).

The publication of this clinical manual reflects recent interest in impulsivity, a construct that cuts across diagnoses and is useful because it appears to bridge clinical phenomena with underlying biological theories (Moeller et al. 2001). *Impulsivity* is defined as "a predisposition toward rapid, unplanned reactions to internal or external stimuli without regard to the negative consequences of these reactions to the impulsive individual or others" (Moeller et al. 2001, p. 1784). Not all impulsivity is aggressive, not all aggression is impulsive, and not all impulsive aggression is part of an antisocial pattern. Nonetheless, the antisocial spectrum is an important clinical area of overlap between impulsivity and aggression. Tantrums and fighting are integral to ODD and CD. It is important to examine the role of impulsivity in aggression in childhood because as a biological construct it could be, and in fact often is, amenable to pharmacological treatment. This chapter uses *impulsive aggression* and a preferred synonym (*affective aggression*) to present an alternative approach to the disruptive behavior disorders, one that provides clinically relevant hypotheses that can be refuted or corroborated by future research.

Clinical Characteristics of Antisocial Behavior

Criteria for ODD and CD comprise a list of behaviors that violate social norms (Table 3–1). There is an immoral undertone to these behaviors, as though the core problem is a weak conscience, a profound collapse of the "Golden Rule." Conscience is not a DSM-IV-TR (American Psychiatric Association 2000) concept because it is difficult to operationalize how humans form moral judgments. Yet DSM-IV-TR's definition of a mental disorder requires that something is wrong with the individual that cannot be explained by social factors alone (Richters 1996). Without a construct like conscience, it is impossible to say what this "something" is. One way out of this conundrum is to isolate the component that one can imagine being dys-

Table 3–1. Disruptive behavior disorders: DSM-IV-TR diagnostic criteria

313.81 Oppositional Defiant Disorder

A. A pattern of negativistic, hostile, and defiant behavior lasting at least 6 months, during which four (or more) of the following are present:

 (1) often loses temper

 (2) often argues with adults

 (3) often actively defies or refuses to comply with adults' requests or rules

 (4) often deliberately annoys people

 (5) often blames others for his or her mistakes or misbehavior

 (6) is often touchy or easily annoyed by others

 (7) is often angry and resentful

 (8) is often spiteful or vindictive

 Note: Consider a criterion met only if the behavior occurs more frequently than is typically observed in individuals of comparable age and developmental level.

B. The disturbance in behavior causes clinically significant impairment in social, academic, or occupational functioning.

C. The behaviors do not occur exclusively during the course of a psychotic or mood disorder.

D. Criteria are not met for conduct disorder, and, if the individual is age 18 years or older, criteria are not met for antisocial personality disorder.

312.9   Disruptive Behavior Disorder Not Otherwise Specified

This category is for disorders characterized by conduct or oppositional defiant behaviors that do not meet the criteria for conduct disorder or oppositional defiant disorder. For example, include clinical presentations that do not meet full criteria either for oppositional defiant disorder or conduct disorder, but in which there is clinically significant impairment.

Conduct Disorder

A. A repetitive and persistent pattern of behavior in which the basic rights of others or major age-appropriate societal norms or rules are violated, as manifested by the presence of three (or more) of the following criteria in the past 12 months, with at least one criterion present in the past 6 months:

 Aggression to people and animals

 (1) often bullies, threatens, or intimidates others

 (2) often initiates physical fights

 (3) has used a weapon that can cause serious physical harm to others (e.g., a bat, brick, broken bottle, knife, gun)

Table 3–1.   Disruptive behavior disorders: DSM-IV-TR diagnostic criteria *(continued)*

Conduct Disorder *(continued)*

    (4)   has been physically cruel to people

    (5)   has been physically cruel to animals

    (6)   has stolen while confronting a victim (e.g., mugging, purse snatching, extortion, armed robbery)

    (7)   has forced someone into sexual activity

Destruction of property

    (8)   has deliberately engaged in fire setting with the intention of causing serious damage

    (9)   has deliberately destroyed others' property (other than by fire setting)

Deceitfulness or theft

    (10)   has broken into someone else's house, building, or car

    (11)   often lies to obtain goods or favors or to avoid obligations (i.e., "cons" others)

    (12)   has stolen items of nontrivial value without confronting a victim (e.g., shoplifting, but without breaking and entering; forgery)

Serious violations of rules

    (13)   often stays out at night despite parental prohibitions, beginning before age 13 years

    (14)   has run away from home overnight at least twice while living in parental or parental surrogate home (or once without returning for a lengthy period)

    (15)   is often truant from school, beginning before age 13 years

B.   The disturbance in behavior causes clinically significant impairment in social, academic, or occupational functioning.

C.   If the individual is age 18 years or older, criteria are not met for antisocial personality disorder.

    Code based on age at onset:

        312.81   **Conduct Disorder, Childhood-Onset Type:** onset of at least one criterion characteristic of conduct disorder prior to age 10 years

        312.82   **Conduct Disorder, Adolescent-Onset Type:** absence of any criteria characteristic of conduct disorder prior to age 10 years

        312.89   **Conduct Disorder, Unspecified Onset:** age at onset is not known

Table 3–1.   Disruptive behavior disorders: DSM-IV-TR diagnostic criteria *(continued)*

Conduct Disorder *(continued)*

Specify severity:

Mild: few if any conduct problems in excess of those required to make the diagnosis **and** conduct problems cause only minor harm to others

Moderate: number of conduct problems and effect on others intermediate between "mild" and "severe"

Severe: many conduct problems in excess of those required to make the diagnosis **or** conduct problems cause considerable harm to others

Source.   Reprinted from American Psychiatric Association: *Diagnostic and Statistical Manual of Mental Disorders,* 4th Edition, Text Revision. Washington, DC, American Psychiatric Association, 2000. Copyright 2000, American Psychiatric Association. Used with permission.

functional on the biological level and redirecting the nosology toward that construct. The clearest candidate for that role is aggression.

Oppositional Defiant Disorder

Children with ODD defy legitimate authority (e.g., reasonable parents and teachers). The pathology of the disorder (tantrums, swearing, stubbornness) is easy to recognize, although whether it crosses a clinical threshold may not be. Such children act out more with people they know well than with those they do not know, and the seriousness may not be evident in an office consultation. Mood lability is often present and contributes to what parents often call a "Jekyll and Hyde phenomenon"; they feel they have two different children depending on whether their child is irritable or not. For this reason, these children are often diagnosed with "juvenile bipolar disorder," even in the absence of classic mania (Donovan et al. 2003; Leibenluft et al. 2003).

Conduct Disorder

CD describes a more pervasive instantiation of the antisocial tendency. The problem is violation of basic rights of others or major age-appropriate societal norms. It is often preceded developmentally by ODD. DSM-IV-TR (Table 3–1) proposes four categories of conduct problems: 1) aggression toward people and animals, 2) destruction of property, 3) deceitfulness/theft, and 4) serious rule violations. In the first category, cruelty and victimization (starting fights, rape, torture, and use of weapons)—not necessarily impulsivity—is evident. The element of deliberation is also present in the second category as "deliberate fire setting with the intention of causing serious damage" (American Psychiatric Association 2000, p. 94). The third category also implies some deliberation to break and enter, con people, or forge signatures. The last category, rule violations, involves staying out late, running away, and truancy. It is clear that none of these behaviors logically entails an impulsive mind. Furthermore, if there is a connection between impulsivity and these behaviors, an intervening step is needed, a matter that is explored further in the section "The Intervening Step," later in this chapter.

Drawing primarily on a multiwave follow-up study of children born in Dunedin, New Zealand, in 1973 (Moffitt 1993b), DSM-IV-TR endorses a separation of CD into early-onset (first symptom before age 10 years) and late-onset types. Early-onset CD has high comorbidity with ADHD, male predominance, and a range of other developmental delays. Late-onset CD is a heterogeneous disorder and even includes some adolescents who are simply delinquent but not psychiatrically impaired (Moffitt 1993b).

A Working Theory of Aggression

If the nosology is to be directed away from intuitions about conscience and toward aggression, a theory of aggression is needed. Mammalian models suggest normal aggression is *affective* or *predatory*. Affective aggression typically occurs intraspecies and involves vocalizations and sympathetic arousal. Predatory aggression is without significant arousal and generally is interspecies (Volavka 1995). Separate neural circuits underlie the respective responses (Panksepp 1998). Vitiello and Stoff (1997) examined evidence from clinical observations, experimental laboratory paradigms, and cluster/factor analyses in humans and found evidence of an impulsive-reactive-hostile-affective subtype of aggression and controlled-proactive-instrumental-predatory subtype, although in individual patients these often co-occur.

It is not obvious how impulsive aggression leads to an intent to hurt people, but it is obvious how predatory aggression leads to that outcome. Unleashed predatory aggression almost logically entails victimization of people. The behaviors described in the CD criteria could easily be the work of a cold, calculating predatory mind (or "psychopath"). Barry et al. (2000) compared callous, unemotional conduct-disordered children with impulsive conduct-disordered children and concluded that "impulsivity and antisocial behavior alone are insufficient to document persons who fit the construct of psychopathy" (p. 335). Much of the biological research on antisocial spectrum problems has emphasized phenomena such as low galvanic skin conductance and low heart rate, signs of the low sympathetic arousal (Ortiz and Raine 2004) that accompanies normal predatory behavior (Panksepp 1998). However deep this line of research may go, it is unlikely to reveal a role for psychopharmacology.

The situation with nonpredatory aggression is very different. Here, a deeper understanding of the biology may well inform psychopharmacological interventions. Pathological affective aggression (or impulsive aggression) is usually taken as the model of pharmacologically treatable aggression, because it entails a subjective experience of anger (Panksepp 1998), is often ego dystonic, and exists in a variety of "organic" states (intoxication, seizures, dementia, medical illnesses; Tardiff 1998).

In contrast to predatory aggression, a variety of pharmacological agents are used with varying but often dramatic success (Bassarath 2003) in affective aggression. This implies that clinical practice already suggests a deeper understanding of the phenomenon than laboratory experiments alone. Pathological affective aggression must be biologically heterogeneous, because there is no other parsimonious explanation for the fact that radically different compounds (stimulants, antipsychotics, antidepressants, beta-blockers, alpha-adrenergic downregulators, and mood stabilizers) sometimes work after others have failed to help or even worsened the clinical situation. Also, in contrast to predatory aggression, affective aggression is not inherently antisocial. It requires social input to lead to antisocial spectrum pathology. Therefore, intervention prior to or concomitant with the social input could theoretically alter the course of the development of antisocial pathology in children and adolescents (Donovan et al. 2004b).

The Intervening Step: From Impulsive Aggression to an Antisocial Pattern

Social factors are important in the genesis of antisocial behavior. High-crime neighborhoods, family discord, harsh punishment, lack of supervision, and access to substances of abuse are all implicated in the development of antisocial

spectrum problems (Rutter 2003). Environmental factors are especially important in adolescent-onset conduct problems, and their mediation can be modeled with sociological concepts alone (Moffitt 1993a). For some adolescent
delinquents, even when psychiatric issues are involved, they may be initially
unrelated to aggression. Aggression may be absent in childhood only to emerge
in the context of substance use and deviant peers (Wilson and Steiner 2002).

For early-onset antisocial problems, a more psychological model is required.
Loosely framed, the question is what reciprocal interactions between a biological factor (affective/impulsive aggression) and the daily environment (a social
factor) erode the developing moral sense in a child. Theories addressing this
question emphasize repeated daily interactions that inculcate a view of what
behaviors make sense in the microenvironment in which the child finds him-
or herself (Dishion et al. 1995b; Ialongo et al. 1996; Kellam et al. 1998).

Coercion theory proposes that a tendency to throw tantrums may be biologically based, but the child quickly learns that contingent rage is a powerful
way to control the microenvironment and comes to value tantrums for their
own sake. Strictly speaking, this is a negative reinforcement paradigm (Dishion et al. 1995b). The demand for socialized behavior is annoying to the
child, who would prefer to do whatever he or she wants. After the parent
makes a demand (clean your room), the child throws a tantrum. The child
and parent argue, and the demand to clean the room is forgotten. The tantrum has been reinforced, because the net result is that the child got out of
cleaning the room. Repeated over thousands of interactions in expanding
contexts, this pattern teaches the child that coercion is adaptive in the short
term (Chilcoat et al. 1995; Dishion et al. 1995b). Attachment explains why
coercion is not universal—why children and parents seek ways to relate that
are adaptive in the long term, even though coercion may work in the short-
term, and why children accept limits and adults try to provide them (Dishion
et al. 1995b). As attachment behaviors improve, coercion decreases.

Also relevant to the pathogenesis of an antisocial attitude from impulsive
aggression is Kellam and colleagues' (1998) focus on the consequences of educational tracking. Social fields have individuals who are "natural raters" of a
child's mastery of the life task that is the focus of that social field. School presents potentially conflicting life tasks (learning and socialization) with different raters (the teacher and the peer group). Classmates may be reinforcing
aggression while the teacher is trying to teach. A child who cannot sit still and

comply with the teacher will be at risk for long-term aggressive behavior if tracked into a classroom with other aggressive children, because these "natural raters" will reinforce the child's innate aggressive tendency. Kellam found that as early as the first grade, schools segregated ("tracked") aggressive children into the same classroom; thus "tracking" made aggression the social norm, homogenized different types of aggression, and had a profound antisocial affect on development (Ialongo et al. 1996; Kellam et al. 1998). Special education is an extreme form of tracking. It would be highly desirable to limit educational tracking (Dishion et al. 1995a). If a child is tracked because of affective (impulsive) aggression, then successful pharmacological treatment of this aggression could allow the child to be mainstreamed and learn with normal peers, promoting prosocial behavior (Kellam 1999).

Subdividing Affective (Impulsive) Aggression

Aggression is easier to operationalize than conscience. Aggression comes in two main types: predatory and affective (impulsive). Unbridled predatory aggression leads directly to antisocial behavior. Affective (impulsive) aggression requires an intermediate step, a complex form of pathological reciprocal social learning, to lead to antisocial behavior. The child's aggression distorts the environment and the environment distorts the child's moral sense; the child's psychopathology helps create the social pathology that promotes the psychopathology. It is also important to know how treatable the biological contribution is, because the effects are cumulative. To address treatment, it is necessary to subdivide affective aggression, starting with observations from clinical research (Table 3–2).

Clinical practice suggests that at least two cognitive and two mood states are associated with pathological affective aggression. One cognitive form involves pure impulsivity: hitting first, without thinking. This pattern was first described by Bradley in 1937. Although children are often diagnosed with ADHD, the criteria for ADHD are neither necessary nor sufficient in order for aggression to improve with stimulants. What seems essential is the impulsive component (Klein et al. 1997). Another cognitive form of pathological aggression commonly seen in abused children is sometimes called "psychosis not otherwise specified" or borderline psychotic rage. These children and adolescents misinterpret reality in a paranoid direction, without being floridly

Table 3–2. Proposed aggressive disorders nosology: medication implications and relation to antisocial behavior

Major division	Subdivision	Second subdivision	Implications for first medication choice	Relation to antisocial behavior
Predatory	None	None	None	Direct
Affective	Cognitive	Impulsive	Stimulant	Indirect
Affective	Cognitive	Paranoid	Low-dose antipsychotics	Indirect
Affective	Mood	Mixed irritable (outer- and inner-directed)	Serotonin reuptake inhibitors	Indirect
Affective	Mood	Outer-directed irritable	Anticonvulsants and mood stabilizers	Indirect

psychotic, and they often respond to low-dose antipsychotics (Campbell et al. 1992). Impulsivity and borderline psychosis may be considered cognitive distortions leading to affective aggression.

There are at least two mood states associated with affective aggression. One seems to involve some degree of autoaggression (Hawton et al. 2002), with negative self-attribution and a mixed irritable-dysphoric state. This state in children and adolescents has not been explored, but adults with these problems benefit from serotonin reuptake blockers (Coccaro and Kavoussi 1997).

Finally, some children have chronic irritability and affective storms (Biederman 1995). It is not settled (Biederman et al. 1998) whether this is a variant of bipolar disorder, but it is clear that the antisocial spectrum (Biederman et al. 1998; Kovacs and Pollock 1995) and substance abuse risk (Biederman et al. 2000) are high in these children. Sullen, withdrawn behavior or loud, intrusive behavior is common, but depression, anxiety, or autoaggression (e.g., wrist cutting) is very rare. The moods shift from normal to irritable, and irritability drives the aggression. Subjects do not meet National Institute of Mental Health criteria (Leibenluft et al. 2003) for juvenile bipolar disorder (Donovan et al. 2004a). An alternative to the bipolar conceptualization is that these children and adolescents have a mood disturbance characterized by outer-directed irritability. Although this disturbance was first defined in adults (Snaith and Taylor 1985; Snaith et al. 1978), subsequent work suggests that its features also characterize a group of explosive youth who improve when given the mood stabilizer/anticonvulsant divalproex (Donovan et al. 2003).

Clinical Phenomenology of Affective (Impulsive) Aggression

The following case examples simplify social factors to illustrate different types of affective aggression. Only clinical vignettes can capture the anguish of raising children and adolescents with impulsive aggression. Because these stories are taken from outpatient clinical research and private practice, the families tend to be well-intentioned. This brings out the distortion this aggression creates in family life.

Certain elements in the environment come through despite the focus on medication. It is very important to involve the school, all caretakers, community organizations, and probation officers. It is also important to structure as much of the day and weekend as possible. Unstructured time, such as the school bus ride, homeroom time, hanging out with peers, and weekends, brings out the pathology.

Aggression Driven by Stimulant-Responsive Impulsivity

Janet was 6 years old, the only child of lower-middle-class parents. She fidgeted and interrupted constantly. Her mother had difficulty arranging play dates because Janet would hit other children without thinking. Embarrassed and frustrated, her mother often yelled at her to think before she acted, but Janet would seem to ignore her, which led to time-outs and corporal punishment. Janet began to deliberately annoy her parents. In kindergarten, she demanded her teacher's attention; when she did not get it, she would provoke other children. She cut into line, and when her peers objected, she pushed and slapped them. Constantly in trouble at school, she had alienated her friends and could not work in a group without starting a verbal or physical fight. Diagnosed with ADHD, Janet was given stimulant medication that eliminated the impulsive aggressive behavior and helped reverse the negative disciplinary situation.

This kind of affective aggression is driven by pure impulsivity in the sense of lack of judgment in how to react to environmental input. It moves toward antisocial behavior, because it provokes angry responses. The child identified with the adult response and impulsively administered it to others: Janet slapped other children as she herself had been slapped. She cannot and eventually does not want to inhibit the impulse. The efficacy of stimulants in this type of aggression should help to break the budding vicious circle.

Aggression Driven by Impulsivity and Irritability

Michael was 11 years old. His mother wanted help with his explosive temper and irritable mood. He always seemed to be irritable, even as a child. His father had a terrible temper, but she divorced him when Michael was an infant, and Michael had had no contact with him since. Michael started fights in kindergarten and was placed in special education in first grade for emotional disturbance. At home, he scowled at his mother but was afraid of her. Lately, he had been having explosive episodes at home; he punched holes in the wall and destroyed a television screen. He had never been arrested. His mother worked for child protective services, and his grandmother provided much of his care during the years he was growing up. In addition to his explosive temper, Michael had had reading delays, but he was currently reading on a fourth-grade level. He entered a treatment study of the mood stabilizer/anticonvulsant divalproex and placebo. He was observed on and off medication because it was a two-phase study. On placebo, his baseline behavior changed slightly with supportive treatment. On active medication, Michael's temper and irritability markedly improved, but he would not sit still. Instead of defying his mother, he acted in a silly manner while fidgeting. Addition of stimulant medication normalized this. Parent management training was available through the mother's work, and she had tried it many times without success; in the ensuing 6 weeks, parent training was far more successful than it had been in the placebo period. Michael was discharged much improved.

This clinical vignette illustrates several features of impulsive aggression. Such children are often in special education. Their relations with their parents and teachers are often hostile and coercive, although here the mother and child were at a stalemate. The mother used her parent training to create counter-coercive measures, but their relationship was devoid of pleasure. There is significant comorbidity with other developmental disorders, in this case a reading delay. This child had both a mood disturbance and ADHD, and the pathologies were distinct and responded separately to different pharmacological interventions. Treatment involves doing many things at once, but addressing the biology of the problem makes psychotherapeutic interventions more productive.

Aggression Driven by Paranoia

At age 6 years, Angel was already in serious trouble. He had been in three foster homes and had been physically and sexually abused prior to these placements. He was deeply suspicious of people and their intentions and pummeled children at school on minimal or no provocation. His grandmother finally obtained custody and tried to care for him. However, constant calls from the school about his aggressive behavior led her to regret her decision to take on this problem child. She described him as intensely jealous of the other children in the house, but it went beyond that. If another child made direct eye contact with him in a hostile or ambiguous way, he would attack with a fury that amazed and frightened his grandmother. He was given long-acting methylphenidate with minimal improvement. Time-outs were also only marginally helpful. The attacks occurred on a daily basis at home and at school. A kitchen knife was found under his bed. The school placed him in special education for his emotional disturbance. Although the violent episodes were reduced in the new school environment, they still occurred, especially on the school bus. The episodes seemed to come out of the blue, without any signs of mood disturbance or hyperactivity. It was as though he were paranoid, although there was no evidence that he was hallucinating. This child improved on a low dose of the antipsychotic medication risperidone. His play still contained elements of surprise, fear, and attack, but he was less inclined to act on these scenarios.

Like children with ADHD, Angel's aggression seemed to spring from cognitive processing problems, but here the problem was not so much a lack of planning as a paranoid distortion of the outside world. He thought about what he was doing, but his thinking was distorted. This pattern is common in children who have been subjected to extreme physical abuse.

Aggression Driven by Outer-Directed Irritability

David was 8 years old with fair features. He had been very well behaved in school until the previous month, when he had had a verbal tantrum. At home, similar problems had been occurring for several years. The slightest criticism could send him on a rampage. He fought with his older brother constantly and broke his radio. Several cracks in the wall were evidence of his fury. Time-outs, rewards, and punishments made little impact. One therapist told his worried, dazed mother that no matter how explosive David became, she must insist he complete the task that led to his tantrum or she would be reinforcing the tantrum. She and her husband tried this, but in his rage David destroyed a set of dishes, a toaster, and a window. He told his teacher and principal that his mother was mean to him and kept him from his toys. The parents were afraid of him.

Partly believing the child, the school pressured the parents to see another therapist. This therapist advised the parents to be less strict and "pick their battles." This also did not work because some battles that had to be won could not be won. What was particularly upsetting was the change in the child's demeanor when he went from a normal to an irritable mood. When in a normal mood, he was sweet and loving, and outside observers were quick to blame the parents for the family discord. A longer period of observation revealed a Jekyll and Hyde phenomenon. He could change on a dime. "He's like the wind," his father stated. "How can you direct the wind?" Although David expressed remorse after each episode, he felt no depression or anxiety. Everything was someone, or something, else's fault. If he knocked over a glass, it was the glass's fault for being there. When truly calm, he could acknowledge some responsibility, but when irritable, his thinking was always directed toward blame in the outside world.

His pediatrician prescribed methylphenidate, but the parents stopped it after a week. It did not help with his temper outbursts and made him more irritable when it wore off. At this point, the parents enrolled David in the same study attended by Michael in the earlier case example. David's explosive episodes ended after 2 weeks of divalproex, and his irritability rating improved markedly. When he was switched double-blind to placebo, his irritability returned to baseline, but his explosive aggression remained well below baseline, although much worse than when he was on medication. During the active medication phase, his parents were able to implement some of the many suggestions they received from psychotherapists, but this became difficult during the placebo phase. On medication, his tendency to blame others declined, suggesting this thinking was associated with his irritable mood.

Both Michael and David met criteria for ODD, and Michael had ADHD and some CD features. David did not have any evidence of ADHD, nor did he have any symptoms of mania. He grew marginally worse on stimulants. He had no evidence of depression or anxiety. Instead his mood was characterized by outer-directed irritability and certain cognitions associated with it (i.e., total externalization of blame). This type of thinking diminished between irritable episodes and virtually disappeared on medication, suggesting the thinking was a rationalization of a mood rather than a budding psychopathic character trait. It is clear in David's case that irritability was driving the aggression rather than both being part of a global, epileptoid phenomenon: irritability returned to baseline on placebo but overt aggression did not, suggesting the two were biologically distinct; whatever the biological diathesis in David was, it was something close to irritability. In both cases, there was a clear role for medication. Behavioral control techniques were not working by themselves. These vignettes do not convey the daily struggle of living with an aggressive oppositional/defiant child.

Aggression Driven by Inner-Directed Irritability

Ricky was adopted at birth. His new parents were thrilled to have their first baby and showered him with love and attention. He was fidgety but otherwise pleasant. Around the time he started school, his adoptive parents had a child of their own. The teachers noted he had trouble sitting still and would hit children without thinking. He was diagnosed with ADHD. Stimulants helped him focus and markedly reduced the hitting, but his academic performance was hampered by reading delays. Around age 12 years, he started to take offense at what anyone in his family said. When told he could not go out, he cursed and broke furniture. He started to steal with his friends and lie to his parents. On at least two occasions he came home drunk, once after stealing the family car. His parents learned that several of his friends had been arrested and that two were dead—one had been murdered and the other had suicided. When his parents told him they had decided to place him in a residential treatment facility, he threw a chair at the television set, then went into his room, where he smashed a window and cut his wrists with a piece of glass. Taken to the hospital, he saw a psychiatrist who asked him about his mood and diagnosed major depression. He was given fluoxetine, and his aggressive behavior disappeared. He is enrolled presently in a day treatment center for his mild substance abuse.

Ricky illustrates the need to ask about inner-directed irritability, anxiety, and depression in children with antisocial spectrum problems. His behavior problems were so clear that the possibility of an underlying mood disorder was not explored. This was despite the change in behavior and the suicide of an acquaintance. Ricky's irritability was not the pure outer-directed type found in David. His was mixed with inner-directed anger, low self-esteem, depression, and anxiety. Accepted by a deviant subculture, he began to use substances, channeling his aggression even more in an antisocial direction.

Affective Aggression and Substance Use, Abuse, or Dependence

Neurobehavioral disinhibition, a deficient capacity to control behavior and regulate emotion commensurate with situational demands, is a construct that is found in children at high risk for substance abuse. It is a risk factor not so much for the amount of a substance used but for the transition from use to abuse. Neurobehavioral disinhibition is consonant with impulsivity in the broad sense or with affective aggression because it includes problems with attention, impulsivity, and emotion (irritability) (Tarter et al. 2003). Although research in this area is preliminary, there may be a specific link on the biological level between outer-directed irritability and marijuana use. Cannabis and disruptive behavior disorders was the only drug–adolescent disorders link found in a review of community studies of adolescent drug use (Armstrong and Costello 2002). Marijuana has anticonvulsant properties (Brust et al. 1992), and some explosive adolescents report that marijuana calms them down. Treatment with an anticonvulsant/mood stabilizer (divalproex) reduces marijuana use in these patients (Donovan et al. 1996, 2004c). Conversely, marijuana withdrawal induces irritable aggression (Haney et al. 1999; Kouri et al. 1999).

Marvin is 17 years old and has a bad temper. He was in special education as a child and had been given a trial of methylphenidate during that time at an unknown dosage. He lives with his mother in a lower-middle-class neighborhood. His mother is a calm, almost complacent woman at first glance, although at second glance one sees she is beyond worry. Marvin has two court dates coming up, and he must not mouth off at the judge. He should not be smoking pot with these court dates coming up, but he insists it is the only thing that calms him down. His mother is no stranger to the Brooklyn courthouse where Marvin will appear. Her brothers have received several jail sentences for drug use, but they never had Marvin's temper. In fact, no one on her side of the family has his temper. Marvin's father, whom Marvin has never met, was a different matter. Like Marvin, he exploded all the time.

At age 12 years, Marvin began to experiment with drugs. He tried alcohol but when he smoked his first joint, he felt a sense of calm come over him. He became patient and tolerant for a while. He tried other drugs but never liked what they did to his mind. "I just smoke weed," Marvin explained. Indeed, he smokes five blunts per day, more than his friends. He is in a special school for delinquent adolescents, but he is not psychopathic. "If you piss me off, I will hurt you," he remarks, but he denies looking for trouble. He is much attached to his mother, although he breaks her things and screams at her when he gets angry. Despite the lack of direction to his life, he is not depressed and has never thought of suicide. His violation of rules and use of a weapon in his fights makes him fit criteria for CD, but his aggression has more the quality of a tantrum.

Assessment

Assessment of children and adolescents with impulsive (affective) aggression proceeds like any other psychiatric assessment in that age group. There are areas of emphasis, however. The chief complaint will reveal a great deal about what kind of contract the clinician has with the child and family. Who is in pain? Who sees that there is a problem? The history should focus on risk factors such as age at onset (adolescent or preadolescent), treatment history (diagnoses, psychotherapy/medication, type, amount, duration, and response), developmental history (prenatal maternal smoking, developmental delays, and multiple caregivers), medical history, and family (abuse, divorce) and social (high-crime neighborhood) data. Parents and child should be interviewed separately and together. Permission to contact other important persons should be obtained. Especially important are teachers, parole officers, and substance abuse counselors.

All reviews of this topic stress the importance of *asking about comorbidities.* Impulsive aggressive children and adolescents often have learning disabilities. Most will have met ADHD criteria at some point in their lives. Some will meet full criteria for major depression and suicidal ideation; in addition, homicidal ideation must be specifically addressed. Substance abuse is extremely common in impulsive aggressive adolescents and represents a major complication. Some patients will already meet criteria for borderline personality disorder, minus the age requirement.

The use of standardized rating forms presents a problem, because a teacher or a parole officer may not carefully complete them. A phone call is likely to be more useful, with some rating-form items worked into the interview. Because many impulsive aggressive children have been in special education, a wealth of information is available from committees on special education regarding the child's IQ (performance and verbal), peer relations, and home situation over an extended period of time. Special education committees can also provide funding if residential placement is necessary.

Treatment

Pharmacotherapy

The evidence base for the pharmacology of aggression is thin. Recent recommendations seem to imply that antipsychotic medications are useful for all forms of pathological aggression. However, this is based on studies in mentally disabled populations (Pappadopulos et al. 2003; Schur et al. 2003) and may not be generalizable. An alternative approach was provided earlier in the chapter (see section titled "Subdividing Affective [Impulsive] Aggression") and is summarized in Table 3–2. For stimulants in impulsive aggression, the dose and response patterns follow the guidelines for stimulant use in ADHD. Dosages of methylphenidate of 70 mg or more are needed before declaring treatment failure (Riddle et al. 2001). For borderline psychotic rage, low dosages of antipsychotic medications are especially helpful (Schur et al. 2003). The dosage is not known a priori, and starting low and increasing gradually is preferable to starting with a large dosage and cutting back. Based on studies in adults with impulsive aggression (Coccaro and Kavoussi 1997) as well as clinical experience, it is reasonable to use serotonin reuptake inhibitors because they are often helpful at antidepressant levels for aggression accompanied by mixed depressed, anxious states. These patients must be watched carefully, because clinical experience suggests these agents may relieve anxiety but increase irritability. The addition of a mood stabilizer is often very helpful. For outer-directed irritability alone, dosages of a mood stabilizer equivalent to divalproex of 10 mg/lb are a reasonable target (Donovan et al. 2000; see Table 3–2).

Psychotherapy

For children with mild oppositional behavior or otherwise normal adolescents caught up in an antisocial, substance-using lifestyle, psychosocial interventions may be sufficient. For impulsive aggressive children and adolescents, even if they improve on medication, they still need corrective socializing experiences. It is logical to recommend evidence-based therapies, but one must note that most treatments offered in the community (talk therapy, group therapy) are not those with an evidence base. For ODD and CD, the following types of treatments have empirical support: parent management training alone or in combination with cognitive problem-solving skills training, and multisystemic therapy.

Parent Management Training

Parent management training is based on coercion theory as outlined earlier in the chapter. It seeks to change parent–child interactions in the home by eliminating the reinforcement of antisocial behaviors. The theory is that these behaviors occur so rapidly that it is necessary to demonstrate them in detail, sometimes on videotape. However, if understood, the tantrums, whining, and incessant demands primarily characteristic of ODD will be extinguished through lack of reinforcement. New skills are applied to simple problems before trying to solve more serious behavior problems. Duration of treatment varies with severity. Programs for children with mild oppositional behavior typically last 6–8 weeks. However, typical treatments for clinically referred youth last much longer (12–25 weeks; Kazdin 2000).

Problem-Solving Skills Training

Problem-solving skills training is an extension of cognitive-behavioral therapy into the realm of antisocial spectrum disorders. It works synergistically with parent management training. The key cognition addressed is the attribution of hostile intent to the actions of others. Problem-solving skills training fosters nonaggressive responses (e.g., to perceived provocations by peers) by altering the cognitive processes that underlie antisocial behavior. The program is composed of small groups of children or adolescents and lasts for about 20 sessions. The therapist is a coach who models the skills being taught and provides cues and feedback (Kazdin 2000).

Multisystemic Therapy

Multisystemic therapy is a macrotherapy that formalizes the intuition that with delinquent youth one must do many things simultaneously. Using a family preservation model of treatment delivery, it brings the treatment to the home or the school and makes it available around the clock. Extending the concepts of boundaries and hierarchies from structural family therapy (Minuchin 1974; Minuchin et al. 1967), it encourages the different systems (school, peers, family, probation department) to communicate in a functional way to supervise a delinquent's behavior (Henggeler et al. 1998). If psychiatric treatment is required, its delivery system is also one of the many systems that must be brought into the loop. Multisystemic therapy involves extensive community outreach and is conducted by a team of two to four therapists and their on-site supervisor. They provide each other with group and peer supervision.

Conclusion

The antisocial spectrum is an area of psychopathology in which impulsivity in the broadest sense and aggression overlap. Impulsive aggression is nonpredatory aggression. Because *impulsivity* is often used to refer specifically to impulsive behavior expressed by stimulant-responsive ADHD children and not to all forms of dysregulated behavior, the term *affective aggression* is preferred. This chapter explored how knowledge of affective aggression and its predictable social consequences can be used to see antisocial behavior in a different light. It has proposed an heuristic clinical nosology of aggression based on the way in which various types of medication are used in clinical practice, with the expectation that this nosology will be modified or refuted by future research.

This chapter also addressed the complex psychology of the social experience an explosive child or adolescent creates in the home and the extent to which it can be reversed. Coercion and educational tracking make pathological aggression seem normal to the child. Reversing this requires an integrated approach. Treating the aspect of the pathology that is amenable to pharmacological intervention should facilitate evidence-based psychotherapeutic approaches.

References

American Psychiatric Association: Diagnostic and Statistical Manual of Mental Disorders, 4th Edition, Text Revision. Washington, DC, American Psychiatric Association, 2000

Armstrong TD, Costello EJ: Community studies on adolescent substance use, abuse, or dependence and psychiatric comorbidity. J Consult Clin Psychol 70:1224–1239, 2002

Barry CT, Frick PJ, DeShazo TM, et al: The importance of callous-unemotional traits for extending the concept of psychopathy to children. J Abnorm Psychol 109:335–340, 2000

Bassarath L: Medication strategies in childhood aggression: a review. Can J Psychiatry 48:367–373, 2003

Biederman J: Developmental subtypes of juvenile bipolar disorder. Harv Rev Psychiatry 3:227–230, 1995

Biederman J, Klein RG, Pine DS, et al: Resolved: mania is mistaken for ADHD in prepubertal children. J Am Acad Child Adolesc Psychiatry 37:1091–1099, 1998

Biederman J, Faraone SV, Wozniak J, et al: Parsing the association between bipolar, conduct, and substance use disorders: a familial risk analysis. Biol Psychiatry 48:1037–1044, 2000

Bradley C: The behavior of children receiving benzedrine. Am J Psychiatry 94:577–584, 1937

Brust JC, Ng SK, Hauser AW, et al: Marijuana use and the risk of new onset seizures. Trans Am Clin Climatol Assoc 103:176–181, 1992

Campbell M, Gonzalez NM, Silva RR: The pharmacological treatment of conduct disorders and rage outbursts. Psychiatr Clin North Am 15:69–85, 1992

Chilcoat HD, Dishion TJ, Anthony JC: Parent monitoring and the incidence of drug sampling in urban elementary school children. Am J Epidemiol 141:25–31, 1995

Coccaro EF, Kavoussi RJ: Fluoxetine and impulsive aggressive behavior in personality disordered subjects. Arch Gen Psychiatry 54:1081–1088, 1997

Dishion TJ, Andrews DW, Crosby L: Antisocial boys and their friends in early adolescence: relationship characteristics, quality, and interactional process. Child Dev 66:139–151, 1995a

Dishion TJ, French DC, Patterson GE: The development and ecology of antisocial behavior, in Developmental Psychopathology. Edited by Cicchetti D, Cohen DJ. New York, Wiley, 1995b, pp 421–471

Donovan SJ, Susser ES, Nunes EV: Divalproex sodium for use with conduct-disordered adolescent marijuana users. Am J Addict 5:181, 1996

Donovan SJ, Stewart JW, Nunes EV, et al: Divalproex treatment for youth with explosive temper and mood lability: a double-blind, placebo-controlled crossover design. Am J Psychiatry 157:818–820, 2000

Donovan SJ, Nunes EV, Stewart JW, et al: Outer directed irritability: a distinct mood syndrome in explosive youth with a disruptive behavior disorder? J Clin Psychiatry 64:698–701, 2003

Donovan S, Stewart JW, Nunes EV: Do divalproate-sensitive youth with explosive outbursts meet new broad criteria for juvenile bipolar disorder? Paper presented at the American Academy of Child and Adolescent Psychiatry Annual Meeting, Washington, DC, October 2004a

Donovan S, Nunes EV, Stewart JW: Medication sensitive behavioral dyscontrol in children at risk for adolescent substance abuse. Presented at the College on Problems of Drug Dependence Annual Meeting, San Juan, Puerto Rico, June 2004b

Donovan S, Stewart JW, Nunes EV: Temper, mood and marijuana: a link at the biological level? Presented at the American Academy of Child and Adolescent Psychiatry Annual Meeting, Washington, DC, October 2004c

Earls F, Mezzacappa E: Conduct and oppositional disorders, in Child and Adolescent Psychiatry. Edited by Rutter M, Taylor E. Oxford, England, Blackwell Scientific, 2002, pp 419–436

Haney M, Ward AS, Comer SD, et al: Abstinence symptoms following smoked marijuana in humans. Psychopharmacology 141:395–404, 1999

Hawton K, Rodham K, Evans E, et al: Deliberate self harm in adolescents: self report survey in schools in England. BMJ 325:1207–1211, 2002

Henggeler SW, Schoenwald SK, Borduin CM, et al: Multisystemic Treatment of Antisocial Behavior in Children and Adolescents. New York, Guilford, 1998

Ialongo N, Edelsohn G, Werthamer-Larsson L, et al: The course of aggression in first-grade children with and without comorbid anxious symptoms. J Abnorm Child Psychol 24:445–456, 1996

Kazdin AE: Treatments for aggressive and antisocial children. Child Adolesc Psychiatr Clin N Am 9:841–858, 2000

Kellam SG: The influence of the first-grade classroom on the development of aggressive behavior. Phi Delta Kappa Center for Evaluation, Development, and Research Bulletin, 1999

Kellam SG, Ling X, Merisca R, et al: The effect of the level of aggression in the first grade classroom on the course and malleability of aggressive behavior into middle school. Dev Psychopathol 10:165–185, 1998

Klein RG, Abikoff H, Klass E, et al: Clinical efficacy of methylphenidate in conduct disorder with and without attention deficit hyperactivity disorder. Arch Gen Psychiatry 54:1073–1080, 1997

Kouri EM, Pope HG Jr, Lukas SE: Changes in aggressive behavior during withdrawal from long-term marijuana use. Psychopharmacology 143:302–308, 1999

Kovacs M, Pollock M: Bipolar disorder and comorbid conduct disorder in childhood and adolescence. J Am Acad Child Adolesc Psychiatry 34:715–723, 1995

Kutcher S, Aman M, Brooks SJ, et al: International consensus statement on attention-deficit/hyperactivity disorder (ADHD) and disruptive behaviour disorders (DBDs): clinical implications and treatment practice suggestions. Eur Neuropsychopharmacol 14:11–28, 2004

Leibenluft E, Charney DS, Towbin KE, et al: Defining clinical phenotypes of juvenile mania. Am J Psychiatry 160:430–437, 2003

Loeber R, Burke JD, Lahey BB, et al: Oppositional defiant and conduct disorder: a review of the past 10 years, part I. J Am Acad Child Adolesc Psychiatry 39:1468–1484, 2000

Minuchin S: Families and Family Therapy. Cambridge, MA, Harvard University Press, 1974

Minuchin S, Montalvo B, Guerney BG, et al: Families of the Slums: An Exploration of Their Structure and Treatment. New York, Basic Books, 1967

Moeller FG, Barratt ES, Dougherty DM, et al: Psychiatric aspects of impulsivity. Am J Psychiatry 158:1783–1793, 2001

Moffitt TE: Adolescence-limited and life-course-persistent antisocial behavior: a developmental taxonomy. Psychol Rev 100:674–701, 1993a

Moffitt TE: The neuropsychology of conduct disorder. Dev Psychopathol 5:135–151, 1993b

Ortiz J, Raine A: Heart rate level and antisocial behavior in children and adolescents: a meta-analysis. J Am Acad Child Adolesc Psychiatry 43:154–162, 2004

Panksepp J: Affective Neuroscience: The Foundation of Human and Animal Emotions. New York, Oxford University Press, 1998

Pappadopulos E, MacIntyre JC, Crismon ML, et al: Treatment recommendations for the use of antipsychotics for aggressive youth (TRAAY), part II. J Am Acad Child Adolesc Psychiatry 42:145–161, 2003

Richters JE: Disordered views of aggressive children: a late twentieth century perspective. Ann N Y Acad Sci 794:208–223, 1996

Riddle MA, Kastelic EA, Frosch E: Pediatric psychopharmacology. J Child Psychol Psychiatry 42:73–90, 2001

Rutter M: Crucial paths from risk indicator to causal mechanism, in Causes of Conduct Disorder and Juvenile Delinquency. Edited by Lahey B, Moffitt T, Caspi A. New York, Guilford, 2003, pp 3–24

Schur SB, Sikich L, Findling RL, et al: Treatment recommendations for the use of antipsychotics for aggressive youth (TRAAY), part I: a review. J Am Acad Child Adolesc Psychiatry 42:132–144, 2003

Snaith RP, Taylor CM: Irritability: definition, assessment and associated factors. Br J Psychiatry 147:127–136, 1985

Snaith RP, Constantopoulos AA, Jardine MY, et al: A clinical scale for the self-assessment of irritability. Br J Psychiatry 132:164–171, 1978

Tardiff K: Unusual diagnoses among violent patients. Psychiatr Clin North Am 21:567–576, 1998

Tarter RE, Kirisci L, Mezzich A, et al: Neurobehavioral disinhibition in childhood predicts early age at onset of substance use disorder. Am J Psychiatry 160:1078–1085, 2003

Vitiello B, Stoff D: Subtypes of aggression and their relevance to child psychiatry. J Am Acad Child Adolesc Psychiatry 36:307–315, 1997

Volavka J: Neurobiology of Violence. Washington, DC, American Psychiatric Press, 1995

Waschbusch DA: A meta-analytic examination of comorbid hyperactivity-impulsive attention problems and conduct problems. Psychol Bull 128:118–150, 2002

Wilson JJ, Steiner H: Conduct problems, substance use and social anxiety: a developmental study of recovery and adaptation. Clin Child Psychol Psychiatry 7:235–247, 2002

4

Self-Injurious Behaviors

Daphne Simeon, M.D.

Phenomenology

Classification and Diagnoses

Self-injurious behaviors (SIBs) perplex and challenge clinicians in their blatant call to be noticed, understood, and treated. *Self-injurious behavior* can be defined as any behavior involving the deliberate infliction of direct physical harm to one's own body without any intent to die as a consequence of the behavior. SIBs are largely underrepresented in the current DSM classification system. DSM-IV-TR (American Psychiatric Association 2000) offers a few diagnoses under which many, but not all, SIBs can be "fitted": trichotillomania or impulse-control disorders not otherwise specified (both under Axis I impulse-control disorders); Axis II borderline personality disorder (BPD) under the criterion "recurrent suicidal behavior, gestures, or threats, or self-mutilating behavior" (p. 710); and stereotypic movement disorder with self-injurious behavior (disorders of infancy, childhood, or adolescence).

More recently, Simeon and Favazza (2001) proposed a phenomenologically based and clinically relevant comprehensive schema for the classification of all SIBs. They proposed four major categories of SIB: stereotypic, major, compulsive, and impulsive. *Stereotypic SIBs* refer to highly repetitive, monotonous, fixed, often rhythmic, seemingly highly driven, and usually contentless (i.e., devoid of thought, affect, and meaning) acts that can range widely in self-inflicted tissue injury from mild to severe or even life-threatening at times. These appear more strongly biologically driven than other types of SIBs and are frequently associated with mental retardation, autism, and syndromes such as Lesch-Nyhan, Cornelia de Lange's, and Prader-Willi. SIBs are quite common in individuals with mental retardation, with estimates ranging from 3% to 46% (Bodfish et al. 1995; Winchel and Stanley 1991). These syndromes are outside the range of behaviors commonly encountered by nonspecialized clinicians; they are not further discussed in this chapter.

Major SIBs include dramatic and often life-threatening forms of self-injury and involve major and often irreversible destruction of body tissue such as castration, eye enucleation, and amputation of extremities. They are most frequently associated with psychotic states such as schizophrenia but also with intoxications, neurological conditions, bipolar disorder, severe personality disorders, and transsexualism. Common themes of major SIBs involve sin, sexual temptation, punishment, and salvation (Clark 1981; DeMuth et al. 1983). Religious delusions are quite common (Nakaya 1996).

Compulsive SIBs include repetitive, often ritualistic behaviors that typically occur multiple times daily, such as trichotillomania (hair pulling), onychophagia (nail biting), and skin picking or skin scratching (neurotic excoriations). Of these, trichotillomania is by far the most extensively investigated and the only one diagnostically classified as a discrete disorder in DSM-IV-TR. Compulsive SIBs other than hair pulling, such as skin picking and nail biting, appear to be quite common but have received much less attention in the psychiatric literature. These behaviors are discussed in Chapter 7, "Trichotillomania."

Impulsive SIBs are the topic of this chapter. The most common behaviors in this category include skin cutting, skin burning, and self-hitting. These behaviors may be broadly conceptualized as acts of impulsive aggression, not unlike impulsive suicide attempts, where the target of the aggression is the self. These behaviors frequently permit those who engage in them to obtain rapid but short-lived relief from a variety of intolerable states, serving a morbidly pathological but life-sustaining function. They are highly complex in their determinants, motivations, and precipitants and need to be thoroughly understood at a descriptive and motivational level on an individual basis before treatment effectiveness can be maximized.

The distinction between compulsive and impulsive repetitive self-injury is not always easy to make. Impulsive SIBs are at times so habitual and repetitive that they can occur on a daily basis without major precipitants, becoming in a sense "compulsions." Indeed, there is some evidence that patients with impulsive SIBs who have obsessional traits are more likely to engage in repetitive self-injury (Gardner and Gardner 1975; McKerracher et al. 1968). A more recent study found that when comparing two groups of patients with BPD, one group that mutilated and one that did not, the former had more obsessive-compulsive symptoms in the absence of more elevated general psychopathology, depression, or anxiety (McKay et al. 2000). Thus, it is probably more accurate to conceptualize impulsive self-injury as encompassing some obsessive-compulsive traits, just as compulsive self-injury may encompass some impulsive traits. Both types of traits facilitate the perpetuation of SIBs via the difficulty in controlling impulses and the tendency to repeat.

Despite the absence of epidemiological data, it has been indirectly calculated that the annual prevalence of impulsive self-injury may be at least 1 in 1,000 people (Favazza 1996). It is more common in females and typically begins in adolescence or early adulthood, although it has been described as early as latency (Green 1978) and preschool (Rosenthal and Rosenthal 1984). Impulsive SIB is more commonly associated with certain disorders such as BPD (Gardner and Cowdry 1985; Schaffer et al. 1982), antisocial personality disorder (Virkkunen 1976), posttraumatic stress disorder (Greenspan and Samuel 1989; Pitman 1990), dissociative disorders (Coons and Milstein 1990; Simeon et al. 1997), and eating disorders (Favaro and Santonastaso 1998; Favazza et al. 1989; Garfinkel et al. 1980; Mitchell et al. 1986; Parkin and Eagles 1993). Of all these diagnoses, the one that most commonly springs to most professionals' minds in association with SIB is BPD, yet it is important to remember that BPD should not be automatically assumed. For example, Axis I diagnoses of substance abuse, posttraumatic stress disorder, and intermittent explosive disorder have been found to be significantly related to self-mutilation independent of borderline and antisocial personality disorder (Zlotnick et al. 1999).

Description

Five descriptive stages have been delineated in impulsive SIB (Leibenluft et al. 1987). The precipitating event often involves real or perceived loss, rejection, or abandonment. It is followed by the escalation of various types of intolerable affects. After failed attempts to forestall the self-injury, the behavior is executed, typically followed by short-lived emotional relief. Individuals describe various self-states and associated motivations leading up to the self-injury (Favazza 1989, 1996; Gardner and Cowdry 1985; Graff and Mallin 1967; Kafka 1969; Leibenluft et al. 1987; Pao 1969). These can include release of unbearable mounting tension; discharge of rage directed at hated parts of the self; self-punishment; lifting of dissociation so as to feel more alive; regaining a sense of control or omnipotence; self-soothing; reconfirming self boundaries; communicating with or controlling others; experiencing sexual excitement or euphoria; relieving intolerable aloneness, alienation, hopelessness, or despair; combating other desperate affects or thoughts; and expression of conflictual dissociative states.

The relationship between impulsive SIBs and suicide attempts is an important one to appreciate. There is evidence that the two conditions are quite distinct from each other, despite their common co-occurrence in patients with certain types of pathologies. The incidence of suicidal ideation during self-mutilation has been found to vary from 28% to 41% (Gardner and Gardner 1975; Pattison and Kahan 1983), yet this need not imply suicidal intent but rather designate the presence of intolerable affective states. In a large cohort of 141 chronically hospitalized patients with BPD, 10 had histories of self-injury alone, whereas 20 had histories of both self-injury and suicide attempts (Stone 1990). A 15-year follow-up showed that a history of self-injury alone was not a predictor of future suicide, whereas a history of prior suicide attempts did predict future suicide. At the same time, one should not underestimate true suicide intent when this is present, misguided by the knowledge that a particular individual is habitually self-mutilating. One study compared the characteristics of suicide attempts in two BPD groups, a self-mutilating and a nonmutilating group. The two groups did not differ in the objective lethality of their attempts; however, the mutilating patients were more depressed, anxious, and impulsive and tended to underestimate the lethality of their attempts (Stanley et al. 2001).

Relationship to Impulsive Aggression

Various studies have clearly demonstrated both the "impulsive" and "aggressive" nature of impulsive SIBs. A very short time lag has been reported between the urge to self-injure and the act itself (Bennum 1983; Favazza and Conterio 1989; Gardner and Gardner 1975). Simeon et al. (1992) found a significant correlation between the severity of self-mutilation and an independent measure of impulsivity in a BPD sample. With respect to aggression, a notable minority of self-injuring individuals, 10%–45%, are aware of conscious anger toward others leading up to the acts of self-injury (Bennum 1983; Gardner and Gardner 1975; Roy 1978). Simeon et al. (1992) reported that, compared with nonmutilating control subjects matched for personality disorder diagnoses, self-mutilating individuals had histories of greater lifetime aggression and sociopathy, and self-mutilation severity correlated significantly with chronic anger. Otto Kernberg's work has traditionally emphasized self-injury as a revengeful enactment in an attempt to omnipotently control the "other" (Kernberg 1987).

Relationship to Childhood Trauma

A history of trauma is another major factor to thoroughly explore whenever impulsive SIBs are encountered. The traumatic experiences usually occurred in childhood, although adult traumata such as combat or rape have also been described in association with self-injury (Greenspan and Samuel 1989; Pitman 1990). A large study of "habitual female self-mutilators" reported childhood abuse in 62% of the subjects. Of these, 29% reported both sexual and physical abuse, 17% reported only sexual abuse, and 16% reported only physical abuse (Favazza and Conterio 1989). Another study compared female incest survivors who did with those who did not self-mutilate and found that those who engaged in SIB had experienced incest of greater duration and frequency, involving a parent perpetrator or a greater number of older offenders (Turell and Armsworth 2000). The loss of a parent at a young age, through death or parental separation, has also been associated with SIB (Kahan and Pattison 1984; Walsh and Rosen 1988). Appallingly, self-mutilation has been described even in preschool children who have suffered abuse or neglect (Rosenthal and Rosenthal 1984). In adolescent inpatients, self-mutilation was predicted by female gender and by histories of sexual abuse and emotional neglect (Lipschitz et al. 1999).

Research supports that above and beyond abuse, neglect can strongly contribute to the genesis and the treatment-resistant perpetuation of SIB (Dubo et al. 1997; van der Kolk et al. 1991). One comprehensive study teased out the contribution of various factors to the genesis and perpetuation of self-destructive behaviors by following 74 individuals with personality disorders over a 4-year period (van der Kolk et al. 1991). A portion of this group had a history of self-mutilation, and within this SIB group there was an 89% incidence of major disruptions in parental care and a 79% incidence of childhood traumas such as physical abuse, sexual abuse, or witnessing domestic violence. Sexual abuse most strongly predicted self-injury, which was also associated with younger age at the time of the abuse as well as with childhood chaos, separations, and neglect. Interestingly, neglect and separation from caregivers predicted continuation of the self-injury in the face of treatment efforts, leading the authors to postulate that such traumas impaired the capacity to form trusting stable bonds that in turn could facilitate treatment change. Another study of inpatients with BPD compared with control subjects with personality disorders similarly found that both parental sexual abuse and emotional neglect were significantly related to self-mutilation (Dubo et al. 1997).

The experience of heightened dissociation leading to self-injury is commonly described by patients. A powerful link between dissociation, childhood abuse, and SIBs has been reported (Brodsky et al. 1995). Dissociation and self-mutilation have been found to be significantly related even when controlling for BPD diagnosis and childhood abuse histories (Zlotnick et al. 1999). An interesting empirical link between alexithymia and self-mutilation suggests that the inability to verbally capture overwhelming affective states may in and of itself be a risk factor for SIB (Zlotnick et al. 1996). Yet other studies have failed to show a link between trauma, dissociation, and self-injury. In two studies comparing self-mutilating with nonmutilating individuals, the two groups did not differ in abuse, separation histories, or parental bonding disturbances (Zweig-Frank et al. 1994a, 1994b). Another type of childhood trauma that less readily comes to mind when encountering SIBs is early invasive physical trauma, mutilation, or surgery (Rosenthal et al. 1972).

Neurobiology

Research into neurobiological processes that may underlie impulsive SIB has been very limited. Therefore, much of what we know or hypothesize is indirectly extrapolated from studies of related entities, such as impulsive aggression or suicide. The most commonly implicated neurochemical systems are the serotonergic and endogenous opioid systems. Coccaro et al. (1989) initially demonstrated that blunted prolactin response to fenfluramine, indicative of reduced serotonergic function, was present in subjects with personality disorder compared with control subjects and correlated with histories of suicide attempts and impulsive aggression. Reduced serotonergic function appears to be a familially transmitted trait, because a blunted prolactin response to fenfluramine in probands with a personality disorder has been found to predict impulsivity in their relatives better than impulsive behaviors per se (Kavoussi et al. 1994). There is also a well-established association between low central serotonin, as measured by cerebrospinal fluid 5-hydroxyindole-acetic acid (CSF 5-HIAA) and a history of violent suicide attempts (reviewed by Lester 1995).

The association between reduced serotonergic function and a history of suicidal or impulsive-aggressive behaviors may or may not apply to self-mutilation. Although it makes some sense to hypothesize that a similar association may apply to impulsive SIB, supporting data are limited. In a negative study, Gardner et al. (1990) reported that decreased CSF 5-HIAA in a group with BPD was significantly related to suicide attempts but not to outward-directed aggression or to self-mutilation. However, it is conceivable that the different incidence of suicide attempts between the mutilating and nonmutilating groups may have concealed an association between CSF 5-HIAA and self-mutilation. Lopez-Ibor et al. (1985) found that inpatients with depression and a history of self-injury without suicidal intent had lower CSF 5-HIAA than those without SIB. Another study by Simeon et al. (1992) compared platelet imipramine binding (a peripheral measure of serotonergic function) and CSF 5-HIAA in 26 personality disorder patients with SIB and 26 matched personality disorder control subjects who did not engage in SIB. Within the SIB group there was a significant negative correlation between platelet imipramine binding and severity of self-mutilation. In addition, when all suicide attempters were excluded from both groups, there was a 44% reduction in CSF 5-HIAA in the small subsample of self-mutilating patients compared with non–self-mutilating patients.

Another common characteristic of impulsive SIB is the frequently reported total or partial analgesia prior to and during the act (Gardner and

Gardner 1975; Leibenluft et al. 1987). The endogenous opioid system is extensively implicated in pain perception and stress-induced analgesia (Amir et al. 1980; Madden et al. 1977). Russ et al. (1993) reported that pain ratings during a cold pressor test were significantly lower in patients with BPD who reported anesthesia during self-injury compared with those who did feel pain during SIB and with nonpsychiatric control subjects. However, the BPD group reporting analgesia during SIB did not exhibit significantly diminished analgesia during the cold pressor test when pretreated with the opioid receptor antagonist naloxone, thus not lending support to the notion of an endogenous opioid system–mediating mechanism being at play (Russ et al. 1994). In another study of self-injuring individuals who reported analgesia, plasma metenkephalin concentration was significantly higher than that of normal control subjects (Coid et al. 1983). However, the authors of the study suggested that this elevation could have been the result rather than the impetus for repeated SIB. The increased pain threshold of analgesic self-mutilating BPD patients appears to be state-independent, because it has been experimentally demonstrated even in states of calmness; under stress, the pain threshold becomes even further elevated (Bohus et al. 2000).

Treatment

Pharmacotherapy

There is no medication currently approved by the U.S. Food and Drug Administration for the treatment of impulsive SIB, and there are no double-blind, placebo-controlled studies of medications designed specifically to study the treatment of impulsive SIB as the primary outcome variable. Still, there is preliminary evidence that medications can be helpful in managing self-mutilation, and presented in the following discussion are the pertinent case studies, open trials, and controlled trials that examined broader related target symptoms and sometimes SIB.

Serotonin Reuptake Inhibitors

A 12-week open-label trial of 80 mg/day fluoxetine was conducted in 22 outpatients diagnosed with borderline and/or schizotypal personality disorders (Markovitz et al. 1991). Twelve of these patients, all meeting criteria for BPD, were engaging in approximately four incidents of self-mutilation per week prior to beginning treatment. By the final week of the study, only two patients were still engaging in self-mutilation, and at a frequency of less than once per week, resulting in a 97% reduction in self-mutilation scores for the total sample. Similarly, in an open trial of venlafaxine in 45 subjects with BPD treated with an average dosage of 315 mg/day (Markovitz and Wagner 1995), 5 of 7 subjects who were engaging in self-injury at the beginning of the trial had ceased to do so after 12 weeks of treatment.

In yet another comparable open trial by the same group (Markovitz 1995), 23 patients with BPD were treated openly for an initial 12-week period with sertraline 200 mg/day, and about half showed improvement in SIB, anxiety, depression, and suicidality. Of note, half of those who responded had previously failed to respond to fluoxetine, underlining the usefulness of trying more than one selective serotonin reuptake inhibitor (SSRI) in this population, given the variability of responses across SSRIs. The trial was continued to a 1-year duration, and the dosage for nonresponders was increased to more than 300 mg/day. By the completion of the study, depression had decreased, on average, by 56% and self-injurious episodes by 93%.

There has been only one controlled study to date that examined the efficacy of serotonin reuptake inhibitors in the treatment of impulsive aggression (Coccaro and Kavoussi 1997). This study investigated the effect of fluoxetine over a 12-week period in 40 personality disorder subjects with marked impulsive aggression as the major entry criterion and without current major depression. About half of the subjects met Cluster B criteria (one-third of the total had BPD), 40% met Cluster C criteria, and 28% met Cluster A criteria. Compared with placebo, fluoxetine at dosages of 20–60 mg/day led to a consistent and significant decrease in aggression and irritability and an increase in global improvement by the second month of treatment, irrespective of changes in depression or anxiety. Unfortunately, the study did not make separate mention of self-mutilation at baseline or after treatment, although self-injury is one of the items of the primary outcome measure used in the study (Overt Aggression Scale—Modified).

Mood Stabilizers

Cowdry and Gardner (1988) initially reported that carbamazepine led to a dramatic and highly significant decrease in behavioral dyscontrol in BPD but had much more modest effects on mood, and patients subjectively did not feel better on it. This was a double-blind, placebo-controlled, 6-week crossover design comparing alprazolam (average dosage 5 mg/day), carbamazepine (average dosage 820 mg/day), trifluoperazine (average dosage 8 mg/day), and tranylcypromine (average dosage 40 mg/day). Subjects were 16 outpatient females with BPD, with additional inclusion criteria of the presence of prominent behavioral dyscontrol and the absence of current major depression. However, another carbamazepine study involving 20 inpatients with BPD without concurrent depression or concomitant medications yielded negative results (De La Fuenta et al. 1994). After 4 weeks of treatment at standard therapeutic drug levels, carbamazepine was no better than placebo in treating depression, behavioral dyscontrol, or global symptomatology.

More recently, anticonvulsant trials have focused on valproate and, to a lesser extent, on the newer anticonvulsants. Several smaller trials of valproate in BPD have suggested some efficacy but did not specifically focus on SIB (Frankenburg and Zanarini 2002; Hollander et al. 2001; Stein et al. 1995). Finally, a larger, controlled multicenter trial of valproate was recently published that focused on the treatment of impulsive aggression in Cluster B personality disorders (Hollander et al. 2003). Ninety-six outpatients selected for the presence of prominent impulsive aggression and the absence of bipolar I disorder or current major depression were randomized to 12 weeks of treatment with placebo or valproate at an average end dosage of 1,400 mg/day and an end mean blood level of 66 mg/L. About 10% of subjects were receiving concomitant stable dosages of antidepressants, and there was an approximately equal dropout rate of almost half of the subjects in each group. The main finding of the study was a significantly greater decrease in overall aggression (verbal assault, assault against objects, and assault against others) and overall irritability in the last month of treatment for valproate compared with placebo. Again, SIB was one item of the primary outcome measure scale but was not separately analyzed.

With respect to newer anticonvulsants, there is little information on the treatment of self-injury or even behavioral dyscontrol more broadly in individuals with personality disorder. A small open trial of lamotrigine in eight patients with BPD without concurrent major depression (Pinto and Akiskal 1998) reported three patients with a robust response who experienced great improvement in overall functioning and cessation of impulsive behaviors such as promiscuity, substance abuse, and suicidality—there was no explicit mention of SIB. Two case reports described the successful treatment of self-mutilation in BPD using topiramate in two patients with concurrent bipolar I disorder (Chengappa et al. 1999b) and one patient with concurrent bipolar II disorder (Cassano et al. 2001).

Atypical Antipsychotics

Atypical antipsychotics have been minimally investigated in the treatment of SIB, but preliminary case reports look promising. Parenthetically, larger open trials of atypical antipsychotics in BPD patients do appear promising in treating core symptom clusters of the disorder (Frankenburg and Zanarini 1993; Schulz et al. 1999; Zanarini and Frankenburg 2001), but none of these trials specifically addressed SIB. A quetiapine treatment of two female BPD patients with severe self-mutilation reported marked improvement in self-injury as well as in overall functioning (Hilger et al. 2003). Another report described marked improvement in self-mutilation and global functioning in seven female BPD patients with Axis I psychotic disorder comorbidity who were severely impaired and chronically hospitalized and whose illness had previously been refractory to various medication combinations (Chengappa et al. 1999a). Yet another study reported excellent response to olanzapine in three nonpsychotic subjects with dermatitis artifacta that had previously been refractory to multiple treatments; these patients' dermatitis artifacta lesions were more extreme than those of classic self-mutilation (Garnis-Jones et al. 2000). Finally, another case report described two individuals with severe BPD whose self-mutilation responded very well to low-dose (5 mg/day) olanzapine (Hough 2001). These medications, then, merit further study in the treatment of severe self-mutilation.

Opioid Antagonists

A single open-label naltrexone treatment in patients engaging in impulsive SIB has been reported in the literature (Roth et al. 1996). Seven patients with at least two episodes of self-injury in the past month were treated with 50 mg/day of naltrexone for about 10 weeks. To be included, subjects needed to experience analgesia during SIB, followed by emotional relief. Six subjects reported a childhood history of severe sexual abuse. Four of the subjects had personality disorder diagnoses, two were depressed, and one had schizoaffective disorder.

Most subjects were taking concurrent psychotropic medications. It was found that three subjects did not engage in any self-injury while on naltrexone. The remaining subjects experienced less analgesia and less dysphoria reduction when self-injuring while on naltrexone and showed a marked decline in SIB by the end of treatment. Another open trial of naltrexone in 15 women with BPD treated with 25–100 mg/day for at least 2 weeks reported a significant decrease in dissociative symptoms and flashbacks but did not make mention of SIB (Bohus et al. 1999).

Psychotherapy

Of the various psychotherapies, the American Psychiatric Association's (2001) treatment guidelines for BPD cite two types of psychotherapy as having some proof of efficacy: dialectical behavior therapy (DBT) and psychodynamic psychotherapy. SIB in particular is not mentioned. We summarize these two treatment approaches in the following discussion, emphasizing those aspects of this extensive literature that specifically address SIB.

Dialectical Behavior Therapy

DBT (Linehan 1993a, 1993b) is a structured psychotherapy that directly addresses suicide and self-mutilation and has been found effective at reducing the incidence and frequency of all forms of parasuicide in patients with BPD. DBT was originally designed for the treatment of chronically parasuicidal women, although over the years its goals and applications have broadened. Basic DBT is a 1-year outpatient treatment that uses primarily behavioral, cognitive, and supportive techniques. Patients participate in weekly individual psychotherapy and in skills training groups that teach adaptive coping skills in four primary domains: affect regulation, frustration tolerance, interpersonal communication, and reduction of identity confusion (Linehan 1993a, 1993b).

In the first DBT clinical trial (Linehan et al. 1991), 47 chronically parasuicidal women with BPD were randomly assigned to either 12 months of DBT or treatment as usual. It was found that the DBT group was less likely to engage in any form of parasuicide or to drop out of treatment than the control group, underwent less psychiatric hospitalization, and demonstrated overall better functioning. The mean number of self-mutilating acts was somewhat, but not significantly, reduced in the DBT compared with the control group.

The second randomized clinical trial was conducted in substance-abusing women with BPD (M.M. Linehan and L.A. Dimeff, "Extension of Standard Dialectical Behavior Therapy to Treatment of Substance Abusers With Borderline Personality Disorder," unpublished manual, 1996). The DBT group showed a greater decline in drug use, stayed in treatment longer, and made significantly greater gains in overall life adjustment. DBT has become increasingly popular and has been empirically studied in various trials with different borderline spectrum populations (Lawson and Bailey 1993; Miller et al. 1997).

The theory used to explain BPD is based in a dialectical philosophy that synthesizes both biological and environmental principles in the etiology and maintenance of BPD. It is presumed that every dysfunction serves some function and that every individual component of a dysfunctional system must be related to the whole. To truly understand a particular behavior, it must be correctly placed in the total behavioral and environmental context. From this perspective, self-mutilation can be seen as a life-saving event that allows patients to cope with overwhelming life demands while at the same time being destructive and leading to poor coping. The emotional dysregulation underlying self-injury is presumed to result from some degree of biologically determined difficulty with affect regulation coupled with environmental experiences that have invalidated the individual's responses to the world. The resulting difficulty in identifying, trusting, and evaluating emotional experience is in itself reinforcing.

DBT treatment has four stages, with the treatment agenda determined by a hierarchy of DBT goals. In pretreatment, the patient is oriented to the philosophy and structure of DBT, with the goal of making a commitment to pursue the goals of DBT. These goals are clearly described. If a patient is currently engaging in suicidal or self-injurious behavior, the patient must agree that controlling such behavior is a primary goal. Explicit agreement by the patient not to hurt or kill himself or herself while in treatment is necessary before full participation in treatment can commence. For patients who are not ready, the pretreatment phase can be extended until there is commitment to these goals.

Once DBT proper begins, Stage 1 is designed to address all life-threatening behaviors, including suicidality and self-mutilation. The establishment of a strong therapeutic relationship is central to this end and a major goal of this stage. In addition to decreasing SIBs, this stage also aims to decrease behaviors that interfere with treatment compliance, to decrease behaviors that impair a patient's quality of life, and to enhance skills that promote better adaptation such as mindfulness, distress tolerance, emotional regulation, and interpersonal effectiveness. Any self-harming behavior is persistently addressed in individual therapy after each and every occurrence; the behaviors are never ignored or made a secondary priority.

A number of different therapeutic strategies are used in DBT: validation, problem solving, exposure, and skills training. Validation is founded on empathy and is achieved by direct verbal, behavioral, and supportive interventions. Problem solving utilizes a technique known as *behavioral analysis*. This is a structured "chain" approach aimed at identifying problematic behavior, its contexts and cues, and its consequences step by step. Once the chain is laid out, a solution is sought that will lessen the dysfunctional behavior by offering more adaptive alternative responses, modifying maladaptive cognitions that promote such behaviors, and using exposure techniques to diminish negative experiences that interfere with more adaptive solutions. Finally, DBT also directly addresses deficits in adaptive skills that are commonly observed in self-injuring patients. Enhancement of adaptive skills is necessary to ameliorate self-damaging behaviors.

A recent DBT study thoroughly examined the impact of DBT on self-mutilation (Verheul et al. 2003). Fifty-eight women with BPD were assigned to 12 months of DBT or usual treatment in a randomized, controlled study. The main outcome measures were retention in treatment and reduction in suicidal behavior, self-mutilation, and self-damaging impulsive behaviors. The authors found that over the course of 1 year, DBT resulted in significantly diminished treatment attrition, self-mutilation, and impulsivity, whereas the difference in suicide attempts between the two treatments was not significant. The beneficial effects of DBT on self-mutilation did not become apparent until the last 6 months of treatment, at which point the two groups markedly diverged in number of self-mutilation episodes. Severity of self-mutilation at baseline was a major determinant of treatment effectiveness. Subjects were divided into high and low severity of self-mutilation based on the lifetime number of episodes. The high-severity group (median lifetime episodes=61) showed a marked improvement with DBT compared with usual treatment, whereas in the low-severity group (median lifetime episodes=4) treatment type did not have a significant impact. The authors concluded that DBT may be most effective for the severe and high-risk behaviors characteristic of BPD

Underlying sadomasochistic object relations have to be unveiled, and alternative ways of working through such dynamics as well as alternative ways of experiencing relationships will have to be made available. Inquiries into the interpersonal context within which the act was carried out are also important. SIB acts must be tied in to conscious or unconscious communications with significant others in the patient's current life, including communications to the therapist. The transference-countertransference context must always be kept in mind, especially as patients become more engaged in their treatments and more prone to reenact SIB dynamics within the therapeutic relationship. Central to the therapeutic stance are interventions that relieve primitive guilt and shame, strengthen the ego, and maintain compassionate firmness and solid boundaries. The message needs to be conveyed that self-mutilation is not acceptable, yet it does not mean the patient is bad or hopeless.

There also needs to be ongoing emphasis on creatively developing with the patient alternative solutions to the expression and function of the self-injurious acts, even before the underlying dynamics are extensively worked through. Ego-supporting interventions can help patients develop better frustration tolerance and delay mechanisms. Patients should be encouraged to anticipate distressing situations and make concrete plans as to how they can cope with these without engaging in self-injury. They can be encouraged to use various resources rather than remain self-contained in their effort to relieve unbearable states.

In conclusion, we review some empirical evidence supporting the efficacy of psychodynamically oriented interventions for the treatment of SIB. Thirty-eight patients with BPD were randomly assigned to either a partial hospitalization with psychodynamically oriented treatment or standard psychiatric care for 18 months (Bateman and Fonagy 1999). The goal of the study was to examine not only self-damaging behaviors but also, more broadly, reasons for living and symptoms of anxiety and depression that do not appear to respond as effectively to DBT acutely or at follow-up (Linehan et al. 1993). The partial hospitalization treatment included once-weekly individual psychoanalytic psychotherapy, thrice-weekly group analytic psychotherapy, once-weekly psychodrama therapy, and once-weekly community meetings. The control treatment included, as indicated, hospitalizations, nonpsychoanalytic partial hospitalization focused on problem solving, and outpatient community follow-up without formal psychotherapy. The two groups did not differ in concurrent medication management. The study revealed that psychoanalytically oriented partial hospitalization resulted in significant decreases in all outcome measures compared with the control group, which showed limited change or deterioration. More specifically, a decrease in SIB was noted by 6 months and continued to the end of the 18-month treatment. The median number of SIB acts per 6-month period declined from nine to one in the partial hospitalization group compared with a decline from eight to six in the control group. Group differences in SIB were significant by 12 months, and the number of individuals no longer engaging in SIB was significantly greater in the partial hospitalization group by the end of the 18-month treatment.

Furthermore, an 18-month follow-up of this study revealed that patients who had completed the partial hospitalization program maintained their substantial gains and showed further statistically significant continued improvement on most outcome measures compared with the control patients, who remained largely unchanged (Bateman and Fonagy 2001). Specifically with respect to SIB, significantly more such acts were committed during the 18-month follow-up period by the control group than by the partial hospitalization group. Finally, in terms of treatment cost, the partial hospitalization psychoanalytic program was not more costly than the control treatment, because it was offset by fewer inpatient admissions and emergency department visits than in the control group, and there was a tendency for decreasing care costs in the partial hospitalization group during the 18-month follow-up in contrast to the steady costs of the control group (Bateman and Fonagy 2003).

Conclusion

Impulsive self-injury, commonly referred to as *self-mutilation,* is one of the four major categories of SIBs. Although better known within the context of borderline personality pathology, it may also occur with other Axis I and II disorders, including substance use disorders, depression, posttraumatic stress disorder, eating disorders, and dissociative disorders. It can be broadly conceptualized as an act of impulsive aggression, a consequence of early traumatic life experiences, or an attempt to modify intolerable self-states. Serotonergic and endogenous opioid dysfunction have been implicated. Limited data suggest that medication treatment can be helpful, including serotonin reuptake inhibitors, mood stabilizers, opioid antagonists, and atypical neuroleptics. Long-term psychotherapy is a necessary treatment component. DBT and psychoanalytically oriented psychotherapy are the best-studied efficacious modalities. Additional general management and supportive interventions such as hospitalizations, structured day settings, and family treatment may also be periodically indicated.

References

American Psychiatric Association: Diagnostic and Statistical Manual of Mental Disorders, 4th Edition, Text Revision. Washington, DC, American Psychiatric Association, 2000

American Psychiatric Association: Practice Guideline for the Treatment of Patients with Borderline Personality Disorder. Am J Psychiatry 158(suppl):44–46, 2001

Amir S, Brown ZW, Amil A: The role of endorphins in stress: evidence and speculations. Neurosci Behav Rev 4:77–86, 1980

Bateman A, Fonagy P: Effectiveness of partial hospitalization in the treatment of borderline personality disorder: a randomized controlled trial. Am J Psychiatry 156:1563–1569, 1999

Bateman A, Fonagy P: Treatment of borderline personality disorder with psychoanalytically oriented partial hospitalization: an 18-month follow-up. Am J Psychiatry 158:36–42, 2001

Bateman A, Fonagy P: Health service utilization costs for borderline personality disorder patients treated with psychoanalytically oriented partial hospitalization versus general psychiatric care. Am J Psychiatry 160:169–171, 2003

Bennum I: Depression and hostility in self-mutilation. Suicide Life Threat Behav 13:71–84, 1983

Bodfish JM, Crawford TM, Powell SB, et al: Compulsions in adults with mental retardation: prevalence, phenomenology and comorbidity with stereotypy and self-injury. Am J Ment Retard 100:183–192, 1995

Bohus MJ, Landwehrmeyer B, Stiglmayr CE, et al: Naltrexone in the treatment of dissociative symptoms in patients with borderline personality disorder: an open-label trial. J Clin Psychiatry 60:598–603, 1999

Bohus M, Limberger M, Ebner U, et al: Pain perception during self-reported distress and calmness in patients with borderline personality disorder and self-mutilating behavior. Psychiatry Res 95:251–260, 2000

Brodsky BS, Cloitre M, Dulit RA: Relationship of dissociation to self-mutilation and childhood abuse in borderline personality disorder. Am J Psychiatry 152:1788–1792, 1995

Cassano P, Lattanzi L, Pini S, et al: Topiramate for self-mutilation in a patient with borderline personality disorder. Bipolar Disord 3:161, 2001

Chengappa KNR, Ebeling T, Kang JS, et al: Clozapine reduces severe self-mutilation and aggression in psychotic patients with borderline personality disorder. J Clin Psychiatry 60:477–484, 1999a

Chengappa KNR, Rathore D, Levine J, et al: Topiramate as add-on treatment for patients with bipolar mania. Bipolar Disord 1:42–53, 1999b

Clark RA: Self-mutilation accompanying religious delusions. J Clin Psychiatry 42:243–245, 1981

Coccaro EF, Kavoussi RJ: Fluoxetine and impulsive aggressive behavior in personality-disordered subjects. Arch Gen Psychiatry 54:1081–1088, 1997

Coccaro EF, Siever LJ, Klar HM, et al: Serotonergic studies in patients with affective and personality disorders. Arch Gen Psychiatry 47:587–599, 1989

Coid J, Allolio B, Rees LH: Raised plasma metenkephalin in patients who habitually mutilate themselves. Lancet 2:545–546, 1983

Coons PM, Milstein V: Self-mutilation associated with dissociative disorders. Dissociation 3:81–87, 1990

Cooper AM: The narcissistic-masochistic character, in Masochism: Current Psychoanalytic Perspectives. Edited by Glick RA, Meyers DI. Jersey City, NJ, The Analytic Press, 1988, pp 117–138

Cowdry RW, Gardner DL: Pharmacotherapy of borderline personality disorder: alprazolam, carbamazepine, trifluoperazine, and tranylcypromine. Arch Gen Psychiatry 45:111–119, 1988

De La Fuenta JM, Lotstra F: A trial of carbamazepine in borderline personality disorder. Eur Neuropsychopharmacol 4:479–486, 1994

DeMuth GW, Strain J, Lombardo-Mahar A: Self-amputation and restitution. Gen Hosp Psychiatry 5:25–30, 1983

Dubo ED, Zanarini MC, Lewis RE, et al: Childhood antecedents of self-destructiveness in borderline personality disorder. Can J Psychiatry 42:63–69, 1997

Favaro A, Santonastaso P: Impulsive and compulsive self-injurious behavior in bulimia nervosa: prevalence and psychological correlates. J Nerv Ment Dis 186:157–165, 1998

Favazza AR: Why patients mutilate themselves. Hosp Community Psychiatry 40:137–145, 1989

Favazza AR: Bodies Under Siege: Self-Mutilation and Body Modification in Culture and Psychiatry. Baltimore, MD, Johns Hopkins University Press, 1996

Favazza AR: The coming of age of self-mutilation. J Nerv Ment Dis 186:259–268, 1998

Favazza AR, Conterio K: Female habitual self-mutilators. Acta Psychiatr Scand 79:283–289, 1989

Favazza A, DeRosear L, Conterio K: Self-mutilation and eating disorders. Suicide Life Threat Behav 19:352–361, 1989

Frankenburg FR, Zanarini MC: Clozapine treatment of borderline patients: a preliminary study. Compr Psychiatry 34:402–405, 1993

Frankenburg FR, Zanarini MC: Divalproex sodium treatment of women with borderline personality disorder and bipolar II disorder: a double-blind placebo-controlled pilot study. J Clin Psychiatry 63:442–446, 2002

Friedman M, Galsser M, Laufer E, et al: Attempted suicide and self-mutilation in adolescence. Int J Psychoanal 53:179–183, 1972

Gardner AR, Gardner AJ: Self-mutilation, obsessionality and narcissism. Br J Psychiatry 127:127–132, 1975

Gardner DL, Cowdry RW: Suicidal and parasuicidal behavior in borderline personality disorder. Psychiatr Clin North Am 8:389–403, 1985

Gardner DL, Lucas PB, Cowdry RW: CSF metabolites in borderline personality disorder compared with normal controls. Biol Psychiatry 28:247–254, 1990

Garfinkel PE, Moldofsky H, Garner DM: The heterogeneity of anorexia nervosa. Arch Gen Psychiatry 37:1036–1040, 1980

Garnis-Jones S, Collins S, Rosenthal D: Treatment of self-mutilation with olanzapine. J Cutan Med Surg 4:160–162, 2000

Graff H, Mallin R: The syndrome of the wrist cutter. Am J Psychiatry 124:36–42, 1967

Green AH: Self-destructive behavior in battered children. Am J Psychiatry 135:579–582, 1978

Greenspan GC, Samuel SE: Self-cutting after rape. Am J Psychiatry 146:789–790, 1989

Hilger E, Barnas C, Kasper S: Quetiapine in the treatment of borderline personality disorder. World J Biol Psychiatry 4:42–44, 2003

Hollander E, Allen A, Lopez RP, et al: A preliminary double-blind, placebo-controlled trial of divalproex sodium in borderline personality disorder. J Clin Psychiatry 62:199–203, 2001

Hollander E, Tracy KA, Swann AC, et al: Divalproex in the treatment of impulsive aggression: efficacy in Cluster B personality disorders. Neuropsychopharmacology 28:1186–1197, 2003

Hough DW: Low-dose olanzapine for self-mutilation behavior in patients with borderline personality disorder. J Clin Psychiatry 62:296–297, 2001

Kafka JS: The body as transitional object: a psychoanalytic study of a self-mutilating patient. Br J Med Psychol 42:207–212, 1969

Kahan J, Pattison EM: Proposal for a distinctive diagnosis: the deliberate self-harm syndrome (DSH). Suicide Life Threat Behav 14:17–35, 1984

Kavoussi RJ, Liu J, Coccaro EF: An open trial of sertraline in personality disordered patients with impulsive aggression. J Clin Psychiatry 55:137–141, 1994

Kernberg O: The borderline self-mutilator. J Personal Disord 1:344–346, 1987

Klein M: A contribution to the psychogenesis of manic-depressive states (1935), in Essential Papers on Object Relations. Edited by Buckley P. New York, New York University, 1986, pp 40–70

Lawson JE, Bailey BJ: The development of an inpatient cognitive-behavioral treatment program for borderline personality disorder. J Personal Disord 7:232–240, 1993

Leibenluft E, Gardner DL, Cowdry RW: The inner experience of the borderline self-mutilator. J Personal Disord 1:317–324, 1987

Lester D: The concentration of neurotransmitter metabolites in the cerebrospinal fluid of suicidal individuals: a meta-analysis. Pharmacopsychiatry 28:45–50, 1995

Linehan MM: Cognitive-Behavioral Treatment for Borderline Personality Disorder. New York, Guilford, 1993a

Linehan MM: Skills Training Manual for Treating Borderline Personality Disorder. New York, Guilford, 1993b

Linehan MM, Armstrong HE, Suarez A, et al: Cognitive-behavioral treatment of chronically parasuicidal borderline patients. Arch Gen Psychiatry 48:1060–1064, 1991

Linehan MM, Heard HL, Armstrong HE: Naturalistic follow-up of a behavioral treatment for chronically parasuicidal borderline patients. Arch Gen Psychiatry 50:971–974, 1993

Lipschitz DS, Winegar RK, Nicolaou AL, et al: Perceived abuse and neglect as risk factors for suicidal behavior in adolescent inpatients. J Nerv Ment Dis 187:32–39, 1999

Lopez-Ibor JJ, Saiz-Ruiz J, Perez de los Cobos JC: Biological correlations of suicide and aggressivity in major depressions (with melancholia): 5-hydroxyindoleacetic acid and cortisol in cerebral spinal fluid, dexamethasone suppression test and therapeutic response to 5-hydroxytryptophan. Neuropsychobiology 14:67–74, 1985

Madden J, Akil H, Patrick R, et al: Stress-induced parallel changes in central opioid levels and pain responsiveness in the rat. Nature 265:358–360, 1977

Markovitz PJ: Pharmacotherapy of impulsivity, aggression, and related disorders, in Impulsivity and Aggression. Edited by Hollander E, Stein DJ. New York, Wiley, 1995, pp 263–291

Markovitz PJ, Wagner SC: Venlafaxine in the treatment of borderline personality disorder. Psychopharmacol Bull 31:773–777, 1995

Markovitz PJ, Calabrese JR, Schulz SC, et al: Fluoxetine in the treatment of borderline and schizotypal personality disorder. Am J Psychiatry 148:1064–1067, 1991

McKay D, Kulchycky S, Danyko S: Borderline personality and obsessive-compulsive symptoms. J Personal Disord 14:57–63, 2000

McKerracher DW, Loughnane T, Watson RA: Self-mutilation in female psychopaths. Br J Psychiatry 114:829–832, 1968

Miller A, Rathus JH, Linehan MM, et al: Dialectical behavior therapy adapted for suicidal adolescents. Journal of Practical Psychiatry and Behavioral Health 3:78–86, 1997

Mitchell JE, Boutacoff LI, Hatsukami D, et al: Laxative abuse as a variant of bulimia. J Nerv Ment Dis 174:174–176, 1986

Nakaya M: On background factors of male genital self-mutilation. Psychopathology 29:242–248, 1996

Pao PN: The syndrome of delicate self-cutting. Br J Med Psychol 42:195–206, 1969

Parkin JR, Eagles JM: Bloodletting in bulimia nervosa. Br J Psychiatry 162:246–248, 1993

Pattison EM, Kahan J: The deliberate self-harm syndrome. Am J Psychiatry 140:867–872, 1983

Pinto OC, Akiskal HS: Lamotrigine as a promising approach to borderline personality: an open case series without concurrent DSM-IV major mood disorder. J Affect Disord 51:333–343, 1998

Pitman RK: Self-mutilation in combat related post-traumatic stress disorder. Am J Psychiatry 147:123–124, 1990

Rosenthal PA, Rosenthal S: Suicidal behavior by preschool children. Am J Psychiatry 141:520–525, 1984

Rosenthal RJ, Rinzler C, Walsh R, et al: Wrist-cutting syndrome. Am J Psychiatry 128:1363–1368, 1972

Rosiello F: The interplay of masochism and narcissism in the treatment of two prostitutes. Contemporary Psychotherapy Review 8:28–43,1993

Roth AS, Ostroff RB, Hoffman RE: Naltrexone as a treatment for repetitive self-injurious behavior: an open-label trial. J Clin Psychiatry 57:233–237, 1996

Roy A: Self-mutilation. Br J Med Psychol 51:201–203, 1978

Russ MJ, Shearin EN, Clarkin JF, et al: Subtypes of self-injurious patients with borderline personality disorder. Am J Psychiatry 150:1869–1871, 1993

Russ MJ, Roth SD, Kakuma T, et al: Pain perception in self-injurious borderline patients: naloxone effects. Biol Psychiatry 35:207–209, 1994

Schaffer CB, Carroll J, Abramowitz SI: Self-mutilation and the borderline personality. J Nerv Ment Dis 170:468–473, 1982

Schulz SC, Camlin KL, Berry SA: Olanzapine safety and efficacy in patients with borderline personality disorder and comorbid dysthymia. Biol Psychiatry 46:1429–1435, 1999

Simeon D, Favazza AR: Self-injurious behaviors: phenomenology and assessment, in Self-Injurious Behaviors: Assessment and Treatment. Edited by Simeon D, Hollander E. Washington, DC, American Psychiatric Publishing, 2001, pp 1–28

Simeon D, Stanley B, Frances A, et al: Self-mutilation in personality disorders: psychological and biological correlates. Am J Psychiatry 149:221–226, 1992

Simeon D, Gross S, Guralnik O, et al: Feeling unreal: 30 cases of DSM-III-R depersonalization disorder. Am J Psychiatry 154:1107–1113, 1997

Simpson MA: Self-mutilation as indirect self-destructive behavior: "nothing to get so
cut up about," in Faces of Suicide: Indirect Self-Destructive Behavior. Edited by
Farberow NL. New York, McGraw-Hill, 1980, pp 257–283

Stanley B, Gameroff MJ, Michalsen V: Are suicide attempters who self-mutilate a
unique population? Am J Psychiatry 158:427–432, 2001

Stein DJ, Simeon D, Frenkel M: An open trial of valproate in borderline personality
disorder. J Clin Psychiatry 56:506–510, 1995

Stone MH: The Fate of Borderline Patients: Successful Outcome and Psychiatric Practice. New York, Guilford, 1990, pp 61–63

Turell SC, Armsworth MW: Differentiating incest survivors who self-mutilate. Child
Abuse Negl 24:237–249, 2000

van der Kolk BA, Perry JC, Herman JL: Childhood origins of self-destructive behavior.
Am J Psychiatry 148:1665–1671, 1991

Verheul R, Van den Bosch LMC, Koeter MWJ, et al: Dialectical behaviour therapy for
women with borderline personality disorder. Br J Psychiatry 182:135–140, 2003

Virkkunen M: Self-mutilation in antisocial personality disorder. Acta Psychiatr Scand
54:347–352, 1976

Walsh B, Rosen P: Self-Mutilation: Theory, Research and Treatment. New York, Guilford, 1988

Winchel RM, Stanley M: Self-injurious behavior: a review of the behavior and biology
of self-mutilation. Am J Psychiatry 148:306–317, 1991

Zanarini MC, Frankenburg FR: Olanzapine treatment of female borderline personality
disorder patients: a double-blind, placebo-controlled pilot study. J Clin Psychiatry
62:849–854, 2001

Zlotnick C, Shea MT, Pearlstein T, et al: The relationship between dissociative symptoms, alexithymia, impulsivity, sexual abuse and self-mutilation. Compr Psychiatry 37:12–16, 1996

Zlotnick C, Mattia JI, Zimmerman M: Clinical correlates of self-mutilation in a sample
of general psychiatric patients. J Nerv Ment Dis 187:296–301, 1999

Zweig-Frank H, Paris J, Guzder J: Psychological risk factors for dissociation and self-
mutilation in female patients with borderline personality disorder. Can J Psychiatry 39:259–264, 1994a

Zweig-Frank H, Paris J, Guzder J: Psychological risk factors and self-mutilation in male
patients with BPD. Can J Psychiatry 39:266–268, 1994b

5

Sexual Compulsions

Andrea Allen, Ph.D.
Eric Hollander, M.D.

Sexual compulsions have been conceptualized in several compelling ways, most commonly as addictive, impulsive, or compulsive disorders. There is no universal agreement on the nature, or even the definition, of sexual compulsions, but at the core are sexual thoughts, urges, and behaviors that are difficult to resist. Sexual compulsions can be categorized as either paraphilias or paraphilia-related disorders, sometimes referred to as nonparaphilic sexual addictions, with the division between the two based on whether the particular sexual compulsion is outside societal norms, although this boundary is not always easily placed. Whether looking at clinical or forensic populations, it is clear that many individuals have an inability to control their sexual thoughts, urges, and behaviors despite negative consequences.

The paraphilias form a recognized category of disorders in DSM-IV-TR (American Psychiatric Association 2000). These disorders all entail socially deviant sexual thoughts, urges, or behaviors that are generally intense and persistent and either involve nonconsenting persons or lead to distress or impairment in functioning. In contrast, paraphilia-related disorders involve sexual thoughts, urges, and behaviors that are normative but occur with such frequency or intensity that they lead to distress or impairment in functioning (Kafka 1994a, 1997a). None of the paraphilia-related disorders are designated as specific disorders in DSM-IV-TR.

Sexual compulsions can be conceptualized as being on an obsessive-compulsive spectrum (Bradford 2001; Hollander and Wong 1995; Jenike 1989) because, like obsessive-compulsive disorder (OCD), sexual compulsions are characterized by obsessive preoccupations (sexual thoughts, fantasies, and urges) and compulsive, repetitive behaviors (in this case, sexual behaviors). The compulsive sexual behaviors differ somewhat from OCD ritual compulsions. OCD rituals are not pleasurable activities engaged in for their own sake, but rather are neutral or often irritating and unpleasant behaviors that are engaged in to reduce anxiety. These behaviors generally have an element of pleasure, at least initially, although they may lose their pleasurable quality over time; in this regard, they are more similar to addictions and to impulse-control disorders such as pathological gambling.

Sexual obsessions can be a presentation of OCD. Paraphilias and paraphilia-related obsessions can be distinguished from the sexual obsessions that are part of OCD because the latter are characterized by recurrent, intrusive sexual thoughts and/or images that are ego dystonic, are morally repugnant, induce anxiety, and usually lead to avoidance and nonsexual rituals rather than to sexual behaviors (Hollander and Wong 1995). The obsessive thoughts often include the fear or belief that one may actually have somehow committed the feared sexual behavior without knowing it. Therefore, the rituals that accompany sexual obsessions in OCD are repetitive behaviors of a nonsexual nature meant somehow to avoid or undo the distressing sexual thoughts or fears. These rituals can take almost any form. For example, someone with an OCD sexual obsession may have intrusive thoughts of having sexual relations with a stranger he passed on the street and may feel compelled to confess to his wife that he may have had sexual relations with the stranger.

There are no large-scale epidemiological studies for sexual compulsions as there are for other disorders. Although all psychiatric disorders present difficulties for epidemiological surveys, the difficulties for sexual disorders are virtually insurmountable. Obstacles include obtaining funding, creating an atmosphere in which to ask questions, and determining whether one has obtained honest responses about socially unacceptable or even illegal behaviors. Therefore, there are many difficulties in characterizing these disorders and those who have them. What is known is based on smaller-scale studies conducted among both clinical and criminal samples.

Phenomenology

Paraphilias

According to DSM-IV-TR, *paraphilias* are sexual disorders characterized by recurrent, intense, sexually arousing fantasies, urges, or behaviors that involve nonhuman objects, children, other nonconsenting individuals, or the suffering or humiliation of the individual or partner (American Psychiatric Association 2000). For a paraphilia diagnosis, the symptoms need to have existed for a minimum of 6 months and to have caused clinically significant distress or impairment in functioning, or the individual needs to have acted on the urges with a nonconsenting person.

Eight specific paraphilias are recognized in DSM-IV-TR: exhibitionism, fetishism, frotteurism, pedophilia, sexual masochism, sexual sadism, transvestic fetishism, and voyeurism. Other paraphilias discussed in the literature, which would be diagnosed according to DSM-IV-TR as paraphilias not otherwise specified, include telephone scatologia, necrophilia, partialism, zoophilia, coprophilia, klismaphilia, and urophilia (see Table 5–1).

Many paraphilic behaviors are considered criminal; however, it is important to realize that not all sexual criminals meet the criteria for paraphilia. The idea of rape as a paraphilia has been controversial (Kafka 1995), and rape has never been included among the paraphilias or any other diagnostic category in DSM; its inclusion has been considered and rejected. Rape is usually considered a crime of violence rather than a sexual disorder, although a small proportion of rapists would meet criteria for sexual sadism. Additional reasons for not including rape among the paraphilias is that rapists are a very heterogeneous group, rape fantasies and coercive sexual behavior are found in many "normal" males, and rapists are difficult to distinguish from other criminals, which casts doubt on the notion of rape as a specialist crime (Marshall and Eccles 1991; Polaschek et al. 1997). Thus, rape is considered outside the scope of this chapter.

Table 5–1. Paraphilias

DSM-IV-TR diagnosis	Fantasies, urges, and/or behaviors
Exhibitionism	Exposure of one's genitals to an unsuspecting stranger
Fetishism	The use of nonliving objects (e.g., female undergarments)
Frotteurism	Touching and rubbing against a nonconsenting person
Pedophilia	Involving sexual activity with a prepubescent child
Sexual masochism	Involving being humiliated, beaten, bound, or made to suffer
Sexual sadism	Involving psychological or physical suffering or humiliation of another
Transvestic fetishism	Involving cross-dressing (in a heterosexual male)
Voyeurism	Observing an unsuspecting person naked, undressing, or engaged in sexual activity
Paraphilias not otherwise specified	
Coprophilia	Feces
Klismaphilia	Enemas
Necrophilia	Corpses
Partialism	Focusing exclusively on part of a body
Telephone scatologia	Obscene phone calls
Urophilia	Urine
Zoophilia	Animals

It seems likely that paraphilias begin by late adolescence, although the disorders seem to peak between ages 20 and 30 years (Black et al. 1997; Ragan and Martin 2000). Most paraphilias are rarely heard of in women, with the exception of sadomasochism, in which males are nevertheless thought to outnumber females 20:1 (Levine 1999). Some believe that the incidence of female sexual abusers has been underestimated (Marshall and Laws 2003). In any case, almost all systematic research has been done in male-only samples.

Paraphilias are usually experienced as having an impulsive or an obsessive-compulsive quality (Bradford 1994, 1996; Coleman 1990; Kafka 1995, 2000; Stein et al. 1992; Suarez et al. 2002) and can differ dramatically in their severity. Two key aspects of severity are the extent to which the individual feels his thoughts, urges, and behaviors are out of control and whether the imagery or activity is absolutely required for sexual arousal to occur. In the least severe, subclinical cases, the thoughts may be fleeting, the behavior under control, and ordinary sexual behavior possible without any apparent unusual activities, although the individual may be using fantasy to integrate his paraphilia into his sexual activity at least some of the time. At the other extreme, individuals' lives may revolve around paraphilic thoughts and behaviors, the urges may be irresistible, and sexual arousal may be possible only in the context of the paraphilia.

Kafka (1997a) found that these men spent an average of 1–2 hours per day in sexual fantasies, urges, or behaviors related to their unconventional sexual interests. Contrary to common belief, individuals with paraphilias do not tend to repeat the same paraphilic behavior over their life span; rather they tend to have multiple paraphilias and paraphilia-related disorders (Abel and Osborn 1992; Abel et al. 1988; Heil et al. 2003; Kafka 1997a).

In one study (Kafka and Hennen 2002), the typical man attending outpatient treatment for paraphilia was a 37-year-old, white, employed man with some college education and a middle-class income (mean $52,600). Notable minorities of these men had experienced abuse as children (30% total: 17% physical, 18% sexual), had problems in school (41% total: 31% suspended/expelled, 24% repeated a grade, 18% truancy), and had a psychiatric hospitalization (25%).

The most common comorbid lifetime Axis I disorders in men with paraphilias are depression (69% dysthymic disorder, 39% major depression); substance abuse (42%), especially alcohol abuse (32%); attention-deficit/hyperactivity disorder (ADHD, 42%); and anxiety disorders (39%), especially social phobia (20%). Many other disorders are found at rates higher than found in the general population, including OCD (9%) and impulse-control disorder not otherwise specified (31%), especially reckless driving (24%) (Kafka and Hennen 2002). The same disorders were generally prominent in a sample of pedophiles in court-ordered treatment, with the exception of dysthymic disorder, which was much less frequent; importantly, diagnoses of ADHD and reckless driving were not made (Raymond et al. 1999).

Paraphilia-Related Disorders

Paraphilia-related disorders are characterized by sexual thoughts, urges, and behaviors that are accepted as normative but are engaged in with a frequency or intensity that leads to distress or significantly interferes with functioning (Kafka 1997a; Kafka and Hennen 1999, 2003) (Table 5–2). They may be experienced as impulsive or compulsive and are often experienced as being out of the individual's control. The most common paraphilia-related disorders reported in a clinical setting by patients with no paraphilias (Kafka and Hennen 1999) are protracted promiscuity (84%), compulsive masturbation (75%), pornography dependence (63%), phone sex dependence (37%), and severe sexual desire incompatibility (10%). These findings are similar to those found in other research (Kafka 1997a; Kafka and Hennen 2003).

Table 5–2. Paraphilia-related disorders

Compulsive masturbation
Phone sex dependence
Pornography dependence
Protracted promiscuity
Severe sexual desire incompatibility
Sexual chat room dependence

It seems likely that paraphilia-related disorders, like paraphilias, also begin by late adolescence and seem to peak between ages 20 and 30 years (Black et al. 1997; Ragan and Martin 2000). The prevalence of paraphilia-related disorders in the general population has been estimated to be as high as 6% (Black et al. 1997; Ragan and Martin 2000). The ratio of males to females is estimated at approximately 3:1 (Carnes 1998). However, the research done on paraphilia-related disorders also tends to have all male samples, just as with the paraphilias.

Paraphilia-related disorders are not currently recognized in the DSM system, and it has been noted that the format used for substance abuse could be used for these disorders as well. In general, in addition to specific symptoms, the DSM focuses on an assessment of distress or impairment to define a problem or behavior as meeting criteria for pathology. This approach could be taken for paraphilia-related disorders, but Kafka (1997a) has also recommended a specific operational definition based on research findings. Using Kinsey's concept of total sexual outlet (TSO), the total number of orgasms achieved per week by any means (Kinsey et al. 1948), Kafka suggested a TSO of seven per week, persistently for at least 6 months, as the minimum for male hypersexuality or paraphilia-related disorders. In the male population overall, a TSO of one to three is typical (Kafka 1997a; Kinsey et al. 1948). Although population surveys find that heterosexual intercourse is the most common sexual outlet for adults, it seems that for men with paraphilias and paraphilia-related disorders, masturbation is the most common sexual outlet, even among those who are married (Kafka 1997a). This is consistent with Kinsey et al. (1948), who found that masturbation was the primary sexual outlet for men with the highest TSO. This is an important point and reinforces that the TSO is a more sensible and sensitive measure to use in sexual compulsion populations. Unfortunately, most surveys of sexual behavior have focused on the occurrence of certain sexual behaviors, most typically intercourse, and neglected the TSO and the total time spent in sexual activities, which are better ways to quantify paraphilias and paraphilia-related disorders.

In one study (Kafka and Hennen 2002), the typical man in outpatient treatment for paraphilia-related disorders was a 38-year-old, white, employed man who had gone beyond college and had a middle-class income (mean $71,600). Notable minorities of these men had experienced abuse as children (19% total: 3% physical, 16% sexual).

Men with paraphilia-related disorders tend to have multiple additional Axis I disorders. The most common lifetime disorders identified across studies are depression, substance abuse, anxiety disorders, and impulse-control disorders. In a sample of 32 men with paraphilia-related disorders, Kafka and Hennen (2002) found these levels of lifetime diagnoses: depression (72%); substance abuse (38%), especially alcohol abuse (25%); anxiety disorders (38%), especially social phobia (25%); and impulse-control disorder not otherwise specified (16%).

Summary: Comparison of Paraphilias and Paraphilia-Related Disorders

The primary difference between the paraphilias and paraphilia-related disorders is the obvious one: those with paraphilias have socially unacceptable sexual desires and therefore run afoul of the law.

In comparing the sexual thoughts, urges, and behaviors of men with paraphilias with those with paraphilia-related disorders, Kafka and Hennen (2003) found that there were few statistically significant differences between the groups: they had similar TSOs for the past 6 months (6.7 ± 5.6 vs. 6.3 ± 4.6 for paraphilia and paraphilia-related disorder groups, respectively) and their lifetime high (12.0 ± 8.0 vs. 10.7 ± 5.1). However, the age at onset for hypersexual TSO was earlier for the men with paraphilias (20.7 ± 6.4 vs. 23.9 ± 8.6). An interesting difference was found when looking at subgroups: the men with the highest number of sexual disorders (five or more) was made up entirely of paraphilic males, primarily sex offenders, who had a higher TSO and were more sexually preoccupied at baseline.

Kafka and Hennen (2002) found men with paraphilias have more lifetime nonsexual Axis I disorders than those with paraphilia-related disorders (3.4 ± 2.5 vs. 2.5 ± 1.0) and are specifically more likely to have met criteria for childhood ADHD (42% vs. 19%), conduct disorder (23% vs. 0%), and cocaine abuse (18% vs. 3%). In this sample, the men with paraphilias had much more troubled educational and criminal justice histories and were more likely to have been psychiatrically hospitalized than those with paraphilia-related disorders. It is notable that a reanalysis of the data demonstrated that childhood ADHD not only distinguished socially deviant from nondeviant sexual diagnoses but accounted for the major demographic and developmental variables that differentiated the groups; the only remaining statistically significant differences were that the men with paraphilias were more likely to have been arrested and that they had fewer lifetime paraphilia-related disorders.

Men with paraphilia-related disorders are quite similar demographically to those with paraphilias (Kafka and Hennen 2002). They differ primarily in being less likely to have experienced physical abuse, having had less trouble in school, and having slightly higher educational achievement and income.

Pathogenesis

There are strong biological influences on human sexual function, especially the basic phases of sexual desire, arousal, and orgasm (Bradford 2001; Greenberg and Bradford 1997; Kafka 1995, 1997b; Meston and Frohlich 2000). Specific endocrine, neurotransmitter, neuropeptide, and central nervous system influences have been identified. The focus here is on those implicated in the pathology or treatment of sexual compulsions.

Some cases of compulsive sexual behavior have been linked to specific brain abnormalities. These may be the result of general behavioral disinhibition or may be more circumscribed; the sexual behaviors may seem compulsive, impulsive, or automatic in character. By their nature, brain abnormalities resulting from trauma or disease are generally not localized in highly specific brain areas or structures, but it is clear that similar changes in sexual behavior can result from lesions varying in severity and location. Indeed, the complexity of the findings supports the importance of circuits rather than specific structures or locations; the frontostriatal and temporolimbic systems have both been implicated (Stein et al. 2000).

Both paraphilias and paraphilia-related disorders have accompanied frontal abnormalities, and these cases seem to indicate general disinhibition rather than increased sexual desire. There have been many reports of hypersexuality associated with frontal lesions following traumatic brain injury (e.g., Lishman 1968; Miller et al. 1986), but a recent controlled study of aberrant sexual behavior after such an event did not find a relationship with frontal lobe injury (Simpson et al. 2001). It remains clear that disinhibition is one common consequence of frontal lesions, but whether lesions will result in aberrant sexual behavior cannot be predicted at this time based on the injury site or severity alone and may be determined in part by premorbid factors.

The frontal lobe is an appealing candidate for importance in sexual compulsions because the orbital frontal cortex is involved in impulse control in general, social cognition, decision making, working memory, and emotional processing. Thus one can speculate that maladaptive sexual behavior and disinhibition in general following frontal lobe injuries may be due in part to impaired cognitions, including failures in recognition of emotional expressions (Hornak et al. 1996), an inability to generate expectations of others' negative emotional reactions (Blair and Cipolotti 2000), and insensitivity to future consequences (Bechara et al. 1994, 2000). There seem to be differences in presentation depending on the age at which the lesion occurred; the prefrontal cortex is also involved in the acquisition of moral and social knowledge so that injury early in life can lead to impairments in such knowledge as well as in values and related reasoning. Social and moral knowledge learned prior to injury appears to remain intact, although the patient may be unable to behave in accordance with this knowledge (Anderson et al. 1999; Price et al. 1990).

Of course, brain abnormalities occurring from causes other than traumatic brain injury can also result in aberrant sexual behavior. Cases of hypersexual episodes accompanying multiple sclerosis have involved frontal lesions, although patients typically have multiple lesions that are located in different areas of the brain (Gondim and Thomas 2001; Huws et al. 1991).

Striatal dysfunction is implicated in some cases of aberrant sexuality such as those found in Huntington's disease (Rosenblatt and Leroi 2000), in Wilson's disease (Akil and Brewer 1995), and following L-dopa treatment in Parkinson's disease (Uitti et al. 1989), adding to the evidence that frontostriatal circuits are important in sexual behavior. Interestingly, these same circuits seem to play a role in Tourette's disorder, which can present with coprolalia and copropraxia among their complex tics. Patients with Tourette's disorder also have higher-than-expected rates of exhibitionism (Comings and Comings 1985).

A recent case report of a man with acquired pedophilia due to a right orbitofrontal tumor supports the role of this area in specific sexual interests and related behaviors (Burns and Swerdlow 2003). This man had preserved moral knowledge but was unable to control his sexual behavior. His pedophilia disappeared with the removal of the tumor and began to recur with its regrowth; removal again resulted in a disappearance of the pedophilia. A recent neuropsychological study of four pedophiles supports the notion that a striato-thalamo-cortical circuit is involved in the pathophysiology of pedophilia (Tost et al. 2004).

Abnormalities in the temporal lobe have also been implicated in compulsive sexual behavior. The most well known, perhaps, is Klüver-Bucy syndrome, a rare disorder with symptoms including hypersexuality, hyperphagia, emotional blunting, visual agnosia, and memory problems (Gerstenbrand et al. 1983; Hayman et al. 1998; Jha and Patel 2004; Salim et al. 2002; Yoneoka et al. 2004). The hypersexuality and hyperphagia seem to reflect a loss of the ability to discriminate appropriate objects more than an increase in drive per se. This disorder can be caused by bilateral lesions of the temporal lobes, specifically the amygdala or the anterior temporal areas; this can be the result of disease or injury. There is evidence that the syndrome also can result from damage to the limbic circuitry (Carroll et al. 1999).

Some conditions, including epilepsy and dementia, are reported to result in sexually aberrant behavior following lesions in either the frontal or temporal areas. Seizures have been associated with hypersexuality, hyposexuality, paraphilias, and sexual automatisms (Devinsky and Vazquez 1993). Disinhibition has been reported to be caused by partial complex frontal lobe seizures (Boone et al. 1988). Sexual automatisms and other hypersexual episodes as well as hyposexuality have been reported in complex partial temporal lobe seizures (Blumer 1970; Remillard et al. 1983; Shukla et al. 1979), but there is some evidence that at least some of these may have their origins in the frontal lobe (Spencer et al. 1983). Hypersexuality has also been found accompanying dementia related to both frontal- and temporal-lobe abnormalities (Alkhalil et al. 2004).

Although sexual desire has clear environmental/nurture influences, endocrine factors are also implicated. Of particular interest here are the androgens, which play a role in sexual interest and activity in both men and women. Hypogonadal or castrated men experience a rapid loss of sexual interest that is reversed with testosterone therapy. In addition, there is a relationship between testosterone levels and the frequency of sexual thoughts in adolescent males (Halpern et al. 1994; Udry et al. 1985). However, it is important to note that in adult males there appears to be no relationship between sexual interest and testosterone level within a wide range of normal testosterone levels (Schiavi and White 1976; Sherwin 1988). Similarly, women experience a decline in sexual interest following a decline in testosterone due to natural or surgically induced menopause (Sherwin 1991; Sherwin et al. 1985). In contrast, in women, there is little effect of estrogen on sexual interest, whereas estrogens and progesterone seem to have an inhibiting effect on male sexual interest (Meston and Frohlich 2000).

Several neurotransmitters play a role in sexual function. Serotonin (5-HT) is one, as is apparent in the sexual side effects that occur with selective serotonin reuptake inhibitors (SSRIs). The side effects are dose dependent, and the most common are delayed ejaculation, delayed or absent orgasm, and somewhat less consistently, decreased desire and difficulties with arousal (Rosen et al. 1999). The role of serotonin in sexual functioning is complex, and research suggests that activation of some serotonin receptors, such as 5-HT_2, impairs functioning, whereas activation of other receptors, such as 5-HT_{1A}, facilitates functioning (Meston and Frohlich 2000). Nefazodone, an SSRI that is also a 5-HT_2 antagonist, reportedly has fewer adverse sexual effects than other SSRIs (Cyr and Brown 1996; Preskorn 1995). Sexual side effects to SSRIs may be more severe in women than in men (Montejo-Gonzalez et al. 1997), but this has not been established definitively.

The role of dopamine in sexual function has been studied in depth, and it has been established that it plays an important role in several aspects of male sexual functioning (Melis and Argiolas 1995). The mesolimbic-mesocortical system plays a role in arousal, motivation, and reward. The nigrostriatal system is involved in control of sensory-motor coordination. The incertohypothalamic system plays a role primarily in seminal emission and erectile function as well as motivation. The role of dopamine in female sexual behavior is unclear. Epinephrine and norepinephrine are active in the sexual response cycles in both men and women (Meston and Frohlich 2000).

Nitric oxide is critical to vasocongestion and tumescence (Meston and Frohlich 2000). Briefly, nitric oxide production leads to the production of cyclic guanosine monophosphate (cGMP). In men, this causes relaxation of the smooth muscles of the penile arteries and corpus cavernosum, which leads to increased blood flow and erection. In women, it may lead to similar changes in the clitoris. The ability of sildenafil and other related medications to treat erectile dysfunction is due to the ability to prolong the action of cGMP by inhibiting its metabolism.

Kafka (1997b, 2003) proposed a monoamine theory of paraphilic disorders that characterizes them as sexual appetite–related behavior disorders resulting from dysregulation in the biological amines serotonin, dopamine, and norepinephrine. His theory is based on four lines of evidence: 1) these neurotransmitters play a modulatory role in sexual motivation; 2) data from studies of the sexual side effects of certain antidepressants, psychostimulants, and neuroleptics demonstrate that these monoamines influence sexual motivation and consummatory behaviors; 3) data suggest that specific characteristics of paraphilic sexual aggressors (antisocial impulsivity, anxiety, depression, and hypersexuality) are correlated with monoamine dysregulation; 4) pharmacological agents that enhance central serotonin neurotransmission seem to reduce paraphilic arousal and behavioral control. Although there are substantial data from basic research supporting these points and the role of monoamines in aggression and impulsivity as well as sexual motivation and consummation, it has not yet been proven that monoamines play a specific role in the paraphilias (Kafka 1997b, 2003).

Other researchers have identified additional mechanisms as playing significant roles. The neuropeptides (e.g., gonadotropin-releasing hormone, corticotropin-releasing hormone, and thyroid-releasing hormone), which are slower acting than the neurotransmitters, clearly play a role in human sexual behavior and may play a role in sexual compulsions (Bradford 2001). Balyk considers pedophilia to be an obsessive-compulsive spectrum disorder and has proposed a biomedical model for it that includes both the prefrontal cortex–basal ganglia–thalamic circuit implicated in OCD (Baxter 1994) and the behavioral inhibition system (Gray 1982), a septal-hippocampal system that accesses behavioral routines from the temporal lobe.

Treatment

The treatment of paraphilias is of significant public interest due to the serious consequences of these disorders; therefore, a large amount of research has been conducted on their treatment. Although it is widely believed that paraphilias are untreatable, this seems to be due more to the severe consequences of any recurrence, rather than to particularly poor treatment efficacy compared with other disorders.

There are many difficulties in conducting research on sex offenders, including assessment of efficacy, especially in evaluating recidivism; duration of follow-up; sample selection; and lack of comparable control groups (because facilities are loath to leave appropriate offenders untreated) or comparison treatments (Grossman et al. 1999).

In contrast to the paraphilias, research on the treatment of paraphilia-related disorders has lagged considerably.

Pharmacotherapy and Other Medical Treatments

Traditionally, the focus of medical approaches to the treatment of paraphilias, especially those that lead to criminal offenses, has been to reduce the patient's sexual drive. Although men with paraphilias have normal testosterone levels, surgical and pharmacological means of lowering testosterone levels have been found to reduce their paraphilic preoccupations, urges, and activities. These approaches generally have been considered too drastic and too risky to be used in treatment of paraphilia-related disorders.

Surgical techniques for lowering testosterone levels are not often used in the United States but are more accepted in Europe; the techniques include both castration and neurosurgery (stereotaxic hypothalamotomy). These techniques have demonstrated success at reducing recidivism in sexual offenders (Grossman et al. 1999).

The most established pharmacological agents for the treatment of paraphilias are those that reduce sexual urges and behavior by reducing testosterone levels (Gijs and Gooren 1996). The most common pharmacological agents are synthetic progesterones that came into use in the 1960s: medroxyprogesterone acetate in the United States and cyproterone acetate in Canada and Europe. The mechanisms of action of these agents are to increase testosterone reductase activity, to decrease testosterone synthesis by a negative feedback effect on hypothalamic and pituitary hormone secretion, and/or to block the action of testosterone at the receptor level (Bradford 2001; Gijs and Gooren 1996; Maletzky and Field 2003).

Although there have been no large, double-blind, controlled trials of these synthetic progesterones, numerous open-label studies and case reports of men with paraphilias suggest that these medications reduce sexual fantasies, urges, and behavior, including the reduction of recidivism in sex offenders (Grossman et al. 1999). Importantly, in most studies of sexual offenders, participants also were receiving some form of psychological treatment. Usual dosages of medroxyprogesterone acetate are 300–500 mg/week intramuscularly or 50–300 mg/day orally (Bradford 2001; Gijs and Gooren 1996); dosages for cyproterone acetate are 300–600 mg/week intramuscularly or 50–200 mg/day orally (Gijs and Gooren 1996). Unlike surgical techniques for reducing testosterone levels, the effects of these agents are reversible; however, most patients on these medications experience a decrease in normal sexual interest and function, so the treatments are not ideal. These also are not often used in men with paraphilia-related disorders.

Another hormonal approach used in the paraphilias that seems promising is the use of synthetic analogues of gonadotropin-releasing hormones (Bradford 2001; Grossman et al. 1999; Maletzky and Field 2003). These initially increase the production of testosterone but lead to a reduction of circulating testosterone within 1–3 months by inhibiting the secretion of naturally occurring gonadotropins. A number of case reports published since the early 1990s report success in reducing sexual urges and behavior in men with paraphilias (Dickey 1992; Rosler and Witztum 1998; Rousseau et al. 1990; Thibaut et al. 1993).

More recently, SSRIs are becoming a first-line treatment for both paraphilias and paraphilia-related disorders (Bradford 2001; Gijs and Gooren 1996). Initially the SSRIs were tried because of the expectation that their sexual side effects, a problem in most disorders, would be helpful in sexual compulsions. However, research suggests that reduction in symptoms is independent of sexual side effects and is a result of their anti-obsessional effects or a decrease in thoughts and urges (Greenberg and Bradford 1997; Kafka 1997b; Kafka and Prentky 1992). This is important, because an ideal treatment would suppress deviant and out-of-control sexual drives and behaviors but leave normative sexual interests and behavior intact; this is particularly important for patients with paraphilia-related disorders. Sexual side effects including decreased libido, delayed ejaculation, and impotence are somewhat common with SSRIs; however, titrating the dosage may reduce these effects. Given that depression and anxiety disorders are common comorbidities with sexual compulsions, the SSRIs can be an excellent treatment, because they are effective treatments of these disorders as well.

Case reports and open-label studies have shown the SSRIs, including fluoxetine, fluvoxamine, paroxetine and sertraline, to be effective in reducing the symptoms of paraphilia and paraphilia-related disorders (Abouesh and Clayton 1999; Bradford and Gratzer 1995; Bradford and Greenberg 1996; Galli et al. 1998; Greenberg and Bradford 1997; Greenberg et al. 1996; Kafka 1991a, 1991b, 1994a; Kafka and Prentky 1992; Zohar et al. 1994). There is no evidence that the SSRIs differ in efficacy.

Specific paraphilias for which SSRIs have been reported to be effective include exhibitionism (Abouesh and Clayton 1999; Kafka 1994a; Kafka and Prentky 1992; Perilstein et al. 1991); fetishism (Kafka 1994a; Lorefice 1991), masochism (Kafka 1994a; Kafka and Prentky 1992), transvestic fetishism (Kafka 1994a), and voyeurism (Abouesh and Clayton 1999; Azhar and Varma 1995; Emmanuel et al. 1991; Perilstein et al. 1991). SSRIs have also been reported to be effective in these paraphilia-related disorders: compulsive masturbation (Kafka 1994a; Kafka and Prentky 1992), pornography dependence (Kafka 1994a; Kafka and Prentky 1992), and sexual compulsions (Aguirre 1999; Kafka 1994a, 2000b; Kafka and Prentky 1992).

To date, no double-blind, controlled trials have been reported. However, a double-blind, placebo-controlled trial of citalopram in men with sexual compulsions who have sex with men is under way at the Mount Sinai School of Medicine in a joint effort between Eric Hollander's research group from the Compulsive, Impulsive and Anxiety Disorders Program and Jan Morgenstern's substance abuse research group.

It is significant that SSRIs can ameliorate paraphilic and paraphilia-related arousal and activity but leave normative sexual functioning intact in many individuals (Bradford and Greenberg 1996; Greenberg and Bradford 1997; Kafka 1994b, 1995, 1997b; Kafka and Prentky 1992, 1994; Stein et al. 1992); however, there are some sexual side effects experienced by these populations. Nefazodone is thus a promising treatment because it has initial reports of success (Coleman et al. 2000) and does not have the same frequency of sexual side effects found with the other SSRIs (Cyr and Brown 1996; Preskorn 1995). Of interest, nefazodone has demonstrated some efficacy in an open trial of pathological gambling (Pallanti et al. 2002). However, the possibility of liver abnormalities has decreased the use of nefazodone.

The neuroleptic benperidol was used in the 1970s to treat sexual deviancy, but few reports have appeared in the literature on its use or that of other antipsychotics (Gijs and Gooren 1996). The atypical antipsychotics are used to treat sexual compulsions in clinical practice today, although there are no published studies regarding their use.

In addition, particular subgroups may benefit from adjunctive treatments. Of importance because ADHD is a common comorbid disorder in sexual compulsions, Kafka and Hennen (2000), in an open-label trial involving men with sexual compulsions who had a retroactive diagnosis of ADHD and continuing symptoms as adults, were able to decrease symptoms of both disorders by augmenting SSRIs with the psychostimulant methylphenidate. The evidence for the use of mood stabilizers and antiseizure medications in sexual compulsions is mixed. Case studies show support for their use in patients who are identified as either bipolar (Cesnik and Coleman 1989; Coleman and Cesnik 1990; Ward 1975) or impulsive (Varela and Black 2002). However, one open-label trial of divalproex sodium in men with paraphilias and comorbid bipolar disorder showed a significant improvement in the patients' manic symptoms but no reduction in their paraphilic symptoms (Nelson et al. 2001).

Psychotherapy

There is a long history of psychological treatments for paraphilias but not for paraphilia-related disorders. Much of the initial work on treating paraphilias developed out of psychoanalysis, but by the 1960s behavioral psychology began to have an impact on research on sexuality, and our current psychological treatments for paraphilias are based in this tradition (Laws and Marshall 2003). These earlier treatments have been found to be ineffective (Abel et al. 1992; Hanson et al. 2002). Cognitive-behavioral therapy (CBT) is the first treatment approach to have proven efficacy, and it has become the basis of complex treatment programs for pedophilia and other sexual disorders that have criminal consequences. Components that should be included in a CBT treatment program are reducing deviant arousal and increasing appropriate arousal (e.g., aversion therapy, desensitization, reconditioning techniques); improving ability to interact socially, especially in relationships (e.g., social skills, assertiveness, anger management training); increasing victim awareness and empathy (e.g., role playing, exposure to victims' experiences, feedback); correcting the cognitive errors that allow rationalizing of criminal behaviors (e.g., cognitive restructuring); treatment for substance abuse; and, critically important, training in relapse prevention techniques (see reviews by Grossman et al. 1999; Marshall and Laws 2003). Relapse prevention was borrowed from the addictions field and incorporated into the treatment programs for sexual offenders in the 1980s (Pithers et al. 1983). This is essential to the treatment of sexual offenders because, although many measures of efficacy can be used, the key treatment goal with offender populations is the reduction of recidivism. However, recidivism is difficult to assess because few sexual offenses are brought to the attention of the authorities, and it is clear that offenders admit to only a very small proportion of their criminal sexual activities (Abel et al. 1987, 1988).

Research reviews and meta-analyses covering modern programs provide evidence that CBT-based treatment programs reduce recidivism (Gallagher et al. 1999; Grossman et al. 1999; Hall 1995; Hanson et al. 2002; Marshall and Laws 2003). Note that recidivism rates vary dramatically from study to study. In studies that have untreated comparison groups and that use charges or rearrest as the criterion for recidivism, rates range from as low as 8% to 13% for the treated and untreated offenders, respectively (Marques et al. 1994), to rates as high as 39% to 57% (Marshall et al. 1991). One meta-analysis found that CBT programs reduced recidivism from 17.4% to 9.9% (Hanson et al. 2002).

Little research is available regarding psychotherapy for paraphilia-related disorders. The most widely publicized treatments are based on 12-Step programs and include Sexaholics Anonymous, Sex and Love Addicts, and Sexual Compulsives Anonymous as well as inpatient and outpatient treatment programs. There are multiple case studies and reports of therapy techniques, generally with combined CBT and 12-Step approaches, but only one study has been published. This pre/post study of group therapy among sexually compulsive gay and bisexual men (Quadland 1985) focused on changing the problem behaviors, and it was effective in decreasing the targeted behaviors. Whether one views paraphilia-related disorders as addictions or as compulsions, it is likely that 12-Step and CBT approaches will be appropriate therapeutic approaches because they are more effective than other approaches in treating similar disorders such as pathological gambling (Freidenberg et al. 2002; Oakley-Browne et al. 2000; Pietrzak et al. 2003).

Conclusion

There are more similarities than differences between the paraphilias and paraphilia-related disorders, and both share many characteristics with OCD, the prototypical obsessive-compulsive spectrum disorder, as well as with the other impulse-control disorders. The similarities include aspects of the phenomenology, neurobiology, age at onset, clinical course, comorbidity, and treatment response to SSRIs. It is important, given the prevalence and the knowledge base that has been accumulated about paraphilia-related disorders, that they be incorporated specifically into DSM-V. It would be reasonable for paraphilia-related disorders to be grouped with the paraphilias, but perhaps these should not be in a category of sexual disorders; it may be time to consider a different organization based on other, deeper similarities in symptoms—for example, constructs such as the obsessive-compulsive spectrum. Alternatively, they could be placed with the impulse-control disorders.

Based on the data currently available, sexual compulsions can easily be fit either onto the obsessive-compulsive spectrum or into an addiction model. Phenomenologically, sexual compulsions seem similar to the addictions; however, there are also similarities with OCD and even more so with some of the other obsessive-compulsive spectrum disorders. With the most severe sexual compulsions, individuals may feel that their lives are out of control. Their days may revolve around arranging for and carrying out their sexual activities just as a drug addict's life can revolve around obtaining and using drugs. However, this is not unlike those with severe OCD who have to organize their lives

around avoidances and rituals and is perhaps indistinguishable from pathological gamblers who spend their time planning for their next gambling opportunity and managing the many negative consequences of gambling losses. Like-
wise, intrusive thoughts do not distinguish between addictions and obsessions;
they may preoccupy the individual for most of the day and prevent normal
social and work functioning as well as create anxiety. With sexual compulsions,
as their condition progresses, the sexual activity generally becomes less pleasurable and less satisfying; this has the closest parallels with addictions in that the
activity may initially, or in other circumstances, be pleasurable. Yet as time
passes, sexual compulsions—also like impulse-control disorders—become
more similar to OCD, with the behaviors being carried out compulsively to
reduce anxiety or other uncomfortable feelings, relief being brief, and the
behaviors serving to maintain the cycle just as rituals do in OCD. It should be
noted that addictions often follow the same course: initially drugs are sought
for the high they provide, but as the addiction progresses, drugs are sought to
relieve withdrawal symptoms and to feel normal.

Also, the phenomenology may differ from individual to individual, or
from time to time, for a specific individual. For some, sexually compulsive
behaviors may seem to arise from sudden impulse or may be carefully planned
and compulsive. Some paraphilic behaviors can be experienced as impulsive
acts that occur almost unexpectedly when the individual is faced with an
opportunity to act out. An exhibitionist, for example, may not be seeking out
opportunities to expose himself or be generally consumed by fantasies but
rather may be functioning normally with only occasional fantasies. However,
a situation matching a fantasy may cue his paraphilia: he may walk down an
empty street and find a young woman walking toward him and realize he is
exposing himself without having planned for it or stopped to consider the
consequences. In contrast, some paraphilic behavior is elaborately planned
out: pedophiles may organize their lives around providing themselves with
many opportunities to have access to young children and may "groom" individual victims.

Like OCD, sexual compulsions are characterized by repetitive behaviors
and an inability to effectively inhibit the behaviors. Although this is characteristic of all obsessive-compulsive spectrum disorders, it is important to realize
that obsessive-compulsive spectrum disorders vary in the extent to which they
are compulsive versus impulsive. They range from the more compulsive disor-

ders (e.g., OCD, hypochondriasis, body dysmorphic disorder) to the more impulsive (e.g., pathological gambling, compulsive shopping, kleptomania) (Hollander and Wong 1995). Disorders on the compulsive end of the spectrum seem to reflect risk aversion and an overestimation of the likelihood of future harm; the impulsive end seems to reflect risk seeking, acting without realistic consideration of future harm. Additionally, for compulsive disorders, the repetitive behavior is anxiety reducing but not pleasurable; in contrast, for the impulsive disorders, the repetitive behavior has some pleasurable aspects, particularly at the beginning of the disorder and/or at times that it is less severe. Impulsive disorders can also be conceptualized as addictions, yet they differ from traditional addictions most notably in that they do not focus on the intake of psychoactive substances. Sexual compulsions best fit at the impulsive end of the continuum: at the time the sexual activities are carried out, there is an underestimation of the negative consequences of impulsivity, perhaps even a psychological high, along with the inability to control the behavior.

Sexual compulsions have been viewed as either addictions or impulse-control problems (Coleman 1992; Kafka 2000; Ragan and Martin 2000). If they are addictions, the sexual behaviors would be used to self-sooth or self-medicate and the chemicals released to produce pleasure could be considered the addictive substances. However, in sexual compulsions, although orgasm produces pleasure, or at least relief, it is quickly replaced by negative emotions, such as depression and guilt, which become reinforcers and perpetuate the addiction cycle (Kafka 2000). This is the same pattern as with the impulse-control disorders.

Those who resist seeing sexual compulsions as an addiction argue that a sexual compulsion cannot be an addiction because people do not become addicted to sex in the same way that they become addicted to psychoactive substances—that is, there is no physical dependence or withdrawal (Coleman 1992). In addition, sexual compulsions seem to be driven more by anxiety reduction than by sexual desire. In fact, sexually compulsive behaviors are often followed by anxiety reduction or mood change similar to that reported by people with OCD following their ritualized behavior (Black et al. 1997; Coleman 1992).

The phenomenology, the pattern of comorbidities, and the incidence of high-risk behaviors suggest that sexual compulsions are more similar to impulse-control disorders, such as pathological gambling and binge eating, than to the more compulsive disorders on the obsessive-compulsive spectrum, such as OCD and body dysmorphic disorder. Thus, sexual compulsions are on the impulsive, risk-taking end of the spectrum. Like other impulsive disorders, sexual compulsions have many similarities to addictions, and substance abuse is a common comorbidity.

References

Abel GG, Osborn C: The paraphilias: the extent and nature of sexually deviant and criminal behavior. Psychiatr Clin North Am 15:675–687, 1992

Abel GG, Becker JV, Mittelman M, et al: Self-reported sex crimes of nonincarcerated paraphiliacs. J Interpers Violence 2:3–25, 1987

Abel GG, Becker JV, Cunningham-Rathner J, et al: Multiple paraphilic diagnoses among sex offenders. Bull Am Acad Psychiatry Law 16:153–168, 1988

Abel GG, Osborn C, Anthony D, et al: Current treatments of paraphiliacs. Annu Rev Sex Res 3:255–290, 1992

Abouesh A, Clayton A: Compulsive voyeurism and exhibitionism: a clinical response to paroxetine. Arch Sex Behav 28:23–30, 1999

Aguirre B: Fluoxetine and compulsive sexual behavior. J Am Acad Child Adolesc Psychiatry 38:943, 1999

Akil M, Brewer GJ: Psychiatric and behavioral abnormalities in Wilson's disease. Adv Neurol 65:171–178, 1995

Alkhalil C, Tanvir F, Alkhalil B, et al: Treatment of sexual disinhibition in dementia: case reports and review of the literature. Am J Ther 11:231–235, 2004

American Psychiatric Association: Diagnostic and Statistical Manual of Mental Disorders, 4th Edition, Text Revision. Washington, DC, American Psychiatric Association, 2000

Anderson SW, Bechara A, Damasio H, et al: Impairment of social and moral behavior related to early damage in human prefrontal cortex. Nat Neurosci 2:1032–1037, 1999

Azhar MZ, Varma SL: Response to clomipramine in sexual addiction. Eur Psychiatry 10:263–265, 1995

Baxter LR Jr: Positron emission tomography studies of cerebral glucose metabolism in obsessive compulsive disorder. J Clin Psychiatry 55 (suppl):54–59, 1994

Bechara A, Damasio AR, Damasio H, et al: Insensitivity to future consequences following damage to human prefrontal cortex. Cognition 50:7–15, 1994

Bechara A, Damasio H, Damasio AR: Emotion, decision making and the orbitofrontal cortex. Cereb Cortex 10:295–307, 2000

Black DW, Kehrberg LL, Flumerfelt DL, et al: Characteristics of 36 subjects reporting compulsive sexual behavior. Am J Psychiatry 154:243–249, 1997

Blair RJR, Cipolotti L: Impaired social response reversal: a case of acquired sociopathy. Brain 123:1122–1141, 2000

Blumer D: Hypersexual episodes in temporal lobe epilepsy. Am J Psychiatry 126:1099–1106, 1970

Boone KB, Miller BL, Rosenberg L, et al: Neuropsychological and behavioral abnormalities in an adolescent with frontal lobe seizures. Neurology 38:583–586, 1988

Bradford JM: Sexual deviancy. Curr Opin Psychiatry 7:446–451, 1994

Bradford JM: The role of serotonin in the future of forensic psychiatry. Bull Am Acad Psychiatry Law 24:419–422, 1996

Bradford JM: The neurobiology, neuropharmacology, and pharmacological treatment of paraphilias and compulsive sexual behavior. Can J Psychiatry 46:26–33, 2001

Bradford JM, Gratzer TG: A treatment for impulse control disorders and paraphilia: a case report. Can J Psychiatry 40:4–5, 1995

Bradford JM, Greenberg DM: Pharmacological treatment of deviant sexual behavior. Annu Rev Sex Res 7:283, 1996

Burns JM, Swerdlow RH: Right orbitofrontal tumor with pedophilia symptom and constructional apraxia sign. Arch Neurol 60:437–440, 2003

Carnes P: The obsessive shadow. Professional Counselor 13:15–17, 1998

Carroll BT, Goforth HW, Carroll LA: Anatomic basis of Kluver-Bucy syndrome. J Neuropsychiatry Clin Neurosci 11:116, 1999

Cesnik JA, Coleman E: Use of lithium carbonate in the treatment of autoerotic asphyxia. Am J Psychother 43:277–286, 1989

Coleman E: The obsessive-compulsive model for describing compulsive sexual behavior. American Journal of Preventive Psychiatry and Neurology 2:9–14, 1990

Coleman E: Is your patient suffering from compulsive sexual behavior? Psychiatr Ann 22:320–325, 1992

Coleman E, Cesnik J: Skoptic syndrome: the treatment of an obsessional gender dysphoria with lithium carbonate and psychotherapy. Am J Psychother 44:204–217, 1990

Coleman E, Gratzer T, Nesvacil L, et al: Nefazodone and the treatment of nonparaphilic compulsive sexual behavior: a retrospective study. J Clin Psychiatry 61:282–284, 2000

Comings DE, Comings BG: Tourette syndrome: clinical and psychological aspects of 250 cases. Am J Hum Genet 37:435–450, 1985

Cyr M, Brown CS: Nefazodone: its place among antidepressants. Ann Pharmacother 30:1003–1012, 1996

Devinsky O, Vazquez B: Behavioral changes associated with epilepsy. Neurol Clin 11:127–149, 1993

Dickey R: The management of a case of treatment-resistant paraphilia with a long-acting LHRH agonist. Can J Psychiatry 37:567–569, 1992

Emmanuel NP, Lydiard RB, Ballenger JC: Fluoxetine treatment of voyeurism (letter). Am J Psychiatry 148:950, 1991

Freidenberg BM, Blanchard EB, Wulfert E, et al: Changes in physiological arousal to gambling cues among participants in motivationally enhanced cognitive-behavior therapy for pathological gambling: a preliminary study. Appl Psychophysiol Biofeedback 27:251–260, 2002

Gallagher CA, Wilson DB, Hirschfield P, et al: A quantitative review of the effects of sex offender treatment on sexual reoffending. Corrections Management Quarterly 3:19–29, 1999

Galli VB, Raute NJ, McConnville BJ, et al: An adolescent male with multiple paraphilias treated successfully with fluoxetine. J Child Adolesc Psychopharmacol 8:195–197, 1998

Gerstenbrand F, Poewe W, Aichner F, et al: Kluver-Bucy syndrome in man: experiences with posttraumatic cases. Neurosci Biobehav Rev 7:413–417, 1983

Gijs L, Gooren L: Hormonal and psychopharmacological interventions in the treatment of paraphilias: an update. J Sex Res 33:273–290, 1996

Gondim FA, Thomas FP: Episodic hyperlibidinism in multiple sclerosis. Mult Scler 7:67–70, 2001

Gray JA: The Neuropsychology of Anxiety: An Enquiry Into the Functions of the Septo-Hippocampal System. Oxford, U.K., Oxford University Press, 1982

Greenberg DM, Bradford JM: Treatment of the paraphilic disorders: a review of the role of the selective serotonin reuptake inhibitors. Sex Abuse 9:349–360, 1997

Greenberg DM, Bradford JMW, Curry S, et al: A comparison of treatment of paraphilias with three serotonin reuptake inhibitors: a retrospective study. Bull Am Acad Psychiatry Law 24:525–532, 1996

Grossman LS, Martis B, Fichtner CG: Are sex offenders treatable? a research overview. Psychiatr Serv 50:349–361, 1999

Hall GCN: Sexual offender recidivism revisited: a meta-analysis of recent treatment studies. J Consult Clin Psychol 63:802–809, 1995

Halpern CT, Udry JR, Campbell B, et al: Testosterone and religiosity as predictors of sexual attitudes and activity among adolescent males: a biosocial model. J Biosoc Sci 26:217–234, 1994

Hanson RK, Gordon A, Harris AJ, et al: First report of the collaborative outcome data project on the effectiveness of psychological treatment for sex offenders. Sex Abuse 14:169–194, 2002

Hayman LA, Rexer JL, Pavol MA, et al: Kluver-Bucy syndrome after bilateral selective damage of amygdala and its cortical connections. J Neuropsychiatry Clin Neurosci 10:354–358, 1998

Heil P, Ahlmeyer S, Simons D: Crossover sexual offenses. Sex Abuse 15:221–236, 2003

Hollander E, Wong CM: Body dysmorphic disorder, pathological gambling, and sexual compulsions. J Clin Psychiatry 56(suppl):7–12, 1995

Hornak J, Rolls ET, Wade D: Face and voice expression identification in patients with emotional and behavioural changes following ventral frontal lobe damage. Neuropsychologia 34:247–261, 1996

Huws R, Shubsachs AP, Taylor PJ: Hypersexuality, fetishism and multiple sclerosis. Br J Psychiatry 158:280–281, 1991

Jenike MA: Obsessive-compulsive and related disorders: a hidden epidemic. N Engl J Med 321:530–541,1989

Jha S, Patel R: Kluver-Bucy syndrome: an experience with six cases. Neurol India 52:369–371, 2004

Kafka MP: Successful antidepressant treatment of nonparaphilic sexual addictions and paraphilias in men. J Clin Psychiatry 52:60–65, 1991a

Kafka MP: Successful treatment of paraphilic coercive disorder (a rapist) with fluoxetine hydrochloride. Br J Psychiatry 158:844–847, 1991b

Kafka MP: Paraphilia-related disorders: common, neglected and misunderstood. Harv Rev Psychiatry 2:39–40, 1994a

Kafka MP: Sertraline pharmacotherapy for paraphilias and paraphilia-related disorders: an open trial. Ann Clin Psychiatry 6:189–195, 1994b

Kafka MP: Sexual impulsivity, in Impulsivity and Aggression. Edited by Hollander E, Stein DJ. Chichester, U.K., Wiley, 1995, pp 201–228

Kafka MP: Hypersexual desire in males: an operational definition and clinical implications for males with paraphilias and paraphilia-related disorders. Arch Sex Behav 25:505–526, 1997a

Kafka MP: A monoamine hypothesis for the pathophysiology of paraphilic disorders. Arch Sex Behav 26:337–352 1997b

Kafka MP: The paraphilia-related disorders: nonparaphilic hypersexuality and sexual compulsivity/addiction, in Principles of Practice of Sex Therapy. Edited by Lieblum S, Rosen RC. New York, Guilford, 2000, pp 471–503

Kafka MP: The monoamine hypothesis for the pathophysiology of paraphilic disorders: an update. Ann N Y Acad Sci 989:86–94; discussion 144–153, 2003

Kafka MP, Hennen J: The paraphilia-related disorders: an empirical investigation of nonparaphilic hypersexuality disorders in outpatient males. J Sex Marital Ther 25:305–319, 1999

Kafka MP, Hennen J: Psychostimulant augmentation during treatment with selective serotonin reuptake inhibitors in men with paraphilias and paraphilia-related disorders: a case series. J Clin Psychiatry 61:664–670, 2000

Kafka MP, Hennen J: A DSM-IV Axis I comorbidity study of males (n=120) with paraphilias and paraphilia-related disorders. Sex Abuse 14:3349–3366, 2002

Kafka MP, Hennen J: Hypersexual desire in males: are males with paraphilias different from males with paraphilia-related disorders? Sex Abuse 15:307–320, 2003

Kafka MP, Prentky R: Fluoxetine treatment of nonparaphilic sexual addictions and paraphilias in men. J Clin Psychiatry 53:351–358, 1992

Kafka MP, Prentky RA: Preliminary observations of DSM-III-R Axis I comorbidity in men with paraphilias and paraphilia-related disorders. J Clin Psychiatry 55:481–487, 1994

Kinsey AC, Pomeroy WB, Martin CF: Sexual Behavior in the Human Male. Philadelphia, PA, WB Saunders, 1948

Laws DR, Marshall WL: A brief history of behavioral and cognitive behavioral approaches to sexual offenders, part 1: early developments. Sex Abuse 15:75–92, 2003

Levine SB: Paraphilias, in Kaplan and Sadock's Comprehensive Textbook of Psychiatry, 7th Edition. Edited by Kaplan BJ, Kaplan VA. Philadelphia, PA, Lippincott Williams & Wilkins, 1999, pp 1631–1645

Lishman WA: Brain damage in relation to psychiatric disability after head injury. Br J Psychiatry 114:373–410, 1968

Lorefice LS: Fluoxetine treatment of a fetish. J Clin Psychiatry 52:41, 1991

Maletzky BM, Field G: The biological treatment of dangerous sexual offenders, a review and preliminary report of the Oregon pilot Depo-Provera program. Aggress Violent Behav 8:391–412, 2003

Marques JK, Day DM, Nelson C, et al: Effects of cognitive-behavioral treatment on sex offender recidivism: preliminary results of a longitudinal study. Criminal Justice and Behavior 21:28–54, 1994

Marshall WL, Eccles A: Issues in clinical practice with sex offenders. J Interpers Violence 6:68–93, 1991

Marshall WL, Laws DR: A brief history of behavioral and cognitive behavioral approaches to sexual offender treatment, part 2: the modern era. Sex Abuse 15:93–120, 2003

Marshall WL, Eccles A, Barbaree HE: The treatment of exhibitionists: a focus on sexual deviance versus cognitive and relationship features. Behav Res Ther 29:129–135, 1991

Melis MR, Argiolas A: Dopamine and sexual behavior. Neurosci Biobehav Rev 19:19–38, 1995

Meston CM, Frolich PF: The neurobiology of sexual functioning. Arch Gen Psychiatry 57:1012–1032, 2000

Miller BL, Cummings JL, McIntyre H, et al: Hypersexuality or altered sexual preference following brain injury. J Neurol Neurosurg Psychiatry 49:867–873, 1986

Montejo-Gonzalez AL, Llorca G, et al: SSRI-induced sexual dysfunction: fluoxetine, paroxetine, sertraline, and fluvoxamine in a prospective, multicenter, and descriptive clinical study of 344 patients. J Sex Marital Ther 23:176–194, 1997

Nelson E, Brusman L, Holcomb J, et al: Divalproex sodium in sex offenders with bipolar disorders and comorbid paraphilias: an open retrospective study. J Affect Disord 64:249–255, 2001

Oakley-Browne MA, Adams P, Mobberley PM: Interventions for pathological gambling. Cochrane Database Syst Rev CD001521, 2000

Pallanti S, Baldini Rossi N, Sood E, et al: Nefazodone treatment of pathological gambling: a prospective open-label controlled trial. J Clin Psychiatry 63:1034–1039, 2002

Perilstein RD, Lippers S, Friedman LJ: Three cases of paraphilias responsive to fluoxetine treatment. J Clin Psychiatry 52:169–170, 1991

Pietrzak RH, Ladd GT, Petry NM: Disordered gambling in adolescents: epidemiology, diagnosis, and treatment. Paediatr Drugs 5:583–595, 2003

Pithers WD, Marques JK, Gibat CC, et al: Relapse prevention with sexual aggressors: a self control model of treatment and maintenance of change, in The Sexual Aggressor: Current Perspectives on Treatment. Edited by Greer JG, Stuart IR. New York, Van Nostrand Reinhold, 1983, pp 214–239

Polaschek DL, Ward T, Hudson SM: Rape and rapists: theory and treatment. Clin Psychol Rev 17:117–144, 1997

Preskorn SH: Comparison of tolerability of bupropion, fluoxetine, imipramine, nefazodone, paroxetine, sertraline, and venlafaxine. J Clin Psychiatry 56 (suppl):12–21, 1995

Price BH, Daffner KR, Stowe RM, et al: The comportmental learning disabilities of early frontal lobe damage. Brain 113:1383–1393, 1990

Quadland MC: Compulsive sexual behavior: definition of a problem and an approach to treatment. J Sex Marital Ther 11:121–132, 1985

Ragan PW, Martin PR: The psychobiology of sexual addiction. Sexual Addiction and Compulsivity 7:161–175, 2000

Raymond NC, Coleman E, Ohlerking F, et al: Psychiatric comorbidity in pedophilic sex offenders. Am J Psychiatry 156:786–788, 1999

Remillard GM, Andermann F, Testa GF, et al: Sexual ictal manifestations predominate in women with temporal lobe epilepsy: a finding suggesting sexual dimorphism in the human brain. Neurology 33:323–330, 1983

Rosen RC, Lane RM, Menza M: Effects of SSRIs on sexual function: a critical review. J Clin Psychopharmacol 19:67–85, 1999

Rosenblatt A, Leroi I: Neuropsychiatry of Huntington's disease and other basal ganglia disorders. Psychosomatics 41:24–30, 2000

Rosler A, Witztum E: Treatment of men with paraphilia with a long-acting analogue of gonadotropin-releasing hormone. N Engl J Med 338:416–422, 1998

Rousseau L, Couture M, Dupont A, et al: Effect of combined androgen blockade with an LHRH agonist and flutamide in one severe case of male exhibitionism. Can J Psychiatry 35:338–341, 1990

Salim A, Kim KA, Kimbrell BJ, et al: Kluver-Bucy syndrome as a result of minor head trauma. South Med J 95:929–931, 2002

Schiavi RC, White D: Androgens and male sexual function: a review of human studies. J Sex Marital Ther 2:214–228, 1976

Sherwin BB: A comparative analysis of the role of androgen in human male and female sexual behavior: behavioral specificity, critical thresholds, and sensitivity. Psychobiology 16:416–425, 1988

Sherwin BB: The psychoendocrinology of aging and female sexuality. Annu Rev Sex Res 2:181–198, 1991

Sherwin BB, Gelfand MM, Brender W: Androgen enhances sexual motivation in females: a prospective, crossover study of sex steroid administration in the surgical menopause. Psychosom Med 47:339–351, 1985

Shukla GD, Srivastava ON, Katiyar BC: Sexual disturbances in temporal lobe epilepsy: a controlled study. Br J Psychiatry 134:288–292, 1979

Simpson G, Tate R, Ferry K, et al: Social, neuroradiological, medical, and neuropsychological correlates of sexually aberrant behavior after traumatic brain injury: a controlled study. J Head Trauma Rehabil 16:556–572, 2001

Spencer SS, Spencer DD, Williamson PD, et al: Sexual automatisms in complex partial seizures. Neurology 33:527–533, 1983

Stein DJ, Hollander E, Anthony DT, et al: Serotonergic medications for sexual obsessions, sexual addictions, and paraphilias. J Clin Psychiatry 53:267–271, 1992

Stein DJ, Black DW, Pienaar W: Sexual disorders not otherwise specified: compulsive, impulsive, or addictive? CNS Spectrums 5:60–64, 2000

Suarez T, O'Leary A, Morgenstern J, et al: Selective serotonin reuptake inhibitors as a treatment for sexual compulsivity, in Beyond Condoms: Alternative Approaches to HIV Prevention. Edited by O'Leary A. New York, Kluwer Academic/Plenum, 2002, pp 199–220

Thibaut F, Cordier B, Kuhn JM: Effect of a long-lasting gonadotropin hormone releasing hormone agonist in 6 cases of severe male paraphilia. Acta Psychiatr Scand 87:445–450, 1993

Tost H, Vollmert C, Brassen S, et al: Pedophilia: neuropsychological evidence encouraging a brain network perspective. Med Hypotheses 63:528–531, 2004

Udry JR, Billy JO, Morris NM, et al: Serum androgenic hormones motivate sexual behavior in adolescent boys. Fertil Steril 43:90–94, 1985

Uitti RJ, Tanner CM, Rajput AH, et al: Hypersexuality with antiparkinsonian therapy. Clin Neuropharmacol 12:375–383, 1989

Varela D, Black DW: Pedophilia treated with carbamazepine and clonazepam. Am J Psychiatry 159:1245–1246, 2002

Ward NG: Successful lithium treatment of transvestism associated with manic-depression. J Nerv Ment Dis 161:204–206, 1975

Yoneoka Y, Takeda N, Inoue A, et al: Human Kluver-Bucy syndrome following acute subdural haematoma. Acta Neurochir (Wien) 146:1267–1270, 2004

Zohar J, Kaplan Z, Benjamin J: Compulsive exhibitionism successfully treated with fluvoxamine: a controlled case study. J Clin Psychiatry 55:86–88, 1994

6

Binge Eating

Susan L. McElroy, M.D.

Renu Kotwal, M.D.

History of Binge Eating As a Symptom

In 1959, Stunkard identified binge eating, which he defined as the consumption of an "enormous amount of food" in a relatively short period of time, as a form of pathological overeating in some obese persons. Binge eating, however, was not included in the modern psychiatric nomenclature until 1980, with the publication of DSM-III (American Psychiatric Association 1980), where it was defined as the "rapid consumption of a large amount of food in a discrete period of time, usually less than 2 hours" (p. 70). It was listed as a defining component of bulimia, but not anorexia nervosa, and patients could meet criteria for both diagnoses. In DSM-III-R (American Psychiatric Association 1987), the definition of binge eating was changed in that the suggested

2-hour limit was eliminated. In DSM-IV (American Psychiatric Association 1994), binge eating was more narrowly defined by requiring that the amount of food consumed be "definitely" larger and there be a "sense of lack of control over eating." An episode of binge eating was therefore defined by two core features: 1) eating in a discrete period of time (e.g., within any 2-hour period) an amount of food that is definitely larger than most people would eat during a similar period of time and under similar circumstances, and 2) a sense of lack of control over the eating during the episode. Also in DSM-IV, binge eating remained a defining component of bulimia nervosa and became a modifier for anorexia nervosa, which thus became mutually exclusive diagnoses. In addition, binge eating became a defining component for a new eating disorder— binge eating disorder (BED). BED was given as an example of eating disorders not otherwise specified and included as a provisional diagnosis in the DSM-IV appendix to account for persons who engaged in recurrent, uncontrollable, and distressing binge eating but not the compensatory weight loss behaviors of bulimia or anorexia. Of note, in DSM-IV, the "binge eating" in BED was more narrowly defined than that of bulimia nervosa. In addition to consumption of a definitely large amount of food and subjective loss of control over eating, a BED episode of binge eating also required three of the following five behavioral indicators of loss of control: 1) eating much more rapidly than normal; 2) eating until feeling uncomfortably full; 3) eating large amounts of food when not feeling physically hungry; 4) eating alone because of being embarrassed by how much one is eating; and 5) feeling disgusted with oneself, depressed, or very guilty after overeating.

Although not well studied, binge eating may be characteristic of some conditions other than eating disorders. These include neurological disorders, such as Prader-Willi syndrome, hyperphagic short stature syndrome, and some hypothalamic tumors (e.g., craniopharyngiomas) (Gilmour et al. 2001) as well as the hyperphagia associated with some medications, particularly atypical antipsychotics (Theisen et al. 2003).

Despite the history of binge eating as a symptom, considerable debate remains regarding its validity (e.g., Is it really different from normal or passive overeating?) and its definition (e.g., How much is a definitely large amount of food? What is loss of control?) (Pratt et al. 1998; Williamson and Martin 1999). Nonetheless, preliminary research suggests binge eating can be diagnosed with some reliability, particularly when assessed on multiple occasions with multiple probe questions (Wade et al. 2000). Latent class analytic (Bulik et al. 2000a) and taxometric (Williamson et al. 2002) studies have provided empirical support for conceptualizing anorexia, bulimia, and BED as discrete syndromes. Moreover, mounting evidence suggests that genetic factors contribute to binge eating behavior in general (Bulik et al. 1998) and to bulimia (Bulik et al. 2000b, 2003) and BED (Branson et al. 2003) as disorders.

Classification: Is Binge Eating an Impulse-Control Disorder?

Considerable phenomenological literature suggests binge eating meets both historical and DSM definitions of an impulse-control disorder (ICD). Historically, ICDs have been conditions characterized by the inability to control irresistible impulses to perform senseless or harmful behaviors (McElroy and Arnold 2001). In DSM-IV and DSM-IV-TR (American Psychiatric Association 2000) the core feature of an ICD is similarly defined as "the failure to resist an impulse, drive, or temptation to perform an act that is harmful to the person or others."

The historical and modern literatures provide many descriptions of overeating in response to uncontrollable or irresistible impulses. In his work "Les Obsessions et la Psychasthénie," Janet (1903) presented four patients with probable binge eating who had voracious appetites, ate in secret, felt remorse after eating voraciously, and never felt satiety (Pope et al. 1985). In 1957, Hamburger described a "frequently uncontrollable" and "most malignant" "constant craving for food, especially candy, ice cream, and other sweets" (p. 491) among obese patients. In his report "Bulimia Nervosa: An Ominous Variant of Anorexia Nervosa," Russell (1979) defined binge eating as both the "irresistible" and the "powerful and intractable" "urge to overeat" (pp. 429 and 445, respectively). In 1980, Casper et al. defined bulimia as the "uncontrollable rapid ingestion of large amounts of food over a short period of time, terminated by physical discomfort, social interruption, or sleep" (p. 1031). In an early study describing the phenomenology of 34 women with DSM-III bulimia, Pyle et al. (1981) found that 24 (71%) reported an "uncontrollable appetite." In 1982, Abraham and Beaumont described bulimia as "episodes of ravenous overeating" that patients "felt unable to control" (p. 625).

More recently, Beglin and Fairburn (1992) evaluated 243 young women with the Eating Disorder Examination (EDE) to see what the young women understood the term *binge* to mean. The EDE distinguishes four forms of overeating: objective bulimic episodes, subjective bulimic episodes, episodes of objective overeating, and episodes of subjective overeating. The distinction between the four types of overeating is based on the presence or absence of two features: loss of control during the episode (required for both types of bulimic episodes) and the consumption of a large amount of food (required for objective bulimic episodes and episodes of objective overeating). Although mutually exclusive, persons commonly report overeating episodes of more than one type. Beglin and Fairburn (1992) found that subjects were more likely to classify subjective bulimic episodes than episodes of objective overeating as binges, indicating that they placed greater emphasis on loss of control than on the quantity eaten when determining a binge. In a similar study, Telch et al. (1998) asked 60 obese women who met DSM-IV criteria for BED how they defined a binge. Loss of control over eating was the most common feature used to define binge eating, used by 49 (82%) of the women.

Historical descriptions of ICDs indicate that the irresistible impulses and impulsive behaviors of these disorders are often associated with affective disturbances (McElroy and Arnold 2001; McElroy et al. 1996). Similarly, DSM-IV-TR specifies that for most ICDs, "the individual feels an increasing sense of tension or arousal before committing the act and then experiences pleasure, gratification, or relief at the time of committing the act" (American Psychiatric Association 2000, p. 663); afterward, "there may or may not be regret, self reproach, or guilt" (p. 663). Many persons with binge eating similarly describe tension, arousal, or other negative affects with the impulses to binge; relief that may be pleasurable with the act of binge eating; and depressive affects, particularly self-reproach, guilt, or disgust, after the act of binge eating. For example, when Stunkard first described binge eating in 1959, he said it had "an orgiastic quality" and was followed by "severe discomfort and expressions of self-condemnation" (Stunkard 1959). In their study of 34 patients with DSM-III bulimia, Pyle et al. (1981) noted that 24 (71%) reported feeling unhappy prior to binge eating. After binge eating, 29 (85%) reported feeling guilty and 23 (68%) reported feeling worried. In a follow-up study of 275 patients with bulimia by the same investigators (Mitchell et al. 1985), patients were asked to give reasons for their binge eating. The most common reasons were "feel tense, anxious" (83.3%); "crave certain foods" (70.2%); and "unhappy" (67.3%). The feelings described after binge eating were mostly negative: "guilt" (86.5%); "too full" (64.4%); and "worried." Abraham and Beaumont (1982) systematically evaluated the mood disturbances of 32 patients with binge eating. All (100%) said they felt anxious and tense before a binge, and 80% described physical symptoms of anxiety, such as palpitations, tremulousness, and sweating. Thirty-four percent of patients described relief of anxiety during binge eating, and 66% described absence of anxiety after the binge had concluded. In addition, 72% of the patients described relief of "negative mood" during binge eating. Despite the high rates of anxiety and negative mood, all patients described pleasure while bingeing, especially early in the binge. Arnow et al. (1992) similarly evaluated the thoughts and feelings that proceeded, accompanied, and followed binge eating in 19 obese subjects with nonpurging bulimia nervosa. Most subjects (63%) reported that binges typically began with a mood change. All 19 subjects reported negative emotions both before and after bingeing. During a binge, 42% of subjects reported positive emotions, 37% reported negative emotions, and 21% reported no emotions.

In sum, these and other studies suggest that negative affective states tend to occur before binge eating and that the act of bingeing may reduce these negative affective states and possibly induce pleasurable states, but be associated with the induction of other negative affective states. Our group (McElroy et al. 1996) and others (Perugi and Akiskal 2002) have written about how such affective dysregulation has a bipolar quality (McElroy et al. 1996). Indeed, Greenberg and Harvey (1987) found that the interaction between dietary restraint and affective lability, defined as biphasic mood shifts as assessed by the General Behavior Inventory (which identifies persons at risk for bipolar disorder), was a better predictor of the severity of binge eating than the interaction between dietary restraint and depressed mood. Binge eating therefore resembles an ICD in that it is characterized by similarly impaired affect regulation: dysphoria that often has an anxious component occurs with the urge to binge, relief of dysphoria that may be mood elevating occurs with the act of bingeing, and dysphoria that often has a depressive component occurs after the act of bingeing.

Another way binge eating resembles an ICD is in its frequent association with poor insight, denial, or ego-syntonicity (McElroy et al. 1993, 1996).

People who binge eat often do not seek treatment for binge eating per se (Whitaker et al. 1990; Wittchen et al. 1998) or even admit to binge eating upon direct questioning (le Grange et al. 2001). Rather, if they seek treatment, they often do so for the complications of binge eating—most commonly, weight problems and complications of compensatory weight loss behaviors (Dingemans et al. 2002; Mehler 2003; Whitaker et al. 1990). Indeed, although some people find their binge eating extremely distressing, others are not aware that they binge eat. For example, le Grange et al. (2001) evaluated the eating behavior of 42 overweight or obese women with or without BED (as established by clinical interview) using Ecological Momentary Assessment (EMA). EMA assesses individuals at various points throughout the day in their natural environment, thereby reducing recall bias. When binge eating was assessed in these women via EMA, le Grange et al. (2001) found no difference in mean binge frequency between the two groups, in that the group without BED binged just as frequently as the group with BED. Similarly, in a recent factor-analytic study of eating disorder symptoms, obese patients without an eating disorder diagnosis still had significantly higher scores on a binge eating factor than normal-weight control subjects (Williamson et al. 2002).

These observations are consistent with a growing number of studies revealing that patients (Crow et al. 2002; Striegel-Moore et al. 2000) and persons from the community (Kendler et al. 1991; Striegel-Moore et al. 2000; Woodside et al. 2001) with partial syndromes of bulimia and BED have more similarities than differences with patients and persons with full syndromes. Moreover, in community studies, persons with partial syndromes are more similar to those with full syndromes than to those without syndromes (Kendler et al. 1991; Woodside et al. 2001). Thus, there may be a continuum of pathological overeating, with infrequent impulsive and/or compulsive overeating representing the milder end and recurrent DSM-IV-TR binge eating the more severe end. Alternatively, binge eating may exist on a continuum with normal eating, with "passive overeating" representing the least severe form, impulsive and/or compulsive overeating representing an intermediate form, and recurrent DSM-IV-TR binge eating representing the most severe form. Of note, other ICDs such as kleptomania and pathological gambling have been hypothesized to exist along similar severity continua (McElroy et al. 1991a).

Epidemiology

The prevalence of binge eating depends on how broadly or narrowly it is defined. Rates of broadly defined binge eating have ranged from 7.3% (Vollrath et al. 1992) to 20.9% (Cooper and Fairburn 1983) in adult women and from 0% (Vollrath et al. 1992) to 7.8% (Garfinkel et al. 1995) in adult men. Rates of bulimia nervosa have ranged from 1.1% (Garfinkel et al. 1995) to 2.1% (Striegel-Moore et al. 2003) in adult females and have been approximately 0.1% (Garfinkel et al. 1995) in adult males. Rates of BED have ranged from 1.0% (Hay and Fairburn 1998) to 4.6% (Spitzer et al. 1993) in general adult population samples, with rates in females ranging from 2.1% (Striegel-Moore et al. 2003) to 5.3% (Spitzer et al. 1993) and rates in males ranging from 0.8% (D.E. Smith et al. 1998) to 3.1% (Spitzer et al. 1993). Binge eating is also a problem among children and adolescents. A study in 15-year-old students from Norway found a current prevalence rate of 0.4% for girls and 0% for boys for anorexia nervosa, bulimic subtype; 1.1% for girls and 0% for boys for bulimia nervosa; and 1.5% for girls and 0% for boys for BED (Rosenvinge et al. 1999). No cases with current anorexia, restricting subtype were identified. In a recent study of different types of overeating in 4,746 girls and boys from the community (Ackard et al. 2003), 17.3% of girls and 7.8% of boys reported some form of overeating. Specifically, 6.3% of girls and 4.5% of boys described overeating alone; 7.9% of girls and 2.4% of boys described binge eating; and 3.1% of girls and 0.9% of boys met criteria for binge eating syndrome.

Course

In both clinical and community samples, the course of binge eating in bulimia nervosa and BED is variable (Cachelin et al. 1999; Fairburn et al. 2000; Keel and Mitchell 1997), with higher recovery rates possibly seen for BED than for bulimia (Fairburn et al. 2000). Fairburn et al. (2000) compared two community-based cohorts prospectively over a 5-year period—102 persons with bulimia nervosa and 48 with BED. At 5-year follow-up, 51% of the bulimia group had a clinical eating disorder of some form compared with 18% of the BED group.

General Medical Comorbidity

The medical complications of the dieting and starvation of anorexia nervosa and the inappropriate compensatory behaviors of bulimia nervosa are well known (Becker et al. 1999; Mehler 2003). However, binge eating itself is associated with significant medical morbidity. Thus, binge eating is associated with upper and lower gastrointestinal symptoms (Crowell et al. 1994), irritable bowel syndrome (Crowell et al. 1994), and overweight and obesity (Black et al. 1992; Britz et al. 2000; Dingemans et al. 2002). Community studies have found that BED co-occurs with obesity in adults (Cachelin et al. 1999; Fairburn et al. 2000; D. E. Smith et al. 1998) and that both bulimia and BED in young women are associated with childhood obesity (Fairburn et al. 1997, 1998). Clinical studies have shown that patients seeking treatment for BED are often obese (Dingemans et al. 2002; Williamson and Martin 1999). Conversely, it has been estimated that up to 82% of obese persons seeking weight loss treatment report some degree of binge eating behavior (Marcus et al. 1985), with DSM-IV-TR BED occurring in up to approximately 30% of patients in weight control programs (Spitzer et al. 1992, 1993), 70% of persons in Overeaters Anonymous (Spitzer et al. 1992), and up to 50% of patients seeking bariatric surgery (Adami et al. 1995). Moreover, among obese patients, the presence or severity of binge eating may be related to the severity of obesity. Thus, compared with obese patients without binge eating, those with binge eating have higher body weight and/or body mass index (Adami et al. 1995; Marcus et al. 1985; Yanovski et al. 1993) and an earlier age at onset of obesity and dieting (Spitzer et al. 1992, 1993). In addition, relatively high rates of BED have been found in patients with type 2 diabetes (Crow et al. 2001).

Associated Psychopathology

A growing body of literature suggests binge eating is associated with features of impulsivity beyond those stipulated in the historical or DSM-IV-TR definitions of an ICD. In other words, binge eating, like other ICDs, is associated with other impulsive behaviors and traits, characterized by a lack of deliberation and a failure to consider risks and consequences before acting. Thus,

Casper et al. (1980) compared 49 hospitalized female patients with anorexia and bulimia with 56 patients with anorexia alone. Patients with both disorders were more likely to report a strong appetite, to be outgoing during childhood, and to report kleptomania than were those with anorexia alone. Lacey and Evans (1986) evaluated 112 consecutive eating disorder patients and found that 41% had a history of theft, 28% had abused drugs, and 26% had abused alcohol. They concluded that a subset of patients with eating disorders had diffuse problems with impulsivity and suggested these patients be viewed as having a "multi-impulsive personality disorder."

Other studies have since consistently found high rates of impulsive behaviors and/or high measures of impulsivity in patients with binge eating. Fahy and Eisler (1993) compared 37 patients with bulimia nervosa and 29 patients with anorexia nervosa (only four of whom had binge eating) regarding impulsive behaviors other than binge eating and degree of impulsivity as measured by the Impulsiveness Questionnaire. Compared with the anorexia patients, significantly more bulimia patients reported at least one impulsive behavior in addition to binge eating (51% vs. 28%) and had significantly higher impulsivity scores on the questionnaire. There were no differences, however, between bulimia patients with high versus those with low scores. Newton et al. (1993) compared 58 normal-weight female outpatients with bulimia and 27 normal-weight control subjects on frequency of impulsive behaviors and measures of impulsivity. The bulimia patients showed a significantly higher number of impulsive behaviors and a significantly higher total score on the Barratt Impulsiveness Scale (BIS). Moreover, the BIS score correlated with the number of impulsive behaviors ($r=0.32$, $P<0.05$). Wiederman and Pryor (1996) evaluated 217 adult women with DSM-III-R bulimia nervosa for impulsive behaviors and found that 40 (18.4%) reported at least three of the following four impulsive behaviors: drug abuse, stealing, self-injury, and attempted suicide. Nagata et al. (2000) evaluated "multi-impulsivity" in Japanese patients with anorexia nervosa, restricting type ($n=60$); anorexia nervosa, binge-eating/purging type ($n=62$); bulimia nervosa, purging type ($n=114$); and control subjects ($n=66$). Multi-impulsivity (defined by three of the following: heavy regular alcohol use, a suicide attempt, self-mutilation, repeated shoplifting of items other than food, and sexual disinhibition) was significantly more common in bulimia patients (18%) than in binge/purge anorexia patients (11%); patients with anorexia nervosa, restricting type

(2%); and control subjects (2%). In a community study of overeating among adolescents, Ackard et al. (2003) found that 28.6% of girls and 27.8% of boys who met criteria for binge eating syndrome reported that they had attempted suicide. Finally, Fischer et al. (2003) evaluated the relationship among bulimic symptoms and two types of impulsivity: 1) lack of planning (inability to delay action to think of the consequences) and 2) urgency (the tendency to act rashly in the face of negative emotion). Impulsivity and eating disorder scales were administered to two groups of undergraduate women. In both groups, urgency, but not lack of planning, was positively correlated with bulimic symptoms.

In sum, when compared with control subjects and patients with anorexia nervosa, patients with bulimia nervosa and persons from the community with bulimia and BED appear to have higher rates of impulsive behaviors (other than binge eating) and higher ratings of impulsivity. However, when persons with bulimia with high impulsivity are compared with those with low impulsivity, the results are inconsistent; some studies suggest the two groups have comparable eating disorder severity (Fahy and Eisler 1993; Fichter et al. 1994; Nagata et al. 2000; Wiederman and Pryor 1996), and others suggest that high impulsivity is associated with greater eating disorder severity (Newton et al. 1993), greater related psychopathology (Fichter et al. 1994), or poorer outcome (Sohlberg et al. 1989).

Another way in which binge eating resembles an ICD is that it is associated with features of compulsivity as well as impulsivity (Favaro and Santonastaso 1998; McElroy et al. 1993). When Casper et al. (1980) compared 49 patients with anorexia and bulimia with 56 patients with anorexia alone and found that the bulimic patients had more impulsive features, they also found that the bulimic patients had significantly higher scores measuring obsession related to food, somatization, anxiety, and depression. When Newton et al. (1993) compared 58 patients with bulimia with control subjects on measures of impulsivity and other aspects of psychopathology, both the BIS score and the number of impulsive behaviors correlated with measures of bulimia, depression, and obsessionality.

Similarly, deZwaan et al. (1995) compared obese patients with BED ($n=83$) and without BED ($n=99$) using the Eating Disorder Inventory (EDI), the Multidimensional Personality Questionnaire (MPQ), and the Three Factor Eating Questionnaire (TFEQ). The patients with BED showed greater impulsivity on the MPQ and greater disinhibition over eating on the TFEQ as well as greater perfectionism on the EDI. Paul et al. (2002) evaluated the lifetime rate and phenomenology of self-injurious behavior in 376 inpatient women with eating disorders (119 with anorexia, 137 with bulimia, and 120 with eating disorder not otherwise specified) using the Traumatic Life Events Questionnaire, the Dissociative Impulsiveness Scale, and the Yale-Brown Obsessive-Compulsive Scale. The lifetime rate of self-injurious behavior was 34.6%. Although patients with eating disorder not otherwise specified (35.8%) and bulimia nervosa (34.3%) had higher rates of self-injurious behavior than those with anorexia nervosa (rate not reported), the differences were not statistically significant. Patients with bulimia, however, had significantly higher impulsivity scores. Also, patients with self-injury showed significantly greater cognitive impulsivity as well as more obsessive-compulsive thoughts and behaviors than did patients without self-injury.

Further supporting a relationship between binge eating and ICDs are a number of studies finding apparently elevated rates of ICDs in patients with binge eating. Specifically, several studies have reported high rates of kleptomania in patients with eating disorders, ranging from 4% in anorexia nervosa alone (Casper et al. 1980) to 44% in anorexia and bulimia nervosa together (Hudson et al. 1983) to 75% in bulimia nervosa alone (Gerlinghoff and Backmund 1987). More recently, Keel et al. (2000) evaluated 173 women with bulimia at 10-year follow-up with the Structured Clinical Interview for DSM-IV and found that 11 (6.4%) met DSM-IV criteria for an ICD within the previous month. The outcome of bulimia was significantly related to the presence of ICDs (and to mood and substance use disorders) but not to the presence of anxiety disorders: nine (17.3%) patients with active bulimia nervosa symptoms had ICDs as compared with two (1.7%) patients whose bulimia symptoms had remitted.

Conversely, high rates of binge eating have been found in patients with ICDs. For example, 12 (60%) of 20 patients with kleptomania evaluated by our group met lifetime DSM-III-R criteria for bulimia (McElroy et al. 1991b). Similarly, 6 (22%) of 27 subjects (including 20 males) with intermittent explosive disorder also evaluated by our group met lifetime DSM-IV criteria for BED ($n=6$), with ($n=3$) or without ($n=3$) bulimia (McElroy et al. 1998).

Several lines of evidence also link binge eating, like other ICDs (McElroy and Arnold 2001; McElroy et al. 1996), with mood, anxiety, and substance use symptoms and disorders (Holderness et al. 1994; Mitchell and Mussell 1995). First, binge eating behavior (Ackard et al. 2003; Angst et al. 2002; Vollrath et al. 1992), bulimia nervosa (Garfinkel et al. 1995; Kendler et al. 1991; Woodside et al. 2001), and BED (Ackard et al. 2003; D.E. Smith et al. 1998) have all been found to be significantly associated with depressive symptoms and/or depressive disorders in community samples. Binge eating behavior has been associated with hypomania, anxiety disorders, and substance abuse in one community sample (Angst 1998). In addition, bulimia has been associated with anxiety and substance use disorders in community samples (Dansky et al. 2000; Garfinkel et al. 1995). For example, studies of obese persons from the community have shown that those with binge eating (Bulik et al. 2002) or BED (Yanovski et al. 1993) have significantly higher rates of mood, anxiety, and substance use disorders compared with obese persons without binge eating or BED. Second, clinical studies have found high rates of mood, anxiety, and substance use disorders in bulimia nervosa and BED patients (Bellodi et al. 2001; Bushnell et al. 1994; Hudson et al. 1987; Keel et al. 2000; McElroy et al. 2000; Mitchell and Mussell 1995). For example, at least four studies comparing mood pathology in obese patients presenting for weight management with and without binge eating found that the patients with binge eating had higher levels of depressive symptoms and/or disorders than those without binge eating (Hudson et al. 1988; Marcus et al. 1990; Prather and Williamson 1988; Specker et al. 1994). Third, clinical studies have found relatively high rates of bulimia and BED in patients with mood disorder, especially those with bipolar disorder (Krüger et al. 1996; McElroy et al. 2002). Indeed, we and others have hypothesized that binge eating, like other ICDs, may have a relationship with mood disorder in general, and bipolar disorder in particular (McElroy et al. 1996; Perugi and Akiskal 2002).

Yet another possible comorbidity similarity between binge eating and ICDs is their co-occurrence with Axis II disorders. Both bulimia nervosa and BED on the one hand, and various ICDs on the other, have been reported to co-occur with personality disorders with impulsive features. For example, a series of systematic studies using structured interviews showed that approximately one-fourth to one-third of patients with bulimia met criteria for a Cluster B personality disorder (Braun et al. 1994; Skodol et al. 1993; Steiger et al. 1994). In a controlled study, patients with bulimia had significantly higher rates of Cluster B personality disorders than control subjects (Lilenfeld et al. 1998). More recently, Westen and Harnden-Fischer (2001) used Q-sort and cluster-analytic procedures to assess personality profiles of eating disorder patients provided by clinicians. Three categories emerged: a high-functioning/perfectionistic group, a constricted/overcontrolled group, and an emotionally dysregulated/undercontrolled group. All patients classified as emotionally dysregulated/undercontrolled had bulimic symptoms; no member of this category had anorexia nervosa alone.

Family History

Substantial family history data indicate binge eating is familial. Thus, many family history studies have found elevated rates of bulimia nervosa and other eating disorders in the first-degree relatives of probands with bulimia (Kassett et al. 1989; Keck et al. 1990; Lilenfeld et al. 1998). A preliminary study found that relatives of obese probands with BED had almost twice the prevalence of BED as did relatives of non-BED obese probands (Lee et al. 1999). Regarding the coaggregation of BED with other eating disorders, one study found that the prevalence of BED in relatives of probands with bulimia or anorexia was 2.6 times the prevalence among relatives of control probands (Lilenfeld et al. 1998), and another study found a significantly higher prevalence of a parental history of bulimia or anorexia among individuals with BED versus those without BED (Fairburn et al. 1998).

Twin studies of bulimia nervosa suggest that a substantial portion of this familiality is due to genetic factors (Bulik et al. 1998, 2000b). Studies based on the Virginia Twin Registry estimated the heritability of broadly defined bulimia nervosa to be approximately 55% (Kendler et al. 1991). In a subsequent two-part interview study of 1,897 female twins from this same registry (including both members of 854 twin pairs), Bulik et al. (2000b) estimated that the heritability of binge eating was 50% and that of broadly defined bulimia was 60%. By combining information from the two interviews, the estimated heritability of the latent vulnerability to binge eating was 82% and that of broadly defined bulimia was 83%. Of note, the reliability of a lifetime history of binge eating ($\kappa = 34$) and of broadly defined bulimia nervosa ($\kappa = 28$) was low. Bulik et al. (1998) concluded that binge eating and broadly defined bulimia nervosa were highly heritable conditions of low reliability.

In the only study of ICDs in family members of persons with binge eating we found, Hudson et al. (1983) reported that 6 (1.4%) of 420 first-degree relatives of 14 patients with anorexia, 55 patients with bulimia, and 20 patients with both disorders had an ICD. Controlled studies have shown that patients with bulimia nervosa (Hudson et al. 1987, 2001; Kasset et al. 1989; Lilenfeld et al. 1998) and BED (Fairburn et al. 1998; Hudson et al. 1998; Lee et al. 1999; Yanovski et al. 1993) have elevated lifetime prevalence rates of mood and substance use disorders in their first-degree relatives. In one study, bulimia was associated with increased familiality of major depression (Kendler et al. 1996). Controlled studies have also found that patients with bulimia have elevated familial rates of obsessive-compulsive and tic disorders (Bellodi et al. 2001; Lilenfeld et al. 1998).

Family history studies examining cross-transmission of eating disorders with other psychiatric disorders have been mixed. Some have found evidence for independent transmission between bulimia and both substance use and mood disorders (Lilenfeld et al. 1998), whereas others have found evidence for familial coaggregation of eating and mood disorders of a magnitude similar to that of the familial aggregation of mood disorders (Hudson et al. 2001, 2003).

Although the familial psychopathology of ICDs has been far less extensively studied than that of binge eating, preliminary findings suggest some ICDs are also associated with elevated familial rates of mood and substance use disorders (McElroy et al. 1991b, 1996). The familial coaggregation of ICDs with conditions with binge eating has been virtually unexamined.

Neurobiology

Laboratory studies have shown that clinically defined binge eating is associated with objective overeating (Mitchell et al. 1998). Thus, in the laboratory setting, subjects with bulimia nervosa have been shown to eat more when allowed or encouraged to binge eat as compared with control subjects (Hadigan et al. 1992; Kaye et al. 1992). Also in the laboratory setting, obese subjects with BED have been shown to consume significantly more calories when instructed to binge eat as compared with obese subjects without BED (Goldfein et al. 1993; Yanovski et al. 1992).

Biological abnormalities reported in binge eating that have been reported in other ICDs include hypothalamic-pituitary-adrenal (HPA) axis abnormalities and indications of dysfunction of the central serotonin system (Kaye and Strober 1999). Thus, hypercortisolemia and elevated urinary levels of free cortisol have been found in normal-weight patients with bulimia (Mortola et al. 1989). Relatively high rates of dexamethasone nonsuppression have also been reported in bulimia; nonsuppression, however, was associated with low body weight and a history of anorexia (Neudeck et al. 2001).

Regarding central serotonergic function, an initial report found that weight-restored patients with anorexia nervosa and persistent bulimic symptoms had lower probenecid-induced cerebrospinal fluid 5-hydroxyindoleacetic acid (CSF 5-HIAA) accumulation compared with those without bulimic symptoms (Kaye et al. 1984). Subsequent studies in normal-weight patients with bulimia found normal levels of CSF 5-HIAA compared with control subjects, with low levels found in a subset of patients with high binge frequencies (Jimmerson et al. 1992). Other abnormalities reported in bulimia nervosa include blunted prolactin and net cortisol response to *m*-chlorophenylpiperazine (Levitan et al. 1997) and blunted prolactin response to fenfluramine (Jimerson et al. 1992), suggesting impaired central nervous system serotonergic responsiveness.

In the only study that examined an index of central (hypothalamic) serotonergic function in patients with anorexia, bulimia, and BED, a significantly decreased prolactin response to *d*-fenfluramine (suggesting reduced serotonergic activity) was found in underweight women with anorexia and in women with high-frequency bingeing and bulimia but not in women with low-frequency bingeing and bulimia or those with BED (Monteleone et al. 2000). However, in the same study, patients with bulimia and BED had low plasma prolactin levels, as found in other studies of women with bulimia (Jimerson et al. 1997).

Several studies have found that central serotonergic abnormalities persist in persons who have recovered from bulimia. These abnormalities have included increased CSF 5-HIAA concentrations (with normal levels of CSF homovanillic acid and methoxyhydroxyphenylglycol) (Kaye et al. 1998), altered serotonin-2A receptor activity (Kaye et al. 2001a), and the induction of subjective loss of control over eating, binge eating, and depressive symptoms following acute trytophan depletion (K.A. Smith et al. 1999). These findings have led some authorities to conclude that a disturbance of central serotonergic function in bulimia nervosa is trait related and contributes to its pathophysiology (Kaye et al. 1998, 2001a).

Of note, neurobiological differences beyond those relating to the HPA axis and serotonergic function have been described between both anorexic and obese women with and without binge eating. In a single photon emission computed tomography examination study that investigated the effect of imagining food on regional cerebral blood flow (rCBF) in patients with anorexia with and without "habitual binge/purge behavior" and healthy control subjects, only those patients with anorexia and binge/purge behavior showed significant increases in the rCBF of the right cortices after imagining food (Narvo et al. 2000). In another neuroimaging study, obese binge-eating women were found to have different changes in cerebral blood flow when exposed to food (higher rCBF in right parietal and temporal cortices) as compared with both obese and normal-weight women who did not binge eat (Karhunen et al. 2000). In a study of continuous CSF sampling, an obese woman with chronic binge eating was shown to have no rise in postprandial CSF glucose concentrations as compared with four control women, leading the authors to hypothesize that binge eating may be associated with defective glucose transport across the blood–brain barrier (Geracioti et al. 1995). In addition, using positron emission tomography, Wang et al. (2003) showed that 10 severely obese subjects had reductions in striatal dopamine D_2 receptors compared with control subjects as well as an inverse relationship between body mass index and dopamine D_2 receptor availability. Although the authors did not mention whether their subjects were binge eaters, they noted that the pathological overeating of obesity resembled pathological gambling and drug addiction and that drug addiction was also characterized by reduced dopamine D_2 receptors (Wang et al. 2001, 2003).

Genetic research has suggested potential candidate genes or chromosomal loci for binge eating. Bulik et al. (2003) found evidence of significant linkage on chromosome 10p in families with bulimia nervosa. Branson et al. (2003) compared 24 severely obese subjects who had melanocortin 4 receptor (*MC4R*) gene mutations with 120 obese subjects without an *MC4R* mutation matched for age, sex, and body mass index. Alpha melanocyte-stimulating hormone acts on MC4R to decrease food intake, and mice and humans with *MC4R* mutations have obesity, hyperphagia, and hyperinsulinemia (Farooqui et al.

2003). All of the *MC4R* gene mutation carriers reported binge eating compared with 14.2% of the obese subjects without mutations ($P<0.001$) and none of the normal-weight subjects without mutations. By contrast, the prevalence of binge eating was similar among carriers and noncarriers of mutations in the leptin-binding domain of the leptin receptor gene.

Treatment Response

The binge eating of bulimia nervosa and BED, like other ICDs (McElroy and Arnold 2001), appears to respond to a variety of psychological and pharmacological treatments. Less is known about the treatment response of binge eating associated with anorexia nervosa and other conditions.

Psychotherapy

Controlled studies have found cognitive-behavioral therapy (CBT) and interpersonal therapy (IPT) to be effective in decreasing binge eating in bulimia nervosa (Agras et al. 1992, 2000; Fairburn and Harrison 2003; Fairburn et al. 1991, 1995) and BED (Agras 2001; Wilfley et al. 2002; Wonderlich et al. 2003), with some evidence of long-term effectiveness for both treatments (Fairburn et al. 1995; Wilfley et al. 2002). Several studies also suggest that self-help manuals, used either alone or with guidance from a therapist, may benefit some patients with bulimia and BED (J.C. Carter et al. 2003; Palmer et al. 2002; Wonderlich et al. 2003). All of these treatments have been shown to be effective in reducing the compensatory weight loss behaviors of bulimia and the associated psychopathology of both bulimia and BED. However, they have been less effective in inducing significant weight loss in BED. By contrast, both the binge eating and overweight of BED may respond to behavioral weight management over the short term (Wonderlich et al. 2003).

Unlike many other ICDs, various psychotherapies have been compared in the treatment of binge eating (Peterson and Mitchell 1999; Whittal et al. 1999). Thus, CBT and IPT have been shown to be comparable in some studies in the treatment of bulimia (Fairburn et al. 1991, 1995) and BED (Wilfley et al. 2002), whereas CBT has been shown to be more effective than behavior therapy, stress reduction, nondirective psychotherapy, focal psychotherapy, and psychodynamic psychotherapy in bulimia (Fairburn et al. 1995; Walsh et al. 1997; Whittal et al. 1999). One multicenter comparison, however, in 220 patients with DSM-III-R bulimia nervosa found CBT superior to IPT after 20 weeks and after 1-year follow-up (Agras et al. 2000). The authors concluded that CBT should be the preferred psychological treatment for bulimia. Although similar comparative data are lacking, preliminary findings suggest that other ICDs may respond better to cognitive-behavioral than to interpersonal psychological treatments (McElroy and Arnold 2001).

Pharmacotherapy

The binge eating of both bulimia nervosa and BED has been reported to respond to various centrally active agents. These include many antidepressants, several centrally active anti-obesity drugs (including two stimulants), several anticonvulsant agents, opiate antagonists, and some novel agents (W. P. Carter et al. 2003; Krüger and Kennedy 2000; Zhu and Walsh 2002). The binge eating of bulimia nervosa has also been reported to respond to lithium, although results of studies are mixed (Hsu et al. 1991; Shisslak et al. 1991).

Regarding antidepressants, the binge eating of both bulimia and BED has been shown to respond to tricyclic antidepressants and selective serotonin reuptake inhibitors (SSRIs) in double-blind, placebo-controlled trials (W. P. Carter et al. 2003; Hudson et al. 1999). The binge eating of bulimia nervosa has also been shown to respond to bupropion (Horne et al. 1988), trazodone (Pope et al. 1989), and phenelzine (Walsh et al. 1988) in double-blind, placebo-controlled trials. In the bulimia trials, purging behavior significantly improved with all antidepressants. In the fluoxetine trials of bulimia, 60 mg was superior to 20 mg in reducing binge eating (and purging) (Fluoxetine Bulimia Nervosa Collaborative Study Group 1992). Also, fluoxetine has been shown to have long-term (up to 52 weeks) efficacy in bulimia (Goldstein et al. 1995; Romano et al. 2002) and to be superior to placebo in bulimia nonresponsive to psychotherapy (Walsh et al. 2000) in controlled trials. In the BED trials, therapeutic weight loss occurred with SSRIs (Arnold et al. 2002; Hudson et al. 1998; McElroy et al. 2000, 2003a), but not with desipramine (McCann and Agras 1990). However, the SSRI trials in BED were only short term (6–9 weeks), and it is therefore unknown whether the antibingeing and weight loss effects of these agents would generalize to longer periods of treatment (W. P. Carter et al. 2003). Regarding other antidepressants in binge eating, a retrospective chart review of 35 patients seeking weight management suggested that the selective serotonin–norepinephrine reuptake inhibitor venlafaxine may reduce binge eating, induce therapeutic weight loss, and improve depressive mood in BED associated with overweight and obesity (Malhotra et al. 2002). Presently, fluoxetine is the only drug approved by the U.S. Food and Drug Administration for binge eating; specifically, it is indicated for the treatment of "binge eating and vomiting behaviors in patients with moderate to severe bulimia nervosa."

Centrally active antiobesity agents (and/or stimulants) reported effective in binge eating include the serotonin-releasing agent *d*-fenfluramine (which has been removed from the market because of safety concerns), the selective serotonin–norepinephrine reuptake inhibitor sibutramine, and the stimulants methylphenidate and *d*-amphetamine. Two controlled studies showed fenfluramine reduced binge eating in bulimia (Blouin et al. 1988) and in BED associated with obesity (Stunkard et al. 1996). In the BED study, however, fenfluramine was not associated with significant weight loss, and by 4 months of treatment, there was no longer a difference between drug and placebo regarding binge frequency. Also, two small placebo-controlled studies of *d*-fenfluramine in bulimia were negative (Fahy et al. 1993; Russell et al. 1988). Two controlled studies have shown sibutramine decreases binge eating in BED (Appolinario et al. 2003; Mitchell et al. 2003); one of these studies suggested the drug also induces therapeutic weight loss and reduces depressive symptoms (Appolinario et al. 2003). The stimulant *d*-amphetamine has been reported to reduce binge eating in patients with bulimia in one controlled study (Ong et al. 1983). Methylphenidate has been reported to reduce binge eating and purging in isolated cases of bulimia (Schweickert et al. 1997; Sokol et al. 1999).

Antiepileptic agents evaluated in binge eating include phenytoin, carbamazepine, topiramate, and zonisamide. Studies have been mixed for phenytoin (reviewed in Hudson and Pope 1988). Early positive open-label reports of phenytoin in patients with compulsive eating binges (Green and Rau 1974; Hudson and Pope 1988) were followed by two small double-blind, placebo-controlled crossover trials. The first ($N=4$) was negative (Greenway et al. 1977) and the second ($N=19$) was marginally positive (Wermuth et al. 1977). There is a small negative controlled study of carbamazepine ($N=6$) in bulimia (Kaplan et al. 1983), and a small positive open study ($N=15$) of zonisamide in BED (McElroy et al. 2004). Two randomized, double-blind trials have shown that topiramate is superior to placebo in reducing binge eating. In a 10-week trial in 69 outpatients with bulimia, topiramate (median dosage, 100 mg/day) significantly reduced the frequency of binge and purge days (days during which at least one binge eating or purging episode, respectively, occurred; Hoopes et al. 2003). Topiramate was also associated with significant improvement in EDI subscales of bulimia/uncontrollable overeating, body dissatisfaction, and drive for thinness; Eating Attitudes Test total scores and subscales of bulimia/food preoccupation and dieting; and Hamilton Rating Scale for Anxiety scores. In a 14-week trial in 61 outpatients with BED and obesity, topiramate (median dosage, 212 mg/day) significantly reduced the frequency of binge eating episodes, number of binge days, body mass indices, and weight (5.9 kg for topiramate versus 1.2 kg for placebo; McElroy et al. 2003b). Topiramate was also associated with significant improvement in obsessive-compulsive symptoms related to binge eating.

Studies of opiate antagonists in binge eating have been mixed, with a failed controlled trial of naltrexone (100–150 mg/day) in bulimia and binge eating with obesity (Alger et al. 1991), a small negative trial of low-dosage naltrexone (50 mg/day) in bulimia (Mitchell et al. 1989), a small positive controlled trial of naloxone in bulimia (Mitchell et al. 1986), several small positive case reports of high-dosage naltrexone (200–300 mg/day) in bulimia (Jonas and Gold 1988), and two positive case reports of naltrexone in BED. The latter were a positive on-off-on case of monotherapy (200 and 400 mg/day) (Marrazzi et al. 1995) and a case of successful fluoxetine augmentation (100 mg/day) (Neumeister et al. 1999). Taken together, these results have led some authorities to suggest that binge eating may respond only to naltrexone dosages greater than those needed to block exogenous opiates (Jonas and Gold 1988).

Lithium has been reported effective in cases of bulimia nervosa with comorbid bipolar disorder (Shisslak et al. 1991) as well as in an open trial in 12 of 14 women with bulimia (Hsu 1984). A subsequent placebo-controlled trial in 91 female patients with bulimia without bipolar disorder showed lithium (mean level, 0.62 mEq/L) was not superior to placebo in decreasing binge eating episodes, except possibly in depressed patients (Hsu et al. 1991). However, nondepressed patients receiving placebo showed just as significant a reduction in binge eating as did nondepressed patients receiving lithium, making this study difficult to interpret.

Novel agents reported effective in binge eating include ondansetron, a

5-HT$_3$ antagonist, in a double-blind, placebo-controlled trial in 29 females with bulimia (Faris et al. 2000) and ipsapirone, a 5-HT$_{1A}$ antagonist, in an open-label trial in 17 patients with bulimia (Geretsegger et al. 1995).

The binge eating of anorexia nervosa has been largely unstudied in psychotherapeutic and pharmacological treatment studies, where the focus has been on weight restoration and/or weight maintenance (Zhu and Walsh 2002). However, in one study, weight-restored patients with anorexia without binge eating maintained their weight to a significantly greater degree with fluoxetine than with placebo (Kaye et al. 2001b). The self-injurious behavior, but not the binge eating, associated with Prader-Willi syndrome has been reported to respond to topiramate (Shapira et al. 2002). Finally, the binge eating of obese BED patients has been reported to respond to bariatric surgery, especially Roux-en-Y gastric bypass, though studies are mixed as to whether binge eating is associated with less favorable response of obesity to surgery (Hsu et al 1996; Mitchell et al. 2001).

Combination Therapy

Five studies have compared CBT with antidepressant medication in the treatment of bulimia. Four studies used a single antidepressant (desipramine, imipramine, or fluoxetine; Agras et al. 1992; Goldbloom et al. 1997; Leitenberg et al. 1994; Mitchell et al. 1990) and the fifth study used two antidepressants sequentially (desipramine followed by fluoxetine if desipramine failed; Walsh et al. 1997). Also, three studies compared CBT alone, an antidepressant alone, and the combination of CBT and an antidepressant (Agras et al. 1992; Goldbloom et al. 1997; Leitenberg et al. 1994), whereas two studies compared CBT plus placebo, an antidepressant alone, a placebo alone, and the combination of CBT and an antidepressant (Mitchell et al. 1990; Walsh et al. 1997). Each study found that CBT alone or CBT plus placebo was superior to an antidepressant alone and not significantly different from the combination in reducing binge and/or purge behavior. These findings have led some authorities to conclude that CBT is more effective than antidepressants for binge eating (Whittal et al. 1999). However, others have noted that the methodological limitations of these studies, including inadequate blinding of CBT and small sample sizes, make such conclusions premature (W. P. Carter et al. 2003). Nonetheless, a meta-analysis of these studies suggested that the combination of CBT and antidepressant medication may be more effective than either treatment alone (Whittal et al. 1999). Similarly, a review of data from seven trials involving a total of 600 patients to assess the effect of CBT plus antidepressants as compared with the effect of either treatment alone reported average remission rates of 42%–49% with the combination versus average remission rates of 23%–36% with any single treatment (Bacaltchuk et al. 2000). These conclusions are consistent with preliminary clinical data for other ICDs, suggesting that combinations of psychological and psychopharmacological treatments may be better than single treatments (McElroy and Arnold 2001).

Conclusion

Although binge eating is currently classified as a form of pathological eating behavior and is a defining component of bulimia nervosa and BED, it meets historical and DSM-IV-TR definitions of an ICD. Binge eating is distinct from other ICDs in some ways, including in its association with other forms of pathological eating behavior, overweight, and obesity. However, binge eating shares phenomenological similarities with ICDs beyond those required for the definition of an ICD, including impulsive features, compulsive features, affective dysregulation, and variable insight. Moreover, binge eating, bulimia, and BED share other features with ICDs. These include similarities regarding associated psychopathology, family history of mental disorders, biological abnormalities, and response to a broad range of available psychological and medical treatments. Viewing binge eating as an ICD may promote novel ways of studying and treating conditions characterized by this behavior.

References

Abraham SF, Beaumont PJV: How patients describe bulimia or binge eating. Psychol Med 12:625–635, 1982

Ackard DM, Neumark-Sztainer D, Story M, et al: Overeating among adolescents: prevalence and association with weight-related characteristics and psychological health. Pediatrics 111:67–74, 2003

Adami GF, Gandolfo P, Bauer B, et al: Binge eating in massively obese patients undergoing bariatric surgery. Int J Eat Disord 17:45–50, 1995

Agras WS: Treatment of binge-eating disorder, in Treatment of Psychiatric Disorders, 3rd Edition. Edited by Gabbard GO. Washington, DC, American Psychiatric Publishing, 2001, pp 2209–2219

Agras WS, Rossiter EM, Arnow B, et al: Pharmacological and cognitive-behavioral treatment for bulimia nervosa: a controlled comparison. Am J Psychiatry 149:82–87, 1992

Agras WS, Walsh T, Fairburn CG, et al: A multicenter comparison of cognitive behavioral therapy and interpersonal psychotherapy for bulimia nervosa. Arch Gen Psychiatry 57:459–466, 2000

Alger SA, Schwalberg MD, Bigaovette JM, et al: Effect of a tricyclic antidepressant and opiate antagonist on binge-eating behavior in normoweight bulimic and obese, binge-eating subjects. Am J Clin Nutr 53:865–871, 1991

American Psychiatric Association: Diagnostic and Statistical Manual of Mental Disorders, 3rd Edition. Washington, DC, American Psychiatric Association, 1980

American Psychiatric Association: Diagnostic and Statistical Manual of Mental Disorders, 3rd Edition, Revised. Washington, DC, American Psychiatric Association, 1987

American Psychiatric Association: Diagnostic and Statistical Manual of Mental Disorders, 4th Edition. Washington, DC, American Psychiatric Association, 1994

American Psychiatric Association: Diagnostic and Statistical Manual of Mental Disorders, 4th Edition, Text Revision. Washington, DC, American Psychiatric Association, 2000

Angst J: The emerging epidemiology of hypomania and bipolar II disorder. J Affect Disord 50:143–151, 1998

Angst J, Gamma A, Sellaro R, et al: Toward validation of atypical depression in the community: results of the Zurich cohort study. J Affect Disord 72:125–138, 2002

Appolinario JC, Bacaltchuk J, Sichieri R, et al: A randomized, double-blind, placebo-controlled study of sibutramine in the treatment of binge eating disorder. Arch Gen Psychiatry 60:1109–1116, 2003

Arnold LA, McElroy SL, Hudson JI, et al: A placebo-controlled trial of fluoxetine in the treatment of binge eating disorder. J Clin Psychiatry 63:1028–1033, 2002

Arnow B, Kenardy J, Agras WS: Binge eating among the obese: a descriptive study. J Behav Med 15:155–170, 1992

Bacaltchuk J, Trefiglio RP, Oliveia IR, et al: Combination of antidepressants and psychological treatments for bulimia nervosa: a systematic review. Acta Psychiatr Scand 101:256–264, 2000

Becker AE, Grinspoon SK, Klibanski A, et al: Eating disorders. N Engl J Med 340:1092–1098, 1999

Beglin SJ, Fairburn CG: What is meant by the term "binge?" Am J Psychiatry 149:123–124, 1992

Bellodi L, Cavallini MC, Bertelli S, et al: Morbidity risk for obsessive-compulsive spectrum disorders in first degree relatives of patients with eating disorders. Am J Psychiatry 158:563–569, 2001

Black DW, Goldstein RB, Mason EE: Prevalence of mental disorders in 88 morbidly obese bariatric clinic patients. Am J Psychiatry 149:227–234, 1992

Blouin AG, Blouin JH, Perez EL, et al: Treatment of bulimia with fenfluramine and desipramine. J Clin Psychopharmacol 8:261–269, 1988

Branson R, Potoczna N, Kral JG, et al: Binge eating as a major phenotype of melanocortin 4 receptor gene mutations. N Engl J Med 348:1096–1103, 2003

Braun DL, Sunday SR, Halmi KA: Psychiatric comorbidity in patients with eating disorders. Psychol Med 24:859–867, 1994

Britz B, Siegfried W, Ziegler A, et al: Rates of psychiatric disorders in a clinical study group of adolescents with extreme obesity and in obese adolescents ascertained via a population based study. Int J Obes Relat Metab Disord 24:1707–1714, 2000

Bulik CM, Sullivan PF, Kendler KS: Heritability of binge eating and broadly defined bulimia nervosa. Biol Psychiatry 44:1210–1218, 1998

Bulik CM, Sullivan PF, Kendler KS: An empirical study of the classification of eating disorders. Am J Psychiatry 157:886–895, 2000a

Bulik CM, Sullivan PF, Wade T, et al: Twin studies of eating disorders: a review. Int J Eat Disord 27:1–20, 2000b

Bulik CM, Sullivan PF, Kendler KS: Medical and psychiatric morbidity in obese women with and without binge eating. Int J Eat Disord 32:72–78, 2002

Bulik CM, Devlin B, Bacanv SA, et al: Significant linkage on chromosome 10p in families with bulimia nervosa. Am J Hum Genet 72:200–207, 2003

Bushnell JA, Wells JE, McKenzie JM, et al: Bulimia comorbidity in the general population and the clinic. Psychol Med 24:605–611, 1994

Cachelin FM, Striegel-Moore R, Elder KA, et al: Natural course of a community sample of women with binge eating disorder. Int J Eat Disord 25:45–54, 1999

Carter JC, Olmsted MP, Kaplan AS, et al: Self-help for bulimia nervosa: a randomized controlled trial. Am J Psychiatry 160:973–978, 2003

Carter WP, Hudson JI, Lalonde JK, et al: Pharmacological treatment of binge eating disorder. Int J Eat Disord 34:574–588, 2003

Casper RC, Eckert ED, Halmi KA, et al: Bulimia: its incidence and clinical importance in patients with anorexia nervosa. Arch Gen Psychiatry 37:1030–1035, 1980

Cooper PJ, Fairburn CG: Binge eating and self induced vomiting in the community: a preliminary study. Br J Psychiatry 142:139–144, 1983

Crow S, Kendall D, Praus B, et al: Binge eating and other psychopathology in patients with type II diabetes mellitus. Int J Eat Disord 30:222–226, 2001

Crow SJ, Agras WS, Halmi K, et al: Full syndromal versus subthreshold anorexia nervosa, bulimia nervosa, and binge eating disorder: a multicenter study. Int J Eat Disord 32:309–318, 2002

Crowell MD, Cheskin LJ, Musial F: Prevalence of gastrointestinal symptoms in obese and normal weight binge eaters. Am J Gastroenterol 89:387–391, 1994

Dansky BS, Brewerton TD, Kilpatrick DG: Comorbidity of bulimia nervosa and alcohol use disorders: results from the national women's study. Int J Eat Disord 27:180–190, 2000

deZwaan M, Bach M, Mitchell JE, et al: Alexithymia, obesity, and binge eating disorder. Int J Eat Disord 17:135–140, 1995

Dingemans AE, Bruna MJ, van Furth EF: Binge eating disorder: a review. Int J Obes Relat Metab Disord 26:299–307, 2002

Fahy T, Eisler I: Impulsivity and eating disorders. Br J Psychiatry 162:193–197, 1993

Fahy TA, Eisler I, Russell GF: A placebo-controlled trial of d-fenfluramine in bulimia nervosa. Br J Psychiatry 162:597–603, 1993

Fairburn CG, Harrison PJ: Eating disorders. Lancet 361:407–416, 2003

Fairburn CG, Jones R, Peveler RC, et al: Three psychological treatments for bulimia nervosa: a comparative trial. Arch Gen Psychiatry 48:463–469, 1991

Fairburn CG, Norman PA, Welch SL, et al: A prospective study of outcome in bulimia nervosa and the long-term effects of three psychological treatments. Arch Gen Psychiatry 52:304–312, 1995

Fairburn CG, Welch SL, Doll HA, et al: Risk factors for bulimia nervosa: a community-based case-control study. Arch Gen Psychiatry 54:509–517, 1997

Fairburn CG, Doll HA, Welch SL, et al: Risk factors for binge eating disorder: a community-based, case-control study. Arch Gen Psychiatry 55:425–432, 1998

Fairburn CG, Cooper Z, Doll HA, et al: The natural course of bulimia nervosa and binge eating disorders in young women. Arch Gen Psychiatry 57:659–665, 2000

Faris PL, Kim SW, Meller WH, et al: Effect of decreasing afferent vagal activity with ondansetron on symptoms of bulimia nervosa: a randomized, double-blind trial. Lancet 355:792–797, 2000

Farooqui IS, Keogh JM, Yeo GSH, et al: Clinical spectrum of obesity and mutations in the melanocortin 4 receptor gene. N Engl J Med 348:1085–1095, 2003

Favaro A, Santonastaso P: Impulsive and compulsive self-injurious behavior in bulimia nervosa: prevalence and psychological correlates. J Nerv Ment Dis 186:157–165, 1998

Fichter MM, Quadflieg N, Rief W: Course of multi-impulsive bulimia. Psychol Med 24:591–604, 1994

Fischer S, Smith GT, Anderson KG: Clarifying the role of impulsivity in bulimia nervosa. Int J Eat Disord 33:406–411, 2003

Fluoxetine Bulimia Nervosa Collaborative Study Group: Fluoxetine in the treatment of bulimia nervosa: a multicenter, placebo-controlled, double-blind trial. Arch Gen Psychiatry 49:139–147, 1992

Garfinkel PE, Lin E, Goering P, et al: Bulimia nervosa in a Canadian community sample: prevalence and comparison of subgroups. Am J Psychiatry 152:1052–1058, 1995

Geracioti TD, Loosen PT, Ebert MH, et al: Fasting and postprandial cerebrospinal fluid glucose concentrations in healthy women and in an obese binge eater. Int J Eat Disord 18:365–369, 1995

Geretsegger C, Greimel KV, Roed IS, et al: Ipsapirone in the treatment of bulimia nervosa: an open pilot study. Int J Eat Disord 17:359–363, 1995

Gerlinghoff M, Backmund H: Stehlen bei anorexia nervosa and bulimia nervosa. Fortschr Neurol Psychiatr 55:343–346, 1987

Gilmour J, Skuse D, Pembrey M: Hyperphagic short stature and Prader-Willi syndrome: a comparison of behavioral phenotypes, genotypes and indices of stress. Br J Psychiatry 179:129–137, 2001

Goldbloom DS, Olmsted M, Davis R, et al: A randomized controlled trial of fluoxetine and cognitive behavioral therapy for bulimia nervosa: short-term outcome. Behav Res Ther 35:803–811, 1997

Goldfein JA, Walsh BT, LaChaussée JL: Eating behavior in binge eating disorder. Int J Eat Disord 14:427–431, 1993

Goldstein DJ, Wilson MG, Thompson VL, et al: Long-term fluoxetine treatment of bulimia nervosa. Br J Psychiatry 166:660–666, 1995

Green RS, Rau JH: Treatment of compulsive eating disturbances with anticonvulsant medication. Am J Psychiatry 131:428–431, 1974

Greenberg BR, Harvey PD: Affective lability versus depression as determinants of binge eating. Addict Behav 12:357–361, 1987

Greenway FL, Dahms WT, Bray GA: Phenytoin as a treatment of obesity associated with compulsive eating. Curr Ther Res 21:338–342, 1977

Hadigan CM, Walsh BT, Devlin MJ, et al: Behavioral assessment of satiety in bulimia nervosa. Appetite 16:219–237, 1992

Hamburger WW: Psychological aspects of obesity. Bull N Y Acad Med 33:771–782, 1957

Hay P, Fairburn C: The validity of the DSM-IV scheme for classifying bulimic eating disorders. Int J Eat Disord 23:7–15, 1998

Hedges DW, Reimherr FW, Hoopes SP, et al: Treatment of bulimia nervosa with topiramate in a randomized, double-blind, placebo-controlled trial, part 2: improvement in psychiatric measures. J Clin Psychiatry 64:1449–1454, 2003

Holderness CC, Brooks-Gunn J, Warren MP: Comorbidity of eating disorders and substance abuse: review of the literature. Int J Eat Disord 16:1–16, 1994

Hoopes S, Reimherr F, Hedges, et al: Part I: topiramate in the treatment of bulimia nervosa: a randomized, double-blind, placebo-controlled trial. J Clin Psychiatry 64:1335–1341, 2003

Horne RL, Ferguson JM, Pope HG, et al: Treatment of bulimia with bupropion: a multicenter controlled trial. J Clin Psychiatry 49:262–266, 1988

Hsu LKG: Treatment of bulimia with lithium. Am J Psychiatry 141:1260–1262, 1984

Hsu LKG, Clement L, Santhouse R, et al: Treatment of bulimia nervosa with lithium carbonate: a controlled study. J Nerv Ment Dis 179:351–355, 1991

Hsu LKG, Betancourt S, Sullivan SP: Eating disturbances before and after vertical banded gastroplasty: a pilot study. Int J Eat Disord 19:23–24, 1996

Hudson JI, Pope HG Jr: The role of anticonvulsants in the treatment of bulimia, in Use of Anticonvulsants in Psychiatry: Recent Advances. Edited by McElroy SL, Pope HG Jr. Clifton, NJ, Oxford Health Care, 1988, pp 141–154

Hudson JI, Pope HG Jr, Jonas JM, et al: Family history study of anorexia nervosa and bulimia. Br J Psychiatry 142:133–138, 1983

Hudson JI, Pope HG Jr, Jonas JM, et al: A controlled family history study of bulimia. Psychol Med 17:883–890, 1987

Hudson JI, Pope HG Jr, Wurtman JJ, et al: Bulimia in obese individuals: relationship to normal-weight bulimia. J Nerv Ment Dis 152:144–152, 1988

Hudson JI, McElroy SL, Raymond NC, et al: Fluvoxamine in the treatment of binge-eating disorder: a multicenter placebo-controlled, double-blind trial. Am J Psychiatry 155:1756–1762, 1998

Hudson JI, Pope HG Jr, Carter WP: Pharmacological therapy of bulimia nervosa, in The Management of Eating Disorders and Obesity. Edited by Goldstein DJ. Totowa, NJ, Humana, 1999, pp 19–32

Hudson JI, Laird NM, Betensky RA, et al: Multivariate logistic regression for familial aggregation of two disorders, II: analysis of studies of eating and mood disorders. Am J Epidemiol 153:506–514, 2001

Hudson JI, Mangweth B, Pope HG, et al: Family study of affective spectrum disorder. Arch Gen Psychiatry 60:170–177, 2003

Janet P: Les Obsessions et la Psychasthénie. Paris, Felix Alcan, 1903

Jimerson DC, Lesem MD, Kaye WH, et al: Low serotonin and dopamine metabolite concentrations in cerebral spinal fluid from bulimic patients with frequent binge episodes. Arch Gen Psychiatry 49:132–138, 1992

Jimerson DC, Wolfe BE, Metzger ED, et al: Decreased serotonin function in bulimia nervosa. Arch Gen Psychiatry 54:529–534, 1997

Jonas JM, Gold MS: The use of opiate antagonists in treating bulimia: a study of low-dose versus high-dose naltrexone. Psychiatry Res 24:195–199, 1988

Kaplan AS, Garfinkel PE, Darby PL, et al: Carbamazepine in the treatment of bulimia. Am J Psychiatry 140:1225–1226, 1983

Karhunen LJ, Vanninen EJ, Kuikka JT, et al: Regional cerebral blood flow during exposure to food in obese binge eating women. Psychiatry Res 99:29–42, 2000

Kassett JA, Gershon ES, Maxwell ME, et al: Psychiatric disorders in the first degree relatives of probands with bulimia nervosa. Am J Psychiatry 146:1468–1471, 1989

Kaye W, Strober M: Neurobiology of eating disorders, in Neurobiology of Mental Illness. Edited by Charney DS, Nestler EJ, Bunney BS. New York, Oxford University Press, 1999, pp 891–906

Kaye WH, Ebert MH, Gwirtsman HE, et al: Differences in brain serotonergic metabolism between nonbulimic and bulimic patients with anorexia nervosa. Am J Psychiatry 141:1598–1601, 1984

Kaye WH, Weltzin TE, McKee M, et al: Laboratory assessment of feeding behavior in bulimia nervosa and healthy women: methods for developing a human-feeding laboratory. Am J Clin Nutr 55:372–380, 1992

Kaye WH, Greeno CG, Moss H, et al: Alterations in serotonin activity and psychiatric symptoms after recovery from bulimia nervosa. Arch Gen Psychiatry 55:927–935, 1998

Kaye WH, Frank GK, Meltzer CC, et al: Altered serotonin 2A receptor activity in women who have recovered from bulimia nervosa. Am J Psychiatry 158:1152–1155, 2001a

Kaye WH, Nagata T, Weltzin TE, et al: Double-blind placebo-controlled administration of fluoxetine in restricting- and restricting-purging-type anorexia nervosa. Biol Psychiatry 49:644–652, 2001b

Keck PE Jr, Pope HG Jr, Hudson JI: A controlled study of phenomenology and family history in outpatients with bulimia nervosa. Compr Psychiatry 31:275–283, 1990

Keel PK, Mitchell JE: Outcome in bulimia nervosa. Am J Psychiatry 154:313–321, 1997

Keel PK, Mitchell JE, Miller KB, et al: Predictive validity of bulimia nervosa as a diagnostic category. Am J Psychiatry 157:136–138, 2000

Kendler KS, MacLean C, Neale M, et al: The genetic epidemiology of bulimia nervosa. Am J Psychiatry 148:1627–1637, 1991

Kendler KS, Eaves LJ, Walters EE, et al: The identification and validation of distinct depressive syndromes in a population-based sample of female twins. Arch Gen Psychiatry 53:391–399, 1996

Krüger S, Kennedy SH: Psychopharmacotherapy of anorexia nervosa, bulimia nervosa and binge-eating disorder. J Psychiatry Neurosci 25:497–508, 2000

Krüger S, Shugar G, Cooke RG: Comorbidity of binge eating disorder and the partial binge eating syndrome with bipolar disorder. Int J Eat Disord 19:45–52, 1996

Lacey JH, Evans DH: The impulsivist: a multi-impulsive personality disorder. Br J Addict 81:641–649, 1986

Lee YH, Abbott DW, Seim H, et al: Eating disorders and psychiatric disorders in the first-degree relatives of obese probands with binge eating disorder and obese non-binge eating disorder controls. Int J Eat Disord 26:322–332, 1999

le Grange D, Gorin A, Catley D, et al: Does momentary assessment detect binge eating in overweight women that is denied at interview? Eur Eat Disord Rev 9:309–324, 2001

Leitenberg H, Rosen JC, Wolf J, et al: Comparison of cognitive-behavior therapy and desipramine in the treatment of bulimia nervosa. Behav Res Ther 32:37–45, 1994

Levitan RD, Kaplan AS, Joffe RT, et al: Hormonal and subjective response to intravenous meta-chlorophenylpiperazine in bulimia nervosa. Arch Gen Psychiatry 54:521–527, 1997

Lilenfeld LR, Kaye WH, Greeno CG, et al: A controlled family study of anorexia nervosa and bulimia nervosa: psychiatric disorders in first degree relatives and effects of proband comorbidity. Arch Gen Psychiatry 55:603–610, 1998

Malhotra S, King KH, Welge JA, et al: Venlafaxine treatment of binge-eating disorder associated with obesity: a series of 35 patients. J Clin Psychiatry 63:802–806, 2002

Marcus MD, Wing RR, Lamparski DM: Binge eating and dietary restraint in obese patients. Addict Behav 10:163–168, 1985

Marcus MD, Wing RR, Ewing L, et al: Psychiatric disorders among obese binge eaters. Int J Eat Disord 9:69–77, 1990

Marrazzi MA, Markham KM, Kinzie J, et al: Binge eating disorder: response to naltrexone. Int J Obes Relat Metab Disord 19:143–145, 1995

McCann UD, Agras WS: Successful treatment of nonpurging bulimia nervosa with desipramine: a double-blind, placebo-controlled study. Am J Psychiatry 147:1509–1513, 1990

McElroy SL, Arnold LM: Impulse-control disorders, in Treatments of Psychiatric Disorders, 3rd Edition, Vol 2. Edited by Gabbard GO. Washington, DC, American Psychiatric Press, 2001, pp 2435–2471

McElroy SL, Keck PE Jr, Pope HG Jr, et al: Kleptomania: clinical characteristics and associated psychopathology. Psychol Med 21:93–108, 1991a

McElroy SL, Pope HG Jr, Hudson JI, et al: Kleptomania: a report of 20 cases. Am J Psychiatry 148:652–657, 1991b

McElroy SL, Hudson JI, Phillips KA, et al: Clinical and theoretical implications of a possible link between obsessive-compulsive and impulse control disorders. Depression 1:121–132, 1993

McElroy SL, Pope HG Jr, Keck PE Jr, et al: Are impulse control disorders related to bipolar disorder? Compr Psychiatry 37:229–240, 1996

McElroy SL, Soutullo CA, Beckman DA, et al: DSM-IV intermittent explosive disorder: a report of 27 cases. J Clin Psychiatry 59:203–210, 1998

McElroy SL, Casuto LS, Nelson EB, et al: Placebo-controlled trial of sertraline in the treatment of binge eating disorders. Am J Psychiatry 157:1004–1006, 2000

McElroy SL, Frye MA, Suppes T, et al: Correlates of overweight and obesity in 644 patients with bipolar disorder. J Clin Psychiatry 63:207–213, 2002

McElroy SL, Hudson JI, Malhotra S, et al: Citalopram in the treatment of binge eating disorder: a placebo-controlled trial. J Clin Psychiatry 64:807–813, 2003a

McElroy SL, Arnold LM, Shapira NA, et al: Topiramate in the treatment of binge eating disorder associated with obesity: a randomized, placebo-controlled trial. Am J Psychiatry 160:255–261, 2003b

McElroy SL, Kotwal R, Hudson JI, et al: Zonisamide in the treatment of binge eating disorder: an open-label, prospective trial. J Clin Psychiatry 65:50–56, 2004

Mehler PS: Bulimia nervosa. N Engl J Med 349:875–881, 2003

Mitchell JE, Mussell MP: Comorbidity and binge eating disorder. Addict Behav 20:725–732, 1995

Mitchell JE, Hatsukami D, Eckert ED, et al: Characteristics of 275 patients with bulimia. Am J Psychiatry 142:482–485, 1985

Mitchell JE, Laine DE, Morley JE, et al: Naloxone but not CCK-8 may attenuate binge-eating behavior in patients with the bulimia syndrome. Biol Psychiatry 21:1399–1406, 1986

Mitchell JE, Christenson G, Jennings J, et al: A placebo-controlled, double-blind cross-over study of naltrexone hydrochloride in outpatients with normal weight bulimia. J Clin Psychopharmacol 9:94–97, 1989

Mitchell JE, Pyle RL, Eckert ED, et al: A comparison study of antidepressants and structured intensive group psychotherapy in the treatment of bulimia nervosa. Arch Gen Psychiatry 47:149–157, 1990

Mitchell JE, Crow S, Peterson CB, et al: Feeding laboratory studies in patients with eating disorders: a review. Int J Eat Disord 24:115–124, 1998

Mitchell JE, Lancaster KL, Burgard MA, et al: Long-term follow-up of patients status after gastric bypass. Obes Surg 11:464–468, 2001

Mitchell JE, Gosnell BA, Roerig JL, et al: Effects of sibutramine on binge eating, hunger, and fullness in a laboratory human feeding paradigm. Obes Res 11:599–602, 2003

Monteleone P, Brambilla F, Bortolotti F, et al: Serotonergic dysfunction across the eating disorders: relationship to eating behavior, purging behavior, nutritional status, and general psychopathology. Psychol Med 30:1099–1110, 2000

Mortola JF, Rasmussen DD, Yen SSC: Alterations of the adreno-corticotropin-cortisol axis in normal weight bulimic women: evidence for a central mechanism. J Clin Endocrinol Metab 68:517–522, 1989

Nagata R, Kawarada Y, Kiriike N, et al: Multi-impulsivity of Japanese patients with eating disorders: primary and secondary impulsivity. Psychiatry Res 94:239–250, 2000

Narvo T, Nakabeppu Y, Saqiyama K, et al: Characteristic regional cerebral blood flow patterns in anorexia nervosa patients with binge/purge behavior. Am J Psychiatry 157:1520–1522, 2000

Neudeck P, Jacoby GE, Florin I: Dexamethasone suppression test using saliva cortisol measurement in bulimia nervosa. Physiol Behav 72:93–98, 2001

Neumeister A, Winkler A, Wöber-Bingöl C: Addition of naltrexone to fluoxetine in the treatment of binge eating disorder. Am J Psychiatry 156:797, 1999

Newton JR, Freeman CP, Munro J: Impulsivity and dyscontrol in bulimia nervosa: is impulsivity an important phenomenon or a marker of severity? Acta Psychiatr Scand 87:389–394, 1993

Ong YL, Checkley SA, Russell GFM: Suppression of bulimic symptoms with methylamphetamine. Br J Psychiatry 143:288–293, 1983

Palmer RL, Birchall H, McGrain L, et al: Self-help for bulimic disorders: a randomized controlled trial comparing minimal guidance with face-to-face or telephone guidance. Br J Psychiatry 181:230–235, 2002

Paul T, Schroeter K, Dahme B, et al: Self-injurious behavior in women with eating disorders. Am J Psychiatry 159:408–411, 2002

Perugi G, Akiskal HS: The soft bipolar spectrum redefined: focus on the cyclothymic, anxious-sensitive, impulse-dyscontrol, and binge-eating connection in bipolar and related conditions. Psychiatr Clin North Am 25:713–737, 2002

Peterson CB, Mitchell JR: Psychosocial and pharmacological treatment of eating disorders: a review of research findings. J Clin Psychol 55:685–697, 1999

Pope HG Jr, Hudson JI, Mialet J-P: Bulimia in the late nineteenth century: the observations of Pierre Janet. Psychol Med 15:739–743, 1985

Pope HG Jr, Keck PE Jr, McElroy SL, et al: A placebo-controlled study of trazodone in bulimia nervosa. J Clin Psychopharmacol 9:254–259, 1989

Prather R, Williamson DA: Psychopathology associated with bulimia, binge eating, and obesity. Int J Eat Disord 7:177–184, 1988

Pratt EM, Niego SH, Agras WS: Does the size of a binge matter? Int J Eat Disord 24:307–312, 1998

Pyle RL, Mitchell JE, Eckert ED: Bulimia: a report of 34 cases. J Clin Psychiatry 42:60–64, 1981

Romano SJ, Halmi KA, Sarkar NP, et al: A placebo-controlled study of fluoxetine in continued treatment of bulimia nervosa after successful acute fluoxetine treatment. Am J Psychiatry 159:96–102, 2002

Rosenvinge JH, Sundgot-Borgen J, Borresen R: The prevalence and psychological correlates of anorexia nervosa, bulimia nervosa and binge eating among 15-year-old students: a controlled epidemiological study. Eur Eat Disord Rev 7:382–391, 1999

Russell G: Bulimia nervosa: an ominous variant of anorexia nervosa. Psychol Med 9:429–448, 1979

Russell GF, Checkley SA, Feldman J, et al: A controlled trial of d-fenfluramine in bulimia nervosa. Clin Neuropharmacol 11(suppl):S146–S159, 1988

Schweickert LA, Strober M, Moskowitz A: Efficacy of methylphenidate in bulimia nervosa comorbid with attention-deficit hyperactivity disorder: a case report. Int J Eat Disord 21:299–301, 1997

Shapira NA, Lessig MC, Murphy TK, et al: Topiramate attenuates self-injurious behaviour in Prader-Willi syndrome. Int J Neuropsychopharmacol 5:141–145, 2002

Shisslak CM, Perse T, Crago M: Coexistence of bulimia nervosa and mania: a literature review and case report. Compr Psychiatry 32:181–184, 1991

Skodol AE, Oldham JM, Hyler SE, et al: Comorbidity of DSM-III-R eating disorders and personality disorders. Int J Eat Disord 14:403–416, 1993

Smith DE, Marcus MD, Lewis CE, et al: Prevalence of binge eating disorder, obesity, and depression in a biracial cohort of young adults. Ann Behav Med 20:227–232, 1998

Smith KA, Fairburn CG, Cowen PJ: Symptomatic relapse in bulimia nervosa following acute tryptophan depletion. Arch Gen Psychiatry 56:171–176, 1999

Sohlberg S, Norring G, Holmgren S, et al: Impulsivity and long-term prognosis of psychiatric patients with anorexia nervosa/bulimia nervosa. J Nerv Ment Dis 177:249–258, 1989

Sokol MS, Gray NS, Goldstein A, et al: Methylphenidate treatment for bulimia nervosa associated with a cluster B personality disorder. Int J Eat Disord 25:233–237, 1999

Specker S, deZwaan M, Raymond N, et al: Psychopathology in subgroups of obese women with and without binge eating disorder. Compr Psychiatry 35:185–190, 1994

Spitzer RL, Devlin M, Walsh T, et al: A multisite field trial of the diagnostic criteria. Int J Eat Disord 11:191–203, 1992

Spitzer RL, Yanovski S, Wadden T, et al: Binge eating disorder: its further validation in a multisite study. Int J Eat Disord 13:137–153, 1993

Steiger H, Thibaudeau J, Leung F, et al: Eating and psychiatric symptoms as a function of Axis II comorbidity in bulimic patients: three-month and six-month response after therapy. Psychosomatics 35:41–49, 1994

Striegel-Moore RH, Dohm FA, Solomon EE, et al: Subthreshold BED. Int J Eat Disord 27:270–278, 2000

Striegel-Moore RH, Dohm FA, Kraemer HC, et al: Eating disorders in white and black women. Am J Psychiatry 160:1326–1331, 2003

Stunkard AJ: Eating patterns and obesity. Psychiatr Q 33:284–295, 1959

Stunkard A, Berkowitz, R, Tanrikut C, et al: *d*-Fenfluramine treatment of binge eating disorder. Am J Psychiatry 153:1455–1459, 1996

Telch CF, Pratt EM, Niego SH, et al: Obese women with binge eating disorder define the term binge. Int J Eat Disord 24:313–317, 1998

Theisen FM, Linden A, Konig IR, et al: Spectrum of binge eating symptomatology in patients treated with clozapine and olanzapine. J Neural Transm 110:111–121, 2003

Vollrath M, Koch R, Angst J: Binge eating and weight concerns among young adults: results from the Zurich Cohort Study. Br J Psychiatry 160:498–503, 1992

Wade TD, Bulik CM, Kendler KS: Reliability of lifetime history of bulimia nervosa: comparison with major depression. Br J Psychiatry 177:72–76, 2000

Walsh BT, Gladis M, Roose SP, et al: Phenelzine vs placebo in 50 patients with bulimia. Arch Gen Psychiatry 45:471–475, 1988

Walsh BT, Wilson GT, Loeb KL, et al: Medication and psychotherapy in the treatment of bulimia nervosa. Am J Psychiatry 154:523–531, 1997

Walsh BT, Agras WS, Devlin MJ, et al: Fluoxetine for bulimia nervosa following poor response to psychotherapy. Am J Psychiatry 157:1332–1334, 2000

Wang G-J, Volkow ND, Logan J, et al: Brain dopamine and obesity. Lancet 357:354–357, 2001

Wang G-J, Volkow ND, Thanos PK, et al: Positron emission tomographic evidence of similarity between obesity and drug addiction. Psychiatr Ann 33:105–111, 2003

Wermuth BM, Davis KL, Hollister LE, et al: Phenytoin treatment of the binge eating syndrome. Am J Psychiatry 134:1249–1253, 1977

Westen D, Harnden-Fischer J: Personality profiles in eating disorders: rethinking the distinction between Axis I and Axis II. Am J Psychiatry 158:547–562, 2001

Whitaker A, Johnson J, Shaffer D, et al: Uncommon troubles among young people: prevalence estimate of selected psychiatric disorders in a nonreferred adolescent population. Arch Gen Psychiatry 47:487–496, 1990

Whittal ML, Agras WS, Gould RA: Bulimia nervosa: a meta-analysis of psychosocial and pharmacological treatments. Behav Ther 30:117–135, 1999

Wiederman MH, Pryor T: Multi-impulsivity among women with bulimia nervosa. Int J Eat Disord 4:359–365, 1996

Wilfley DE, Welch R, Stein RI, et al: A randomized comparison of group cognitive-behavioral therapy and group interpersonal psychotherapy for the treatment of overweight individuals with binge-eating disorder. Arch Gen Psychiatry 59:713–721, 2002

Williamson DA, Martin CK: Binge eating disorder: a review of the literature after publication of DSM-IV. Eat Weight Disord 4:103–114, 1999

Williamson DA, Womble LG, Smeets MAM, et al: Latent structure of eating disorder symptoms: a factor analytic and taxometric investigation. Am J Psychiatry 159:412–418, 2002

Wittchen H-U, Nelson CB, Lachner G: Prevalence of mental disorders and psychosocial impairments in adolescents and young adults. Psychol Med 28:109–126, 1998

Wonderlich SA, de Zwaan M, Mitchell JE, et al: Psychological and dietary treatments of binge eating disorder: conceptual indications. Int J Eat Disord 34:S58–S73, 2003

Woodside DB, Garfinkel PE, Lin E, et al: Comparisons of men with full or partial eating disorders, men without eating disorders, and women with eating disorders in the community. Am J Psychiatry 158:570–574, 2001

Yanovski SZ, Leet M, Yanovski J, et al: Food selection and intake of obese women with binge-eating disorder. Am J Clin Nutr 56:975–980, 1992

Yanovski SZ, Nelson JE, Dubbert BK, et al: Association of binge eating disorder and psychiatric comorbidity in obese subjects. Am J Psychiatry 150:1472–1479, 1993

Zhu AJ, Walsh BT: Pharmacological treatment of eating disorders. Can J Psychiatry 47:227–234, 2002

7

Trichotillomania

Martin E. Franklin, Ph.D.
David F. Tolin, Ph.D.
Gretchen J. Diefenbach, Ph.D.

Trichotillomania is a chronic impulse-control disorder characterized by repetitive pulling out of one's own hair, resulting in noticeable hair loss. In this chapter, we describe the symptoms of trichotillomania in adults and youth as well as its epidemiology and scope. We review the outcome literature on current treatments for trichotillomania and discuss how treatment efficacy might be enhanced via the development of a comprehensive biopsychosocial model of trichotillomania. Toward that end, we provide specific recommendations for research avenues to pursue that will inform the development of such a model. Because trichotillomania is apparently more common than previously believed,

This work was supported in part by a grant from the National Institute of Mental Health (MH61457).

negatively impacts quality of life, and does not appear to be highly responsive to the interventions currently available, expanding knowledge about the nature of trichotillomania is an essential next step in improving long-term outcomes.

Psychopathology

Definitions and Variations of Trichotillomania

DSM-IV-TR (American Psychiatric Association 2000, p. 674) defines *tricho-tillomania* as follows: A) recurrent pulling out of one's own hair that results in noticeable hair loss; B) an increasing sense of tension immediately before pulling or when attempting to resist the behavior; C) pleasure, gratification, or relief when pulling; D) not better accounted for by another mental disorder and not due to a general medical condition (e.g., dermatological condition); and E) causing clinically significant distress or impairment in social, occupational, or other important areas of functioning. Criteria B and C are somewhat controversial in light of data suggesting that a significant minority of individuals who pull their hair do not report experiencing these feelings. Christenson et al. (1991a) reported that in a sample of 60 adult patients, 5% failed to endorse a feeling of tension prior to pulling and 12% did not report gratification or tension release subsequent to pulling; similarly, Schlosser et al. (1994) indicated that 23% of their clinical sample failed to meet the diagnostic criteria of tension and gratification. This issue may be even more pronounced in youngsters who pull; results from a small study by Hanna (1997) on children and adolescents exhibiting pulling behavior found that only half of the sample endorsed both rising tension and relief associated with hair pulling. From these data, Hanna concluded that awareness of internal states and the ability to recognize and report tension and relief may be associated with cognitive development and/or neurobiological changes associated with hair pulling. Indeed, endorsement of these symptoms is more common in older children and adolescents (King et al. 1995). Taken collectively, these findings suggest that the current diagnostic classification of trichotillomania may be overly restrictive, particularly with respect to pediatric samples. Perhaps of greater importance, whether trichotillomania meeting full DSM criteria is taxometrically distinct from trichotillomania meeting partial criteria remains to be examined in studies with sufficient sample sizes to allow for subgroup comparisons. Information from studies of this kind would undoubtedly advance trichotillomania theory and improve our classification system, because as of now it is unclear whether chronic hair pulling is best conceptualized as a single entity or as a symptom with myriad root causes yet to be identified, with little unifying the subtypes theoretically.

On a related note, approximately 75% of adult trichotillomania patients report that most of their hair-pulling behavior takes place "automatically" or outside of awareness, whereas the remaining 25% describe themselves as primarily focused on hair pulling when they pull (Christenson and Mackenzie 1994). However, the distinction between focused and unfocused pulling is complicated by the fact that at least some patients engage in both types of pulling behavior. Compared with unfocused hair pullers, the subset of patients who primarily engage in focused hair pulling are more likely to pull hair from the pubic area and to report shame as a result of their hair pulling (du Toit et al. 2001). Whether these two observations are related to one another is unclear, because the study did not report whether focused hair pullers who do not pull from the pubic region are more ashamed than unfocused hair pullers. Some researchers have postulated that trichotillomania patients who engage primarily in focused hair pulling are more similar to individuals with obsessive-compulsive disorder (OCD) and may be more responsive to pharmacological interventions found effective for OCD (Christenson and O'Sullivan 1996; du Toit et al. 2001). In general, the issue of trichotillomania subtyping is one of both considerable importance and ongoing debate, and no formal subtyping system incorporating affective correlates of pulling has been advanced.

Much less information is available on how trichotillomania presents in children and adolescents, but the little that has been published suggests similarities to adult hair pulling. As with adults, the scalp is the most common pulling site in children and adolescents, followed by eyelashes and eyebrows (Reeve 1999). Hanna (1997) found that 6 of 11 children and adolescents pulled from two or more sites, 3 pulled scalp hair exclusively, and 2 pulled eyelashes exclusively. Almost half of the subjects described having a ritual or routine involved in pulling their hair. The absence of body hair on younger children precludes pulling from certain sites, but clinical work with adolescents appears consistent with the adult data in that pulling from sites other than the face and scalp is also common. When completed, ongoing research regarding the preferred pulling sites of children and adolescents (Franklin et al. 2002; Tolin et al. 2002) will add to this knowledge base.

Epidemiology and Comorbidity

Early clinical studies suggested that trichotillomania was extremely rare (Mannino and Delgado 1969); however, survey research with nonclinical samples has indicated that hair pulling is more common than originally suggested. In studies involving college samples, 10%–13% of students reported hair pulling, with the prevalence of clinically significant pulling ranging between 1% and 3.5% (Christenson et al. 1991b; Rothbaum et al. 1993). A large study of trichotillomania and skin picking using psychometrically sound self-report instruments is under way in a large sample of college freshmen that will extend the literature on trichotillomania's prevalence and shed light on the co-occurrence of these impulse-control disorders (Hajcak et al. 2004). Epidemiological research on trichotillomania is extremely limited both in terms of the number of studies and in terms of methodology. One epidemiological survey of 17-year-old adolescents in Israel suggests a prevalence rate of 1% for current or past hair pulling, with fewer reporting noticeable hair loss or distress from these symptoms (King et al. 1995). However, the generalization of these data to more representative epidemiological research is unclear, and there remains a need for epidemiological research on trichotillomania.

In general, psychiatric comorbidity appears to be quite common among adults with trichotillomania. Christenson et al. (1991a) found that approximately 82% of an adult clinical sample with trichotillomania met criteria for a past or current comorbid Axis I disorder, the most common being affective, anxiety, and addictive disorders. Specifically, of these patients with comorbid disorders, there was a lifetime prevalence rate of 65% for mood disorders, 57% for anxiety disorders, 22% for substance abuse disorders, 20% for eating disorders, and 42% for personality disorders. The most frequently cited comorbid personality disorders are histrionic, borderline, and obsessive-compulsive (Christenson et al. 1992; Schlosser et al. 1994; Swedo and Leonard 1992). In a larger sample of adults seeking treatment for trichotillomania, Christenson (1995) found comorbidity rates of 57% for major depression, 27% for generalized anxiety disorder, 20% for eating disorders, 19% for alcohol abuse, and

16% for other substance abuse. In a mixed sample of children, adolescents, and adults with trichotillomania, Swedo and Leonard (1992) found comorbidity rates of 39% for unipolar depression, 32% for generalized anxiety disorder, 16% for OCD, and 15% for substance abuse.

Only two very small studies regarding comorbidity have been conducted on exclusively pediatric clinical samples. Reeve et al. (1992) and King et al. (1995) found that 7 of 10 and 9 of 15 children with trichotillomania had at least one comorbid Axis I disorder, respectively. Notably, Franklin et al. (2002) and Tolin et al. (2002) reported little comorbidity in their pediatric treatment-seeking samples, which may relate to the critical issue of whether comorbidity develops secondarily in the wake of trichotillomania. Sampling issues most likely underlie these observed differences in that our samples were subject to a telephone screen up front that may have excluded some cases likely to evidence comorbid psychopathology. Nevertheless, if it is indeed the case that children and adolescents with trichotillomania are less comorbid than adults with trichotillomania, perhaps successful early intervention in children and adolescents who have trichotillomania may prove helpful in reducing the rates and severity of later adult psychiatric comorbidity as well as functional impairment associated with the disorder (Keuthen et al. 2002). Much more longitudinal and psychopathology research is needed on this urgent topic.

Functional Impairment and Quality of Life

From a clinical standpoint, it is clear that trichotillomania can significantly impact functioning, especially when onset occurs during the sensitive years of early adolescence (Christenson et al. 1991a). Significant rates of avoidance and distress involving public activities, sexual intimacy, and athletic endeavors have been reported in clinical samples (e.g., Stemberger et al. 2000), and other studies have indicated that many trichotillomania patients spend more than 1 hour/day extracting hair (e.g., Koran et al. 1992; Mansueto 1990). That being said, it was only recently that functional impairment has been systematically evaluated using psychometrically sound instruments. Functional limitations were examined in a cohort of adult hair pullers (N= 58) attending a national trichotillomania conference using survey questions and standardized self-report scales (Keuthen et al. 2002). Seventy-one percent of the sample endorsed trichotillomania-related distress or impairment in social functioning, including decreased contact with friends (40%), decreased dating activity (47%), loss of intimacy (40%), and negative impact on family relationships (50%). In addition, 55% of the sample endorsed trichotillomania-related distress or impairment in occupational functioning, including job avoidance (29%), lateness to work (22%), decreased coworker contact (28%), and decreased career aspirations (34%). Finally, 69% of the sample endorsed avoidance of specific leisure activities. The Medical Outcomes Study 36-Item Short-Form Health Survey (Ware 1993) found quality-of-life impairment on all mental health subscales. Severity of hair pulling was negatively correlated with scores on all four subscales, and, importantly, depression was found to mediate the relationship between trichotillomania and quality of life. Of note, Koran et al. (1996) also reported lowered quality-of-life scores for the same subscales for an OCD sample in comparison with population norms, further suggesting that the effects of trichotillomania on quality of life are far from trivial.

Relationship With Obsessive-Compulsive Disorder, Skin Picking, and Nail Biting

One of the key theoretical debates within the field pertains to whether trichotillomania should be conceptualized as an impulse-control disorder or simply a variant of OCD. Many have likened trichotillomania to OCD, given the apparent formal similarity between the repetitive and perceived uncontrollable nature of hair pulling with that of compulsions and because of the possible selective responsiveness of trichotillomania to serotonin reuptake inhibitors. The classification of trichotillomania as an obsessive-compulsive spectrum disorder is also supported by evidence showing elevated rates of OCD in patients with trichotillomania (Christenson et al. 1991a). Swedo (1993) and Swedo and Leonard (1992) suggested that both OCD and trichotillomania patients see their hair-pulling/compulsive behaviors as unreasonable and describe an irresistible urge and anxiety that cause them to engage in the behaviors and benefit from the accompanying relief. The percentage of trichotillomania patients who fail to endorse criteria in the DSM specifying tension and relief associated with hair pulling, although relatively low, supports some researchers' inclination to conceptualize trichotillomania as a variant of OCD (Jenike 1989; Swedo and Leonard 1992) and not as an impulse-control disorder, at least in adult populations.

Numerous researchers have argued instead that trichotillomania and OCD are separate, distinct diagnoses. Unlike the repetitive and intrusive nature of obsessions in OCD, they propose that trichotillomania is not at all characterized by persistent and intrusive thoughts regarding hair pulling and that hair pulling often occurs outside awareness. The nature of the repetitive behavior in trichotillomania is generally limited to the topography of hair pulling, whereas compulsions in OCD often consist of a variety of behaviors performed to alleviate anxiety. Moreover, individuals with OCD describe their compulsions as unpleasant but necessary to reduce negative affect, whereas most with trichotillomania describe hair pulling as pleasurable or satisfying in some way. Thus, OCD is maintained by negative reinforcement (decrease in negative affect) rather than by positive reinforcement, whereas trichotillomania is more likely to be maintained by positive reinforcement.

In further support of the distinction between the two disorders, phenomenology and epidemiology also differ with respect to OCD and trichotillomania. Age at onset is generally later for OCD than for trichotillomania (Himle et al. 1995; Swedo 1993; Tukel et al. 2001). Additionally, patients with OCD report higher levels of overall anxiety than do those with trichotillomania (Himle et al. 1995; Tukel et al. 2001), and trichotillomania is associated with a broader range of affective states than is OCD (Stanley and Cohen 1999). The proposed difference in conceptualizations of OCD and trichotillomania has critical implications for treatment that lead to the use of disparate cognitive-behavioral therapy (CBT) strategies for each disorder. In CBT for OCD, individuals are encouraged to remain in anxiety-provoking situations to promote habituation. Theoretically, those receiving CBT for trichotillomania might be better served by reducing urges and altering hair-pulling cues (e.g., exiting high-risk situations, using competing response strategies) rather than completing focused exposures without adjunctive efforts to reduce anxiety (as in exposure and ritual prevention for OCD), given that positive rather than negative reinforcement is more likely to underlie trichotillomania behaviors. In order to weaken pulling urges, trichotillomania patients must learn not to positively reinforce urges by pulling; out of this conceptualization comes habit reversal, which is essentially the substitution of an alternative positively reinforcing behavior that is incompatible with pulling.

Although a detailed consideration of other body-focused impulse-control disorders such as skin picking and severe nail biting is beyond the scope of this chapter, many experts (e.g., Christenson and Mansueto 1999) have noted formal similarities among these conditions as well as common co-occurrence. As with trichotillomania, it is important conceptually to determine the function of the behavior in order to decide how to define and treat it. If the skin picking and nail biting appear to be largely negatively reinforcing—that is, reducing anxiety associated with specific obsessional thoughts and/or reducing the likelihood of feared outcomes—they may be better conceptualized as OCD behaviors and addressed accordingly. In our clinical experience these conditions are much more likely to formally resemble trichotillomania as described earlier and thus may very well fit the conceptual model we describe in this chapter. Nevertheless, much more research is needed to determine how these conditions differ in order to say with confidence whether they are all one entity or conceptually distinct conditions that require separate theoretical consideration and treatment approaches.

Treatment

Alarmingly, a review of the literature reveals that only seven randomized trials have been conducted thus far, six of which included a control condition. The treatment literature is generally made up of case studies, with progressively more controlled investigation in recent years. In general, knowledge about trichotillomania treatments is limited by small sample sizes, lack of specificity regarding sample characteristics, nonrandom assignment to treatment, dearth of long-term follow-up data, exclusive reliance on patient self-report measures, and lack of information regarding rates of treatment refusal and dropout.

Pharmacotherapy

Of the six randomized controlled trials evaluating the efficacy of pharmacotherapy conducted to date, five involved the evaluation of serotonin reuptake inhibitors. This may reflect the previously prevailing view that trichotillomania is a variant of OCD and thus ought to be responsive to the same pharmacological agents that have proven successful in ameliorating OCD symptoms.

Swedo et al. (1989) conducted a double-blind crossover study with 14 women and found clomipramine superior to desipramine after treatment. However, long-term response to clomipramine varied widely, with an overall 40% reduction in symptoms maintained at 4-year follow-up (Swedo et al. 1993). Christenson et al. (1991c) failed to demonstrate the superiority of fluoxetine over placebo in a double-blind crossover study; in that trial, neither condition improved hair pulling significantly. Following on from Christenson et al. (1991c), Streichenwein and Thornby (1995) also failed to show any difference between fluoxetine and placebo in reducing hair pulling despite having lengthened the treatment phase and increasing the maximum fluoxetine dose to 80 mg. In the first study that examined the efficacy of pharmacotherapy and an active comparator, Ninan et al. (2000) compared clomipramine, CBT, and placebo. CBT produced greater changes in hair-pulling severity and associated impairment and yielded a significantly higher responder rate; differences between clomipramine and placebo approached but did not achieve statistical significance. Similarly, another randomized, controlled trial found CBT superior to fluoxetine and a waiting-list condition but failed to find a significant treatment effect for fluoxetine (van Minnen et al. 2003). Taken together, results from these controlled studies of serotonin reuptake inhibitors are equivocal at best, although in view of the small sample sizes more controlled research should still be conducted to determine their efficacy more definitively.

Although double-blind discontinuation studies have not been conducted in trichotillomania, accumulating evidence from open studies suggests that treatment response gained from pharmacotherapy may not be maintained in the long run. For example, an uncontrolled study by Pollard et al. (1991) indicated that the majority of a small sample of patients treated with clomipramine lost their treatment gains even while being maintained on a previously therapeutic dose of the drug. In addition, a retrospective study by Iancu et al. (1996) found that of patients receiving treatment with serotonergic drugs, 75% achieved a clinically significant response during the first 2 months, but symptoms returned to pretreatment levels during the third month with continued medication.

As is evident from this review, the trichotillomania pharmacotherapy literature to date is both underdeveloped and equivocal. Serotonin reuptake inhibitors, the class of medication found routinely efficacious in OCD, have generally not yielded promising outcomes in trichotillomania. Perhaps, as we discussed earlier, important differences between OCD and trichotillomania underlie this apparent difference in treatment response. Intriguingly, naltrexone, an opioid-blocking compound thought to decrease positive reinforcement by preventing the binding of endogenous opiates to relevant receptor sites in the brain, has also been found superior to placebo in reducing trichotillomania symptoms (Christenson et al. 1994b). In addition, several case studies have indicated that augmentation of selective serotonin reuptake inhibitors with atypical neuroleptics may be beneficial (Epperson et al. 1999; Stein and Hollander 1992), and a recent open trial suggested that olanzapine may be efficacious as a monotherapy for trichotillomania (Stewart and Nejtek 2003). Clearly there is much more work to be done in the area of pharmacotherapy development and outcome evaluation; the absence of a single randomized, controlled trial in pediatric trichotillomania severely limits treatment recommendations that can be made to parents whose children have this disorder.

Psychotherapy

With respect to behavioral approaches and CBT packages, a variety of specific techniques have been applied, including awareness training, self-monitoring, aversion, covert sensitization, negative practice, relaxation training, habit reversal, competing response training, stimulus control, and overcorrection. Although the state of the CBT literature justifies only cautious recommendations, habit reversal, awareness training, and stimulus control are generally purported as the core efficacious interventions for trichotillomania, with other intervention strategies such as cognitive techniques to be used on an as-needed basis. As emphasized in the following review, however, more research is needed to dismantle the effectiveness of multicomponent behavioral programs and inform the development of more efficacious and durable cognitive-behavioral interventions.

Successful outcome has been reported on several of the aforementioned interventions. However, because the vast majority of the literature consists of uncontrolled case reports or small case series, confident conclusions cannot be drawn about the specificity of the observed reductions. Three randomized trials with adults have been conducted regarding the efficacy of CBT. As mentioned earlier, Ninan et al. (2000) found CBT superior to both clomipramine and placebo at posttreatment, which is the same pattern reported by van Minnen et al. (2003) in their recently completed randomized, controlled trial involving CBT, fluoxetine, and a wait-list condition. In the only published comparison with another psychosocial intervention, Azrin et al. (1980) found that habit reversal was more effective than negative practice; habit-reversal patients reported a 99% reduction in the number of hair-pulling episodes compared with a 58% reduction for negative practice patients. Moreover, the habit-reversal group maintained its gains at 22-month follow-up, with patients reporting an 87% reduction compared with pretreatment rates. Although these results are encouraging, the study's ultimate utility is limited by methodological issues including exclusive reliance on patient self-report, substantial attrition (7 of 19) during the follow-up phase, and the absence of a formal treatment manual to allow for replication.

The significant problem of relapse following CBT approaches, which is certainly a common phenomenon reported clinically, was highlighted in an open study in which patients received nine sessions of CBT involving habit reversal (Lerner et al. 1998). Twelve of 14 patients were classified as responders at posttreatment (>50% National Institute of Mental Health—Trichotillomania Severity Scale [NIMH-TSS] reduction), yet only 4 of 13 met this criterion an average of 3.9 years posttreatment. Keuthen et al.'s (2001) naturalistic follow-up of patients who received state-of-the-art pharmacotherapy or behavior therapy further underscored concern about maintenance of gains. Similarly, Mouton and Stanley (1996) found that whereas four of five patients benefited initially from group habit-reversal therapy, only two patients maintained clinically significant gains at 6-month follow-up.

Generally speaking, the limited and equivocal treatment literature strongly suggests that there is neither a universal nor a complete response to any treatments for trichotillomania. Given that monotherapy with CBT or pharmacotherapy is likely to produce only partial symptom reduction in the long run, these therapies might yield superior improvement when combined. Unfortunately, the absence of any controlled studies examining the efficacy of CBT treatments involving habit reversal, pharmacotherapy, and their combination weakens this claim considerably.

Toward an Empirical Understanding of Trichotillomania

There is a clear need for improved efficacy of psychological and pharmacological treatments for trichotillomania. We suggest that the available treatments are only as good as the empirical model upon which they are based. To date, there has been insufficient experimental study of the psychopathology of hair pulling, which results in critical gaps in our understanding of the factors that cause and/or maintain this behavior. The corollary of this idea is that an enhanced empirical understanding of hair pulling will lead to a more comprehensive biopsychosocial model of trichotillomania, which will in turn inform the next generation of therapeutic interventions (Foa and Kozak 1997).

Figure 7–1 shows a schematic diagram of a preliminary biopsychosocial model of trichotillomania. We stress that this model is preliminary, because the available experimental and descriptive psychopathology research in trichotillomania is relatively sparse. Therefore, the primary aim of this model is heuristic rather than explanatory. Our hope is that it will stimulate new studies on the mechanisms of trichotillomania and will be modified over time as new data become available. In the following sections, we describe each component of the model in detail.

Biological Vulnerability

It is likely that biological vulnerabilities increase the probability that a person will develop trichotillomania. Familial research suggests that trichotillomania may be associated with increased rates of OCD or other excessive habits among first-degree relatives (Bienvenu et al. 2000; King et al. 1995; Lenane et al. 1992). This finding is consistent with the notion of a genetic basis for a spectrum of excessive grooming behaviors that include trichotillomania, although environmental factors such as social learning cannot be ruled out as yet.

Neuroimaging research has demonstrated hyperactivity in the left cerebellum and right superior parietal lobe (Swedo et al. 1991) as well as possible structural abnormalities in the left putamen (O'Sullivan et al. 1997), left inferior frontal gyrus, and right cuneal cortex (Grachev 1997). Furthermore, trichotillomania patients have been shown to make errors in spatial processing (Rettew et al. 1991), divided attention (Stanley et al. 1997), and nonverbal memory and executive functioning (Keuthen et al. 1996), although we note that in the latter study, Bonferroni correction for multiple comparisons would have made these differences nonsignificant. Studies such as these do not necessarily imply that preexisting brain abnormalities cause the symptoms of trichotillomania; it is entirely possible that chronic trichotillomania or its associated features lead to

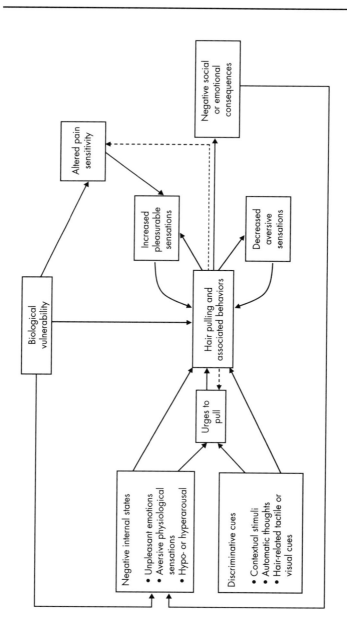

Figure 7–1.   Schematic diagram of a preliminary biopsychosocial model of trichotillomania.

changes in brain structure or function or that both trichotillomania and the brain abnormalities are caused by a third, as yet unknown, variable.

We also suspect that a nonspecific biological vulnerability is manifested in difficulty tolerating discomfort. That is, individuals who feel a need to control or eliminate their uncomfortable emotions or sensations might be at greater risk to develop trichotillomania and perhaps other disorders as well. This notion of "experiential avoidance" has been forwarded as a vulnerability factor for general psychopathology by Hayes and colleagues (e.g., Hayes et al. 1999), and intolerance of aversive states has been noted in anxiety disorders (Ladouceur et al. 2000; Reiss et al. 1986; Tolin et al. 2003). A preliminary investigation of experiential avoidance in trichotillomania suggested that a tendency to avoid unpleasant emotions was related to severity of hair-pulling urges (Begotka et al. 2003). However, the relationship, although significant, was relatively weak. This may relate to the fact that the investigators used a questionnaire that assessed primarily anxiety- and depression-related avoidance rather than an avoidance of physiological arousal or other sensations that may be more directly applicable to trichotillomania. This study also did not use a nonclinical control group; thus, range restriction may have been a factor. Clearly, more research is needed to investigate the relationship between experiential avoidance and hair pulling and, more broadly, to examine whether experiential avoidance is related to biological factors and whether it represents a global diathesis for the development of maladaptive behaviors.

Altered Pain Sensitivity

Individuals with trichotillomania often report that hair pulling is not painful (Christenson et al. 1991b; Sanderson and Hall-Smith 1970) or in many cases that it feels good or pleasurable (Stanley et al. 1992). To our knowledge, no direct tests have been conducted to compare hair-pulling sensations between persons with trichotillomania and those without. However, we suspect that individuals without trichotillomania generally do not derive pleasure from pulling; rather, they are likely to describe it as painful. Thus, it is possible that alterations in pain sensitivity influence the reinforcing quality of pulling behavior. One possible mechanism for such alterations is upregulation of the endogenous opioid system; this model has not been supported by challenge tasks (Frecska and Arato 2002), although some evidence suggests that pulling may decrease with administration of opiate receptor antagonists (Carrion 1995; Christenson et al. 1994b). Intriguingly, dogs with acral lick dermatitis (a potential animal model of trichotillomania) show reductions in evoked sensory nerve action potentials (van Nes 1986), possibly suggesting decreased pain sensitivity. However, trichotillomania patients do not appear to show reduced pain in nonpulling areas such as the fingertips (Christenson et al. 1994a). It may be that pain sensations are not globally altered in trichotillomania but rather are diminished only at the sites of pulling. This may result from habituation of the pain response caused by repeated pulling over time, although pain absence has been noted even in young children with short pulling histories (Chang et al. 1991). To date, no studies of pain tolerance at the preferred pulling site have been conducted. For those patients who do experience pulling-related pain, the pain itself may be reinforcing because it distracts the individual from negative emotional or physiological states (Christenson and Mansueto 1999).

Hair-Pulling Cues

The behavioral model of hair pulling suggests that pulling begins as a normal response to stress but eventually becomes associated with a variety of internal and external cues through conditioning mechanisms (Azrin and Nunn 1973; Mansueto et al. 1997). Descriptive research has indicated that situations associated with hyperarousal (e.g., negative affective states) or hypoarousal (e.g., boredom, fatigue, sedentary activities) are common cues for hair pulling. For example, Christenson et al. (1993) identified two factors of hair-pulling cues: negative affect and sedentary/contemplative cues. The negative affect component was composed of feeling terms (e.g., feeling angry, feeling hurt) and situations associated with negative self-evaluation (e.g., weighing yourself, interpersonal conflicts). The sedentary/contemplative component comprised situations associated with fatigue (e.g., lack of sleep) and directed attention (e.g., reading, television). However the relationship between pulling cues and trichotillomania "subtypes" requires further examination. Physical sensations have also been identified as arousal cues for hair pulling. For example Mansueto (1990) found that a substantial minority of patients reported skin sensitivity (25%), itching (23%), irritation (16%), pressure (14%), and burning sensations (5%) preceding pulling episodes.

Cognitive components are also involved at least to some extent in conceptualizing this disorder, in that cognitions may serve as cues and consequences to the behavioral sequence. In some cases, negative cognitions about the pulling habit itself, such as fear of negative evaluation, may also play a role in the perpetuation of pulling, because these cognitions result in increased negative emotion that in turn may increase urges to pull. Additionally, patients sometimes worry that the urges to pull will never go away or will get stronger until they pull, despite their being able to provide ample evidence to the contrary from their own experience with urges. Belief in the positive effects of hair pulling (e.g., "Hair pulling will make me feel better") or pulling-facilitative thoughts (e.g., "I'll just pull one") may also cue pulling episodes (Gluhoski 1995).

Another category of potential pulling triggers is contextual cues, which may not have originally been associated with pulling or pulling-related feelings or sensations but by the process of associative conditioning have become linked with these factors through repetitive pulling episodes. Common contextual cues for pulling include visual signs that hair is misshapen or unattractive (e.g., asymmetrical hair, gray hair), tactile sensations (e.g., feeling a coarse hair), places or activities where pulling has occurred in the past (e.g., bathroom, bed, watching television), being alone, or the presence of pulling implements (e.g., tweezers). Both arousal and contextual cues may be associated with pulling, either directly or through the mediation of a hair-pulling "urge." Over time, hair-pulling urges that are reinforced by pulling lead to stronger urges to pull, which perpetuates the behavioral cycle.

Reinforcement

As described earlier, hair pulling is often preceded by negative internal states such as unpleasant emotions, aversive physiological sensations, or dysregulated arousal. Hair pulling, in turn, appears to result in a decrease of these states. In retrospective reports, trichotillomania patients report that pulling leads to reduced feelings of tension, boredom, and anxiety, whereas nonclinical hair pullers also report reductions in sadness and anger (Stanley et al. 1995). In these cases, hair pulling is negatively reinforced and is thus functionally somewhat similar to the compulsive behaviors seen in OCD (Tolin and Foa 2001). However, to the extent that hair pulling evokes pleasurable sensations (Stanley et al. 1992), the pulling habit may also be strengthened via *positive* reinforcement (Azrin and Nunn 1973; Mansueto et al. 1997). Pleasure may be obtained not only through pulling but also through associated behaviors such as playing with or inspecting the hair, oral stimulation, or trichophagia (Christenson and Mansueto 1999). Thus, pulling may be maintained by either negative or positive reinforcement. Our clinical observations suggest that some trichotillomania patients may experience one or the other form of reinforcement, or different kinds of reinforcement may be active for the same person at different times. We propose that careful attention to the specific hair-pulling contingencies is critical in developing a functional analysis and planning therapeutic interventions for trichotillomania.

Delayed Consequences of Pulling

Although hair pulling is immediately reinforced via its consequent emotional or interoceptive changes, longer-term negative consequences of pulling also exist. The most obvious delayed consequence of hair pulling is the negative impact on physical appearance, which many hair pullers take great efforts to conceal. Concealment of hair loss can take the form of wigs or special makeup, which can be costly, time consuming, and uncomfortable. Increases in negative emotional states, including guilt, sadness, and anger, also occur after pulling episodes for trichotillomania patients (Diefenbach et al. 2002). Hair pulling has also been associated with negative self-evaluation, frustration over lacking control of pulling behaviors, and low self-esteem (Casati et al. 2000; Soriano et al. 1996; Stemberger et al. 2000). Hair pulling can also lead to negative social consequences. In an experimental study, adolescents viewing videotapes of individuals pulling hair rated hair pullers lower in social acceptability than those who were not pulling hair (Boudjouk et al. 2000). Consequently, hair pullers have reported interpersonal conflicts, social isolation, and loneliness (Casati et al. 2000; Stemberger et al. 2000). However, as with many maladaptive behaviors (e.g., smoking, overeating), the short-term reinforcement value often overpowers the delayed aversive consequences, resulting in continued pulling. In fact, the longer-term consequences may even serve to escalate the pulling cycle by providing a new stimulus cue (e.g., negative self-evaluative thoughts, negative affect) that can prompt additional pulling episodes. Given the importance of pulling resistance and tolerance of subsequent uncomfortable affect to the eventual discontinuation of pulling (through extinction of reinforcing consequences), investigations into interventions that maximize these factors (e.g., acceptance and commitment therapy, motivational interviewing) may be fruitful.

Summary

At present, the experimental and descriptive psychopathology literature in trichotillomania is quite "young," and there is a clear need for additional research in this area. However, preliminary data are converging on a tentative biopsychosocial model in which biologically vulnerable individuals become trapped in cycles of hair pulling that are triggered by internal and contextual discriminative cues and subsequently reinforced because the behavior reduces a variety of negative internal stimuli or elicits positive sensations. This cycle persists despite clear negative social and emotional consequences because such consequences are delayed and thus are outweighed by more immediate and salient reinforcers. We fully expect that additional research will result in the modification of this preliminary model and we hope, in the spirit of Foa and Kozak (1997), that a more comprehensive and empirically informed model will break the apparent "efficacy ceiling" of trichotillomania treatment and lead to more effective interventions.

Future Directions

Several steps can be taken to rectify the dearth of trichotillomania research. A large-scale epidemiological study should be conducted to determine the point and lifetime prevalence rates of the disorder in pediatric and adult samples. Although some small-scale prevalence studies have hinted that trichotillomania is a surprisingly common condition, a larger epidemiological effort would clarify the need to direct resources toward the scientific study of this problem.

Another essential issue to be addressed is the improved assessment of functional impairment measures in trichotillomania. Those who treat patients with trichotillomania know from clinical experience that these patients are often isolated, avoidant of situations in which their alopecia and pulling behavior might be discovered (e.g., swimming, dating), and frequently feel inferior or "weird," but as yet there is little empirical research documenting dysfunction in these important dimensions. Use of existing psychometrically sound measures (e.g., Medical Outcomes Survey) and development of new trichotillomania-specific interference instruments may be used to accompany symptom measures and improve understanding of trichotillomania's impact on hair pullers as well as the effects of treatments.

Longitudinal research is also needed to determine the percentage of people with trichotillomania whose hair pulling remits without intervention; examination of factors associated with maintenance of pulling behavior over time may help determine which hair pullers ought to be targeted for earlier intervention. These types of studies are contingent on the development of psychometrically sound interviews and self-report measures, a process that has already begun in adult trichotillomania (Keuthen et al. 1995; O'Sullivan et al. 1995) and is now under way with younger samples (Diefenbach et al. 2003). Once available, these measures will set the stage for the epidemiological and longitudinal studies described earlier.

Experimental psychopathology studies linking psychological and biological methods would also go a long way toward closing the current knowledge gaps and perhaps would stimulate a more interdisciplinary approach to the treatment of this condition. The prevailing biological theory of dysfunction, namely a serotonin deficit, may require reconsideration given the relatively poor treatment response demonstrated thus far with medications that are selective for that neurotransmitter. It may be especially useful to examine psychological and biological measures while a patient is pulling or resisting urges to pull. For example, psychophysiological research may explore the modulation function of hair pulling to establish a relationship between changes in subjective experiences (e.g., decreased urge, decreased tension) and physiological responding over the hair-pulling cycle. Additionally, studies of pulling site–specific pain tolerance may very well shed light on an ongoing area of controversy, namely whether trichotillomania patients experience pain at the pulling site when pulling and whether there are biological correlates to the subjective experience that may help us better understand trichotillomania.

The meager treatment outcome literature and the equivocal findings from randomized, controlled trials suggest that there is much to do with respect to trichotillomania intervention research. Preliminary evidence suggests that CBT is effective for many trichotillomania patients; however, additional trials comparing CBT with alternative psychological (e.g., supportive counseling) and pharmacological (e.g., serotonin reuptake inhibitor medications, naltrexone) treatments are needed. Given the possible role of experiential avoidance in the etiology and/or maintenance of trichotillomania, the addition of mindfulness/acceptance strategies may also prove fruitful. Next, dismantling research is critical for identifying the efficacious elements of CBT; additional research on which patients respond to which elements would also be helpful in the construction of treatment-planning algorithms. Additional biological research is needed to examine patterns of abnormal neurotransmitter and brain metabolic activity in those with trichotillomania and the effect of specific compounds on these factors. Most research to date has focused on serotonergic medications; however, research into other strategies (e.g., opioid blockers, glutamatergic compounds) may also be useful. Following this, effectiveness research is needed to determine the degree to which CBT and pharmacological algorithms can be successfully implemented in front-line mental health settings with less rigidly selected patients. These research steps will be greatly facilitated by improved theoretical models of trichotillomania based on additional experimental psychopathology findings, epidemiological evidence, and functional impairment data.

References

American Psychiatric Association: Diagnostic and statistical manual of mental disorders, 4th Edition, Text Revision. Washington, DC, American Psychiatric Association, 2000

Azrin NH, Nunn RG: Habit-reversal: a method of eliminating nervous habits and tics. Behav Res Ther 11:619–628, 1973

Azrin NH, Nunn RG, Frantz SE : Treatment of hair pulling (trichotillomania): a comparative study of habit reversal and negative practice training. J Behav Ther Exp Psychiatry 11:13–20, 1980

Begotka AM, Woods DW, Wetterneck CT: The relationship between experiential avoidance and the severity of trichotillomania in a nonreferred sample. Manuscript submitted for publication, 2003

Bienvenu OJ, Samuels JF, Riddle MA, et al: The relationship of obsessive-compulsive disorder to possible spectrum disorders: results from a family study. Biol Psychiatry 48:287–293, 2000

Boudjouk PJ, Woods DW, Miltenberger RG, et al: Negative peer evaluation in adolescents: effects of tic disorders and trichotillomania. Child and Family Behavior Therapy 22:17–28, 2000

Carrion VG: Naltrexone for the treatment of trichotillomania: a case report. J Clin Psychopharmacol 15:444–445, 1995

Casati J, Toner BB, Yu B: Psychosocial issues for women with trichotillomania. Compr Psychiatry 41:344–351, 2000

Chang CH, Lee MB, Chiang YC: Trichotillomania: a clinical study of 36 patients. J Formos Med Assoc 90:176–180, 1991

Christenson GA: Trichotillomania: from prevalence to comorbidity. Psychiatric Times 12:44–48, 1995

Christenson GA, Mackenzie TB: Trichotillomania, in Handbook of Prescriptive Treatments for Adults. Edited by Hersen M, Ammerman RT. New York, Plenum, 1994, pp 217–235

Christenson GA, Mansueto CS: Trichotillomania: descriptive characteristics and phenomenology, in Trichotillomania. Edited by Stein DJ, Christenson GA, Hollander E. Washington, DC, American Psychiatric Press, 1999, pp 1–41

Christenson GA, O'Sullivan RL: Trichotillomania: rational treatment options. CNS Drugs 6:23–34, 1996

Christenson GA, Mackenzie TB, Mitchell JE: Characteristics of 60 adult chronic hair pullers. Am J Psychiatry 148:365–370, 1991a

Christenson GA, Pyle RL, Mitchell JE: Estimated lifetime prevalence of trichotillomania in college students. J Clin Psychol 52:415–417, 1991b

Christenson GA, Mackenzie TB, Mitchell JE, et al: A placebo-controlled, double-blind crossover study of fluoxetine in trichotillomania. Am J Psychiatry 148:1566–1571, 1991c

Christenson GA, Chernoff-Clementz E, Clementz BA: Personality and clinical characteristics in patients with trichotillomania. J Clin Psychiatry 53:407–413, 1992

Christenson GA, Ristvedt SL, MacKenzie TB: Identification of trichotillomania cue profiles. Behav Res Ther 31:315–320, 1993

Christenson GA, Raymond NC, Faris PL, et al: Pain thresholds are not elevated in trichotillomania. Biol Psychiatry 36:347–349, 1994a

Christenson GA, Crow SJ, Mackenzie TB: A placebo controlled double blind study of naltrexone for trichotillomania. Paper presented at the 147th annual meeting of the American Psychiatric Association, Philadelphia, PA, May 1994b

Diefenbach GJ, Mouton-Odum S, Stanley MA: Affective correlates of trichotillomania. Behav Res Ther 40:1305–1315, 2002

Diefenbach GJ, Tolin DF, Franklin ME, et al: The Trichotillomania Scale for Children (TSC): a new self-report measure to assess pediatric hair pulling. Paper presented at the annual meeting of the Association for Advancement of Behavior Therapy, Boston, MA, November 2003

du Toit PL, van Kradenburg J, Niehaus DHJ, et al: Characteristics and phenomenology of hair-pulling: an exploration of subtypes. Compr Psychiatry 42:247–256, 2001

Epperson NC, Fasula D, Wasylink S, et al: Risperidone addition in serotonin reuptake inhibitor-resistant trichotillomania: three cases. J Child Adolesc Psychopharmacol 9:43–49, 1999

Foa EB, Kozak MJ: Beyond the efficacy ceiling? Cognitive behavior therapy in search of theory. Behav Ther 28:601–611, 1997

Franklin ME, Keuthen NJ, Spokas ME, et al: Pediatric trichotillomania: descriptive psychopathology and comorbid symptomatology. Paper presented at the Trichotillomania: Psychopathology and Treatment Development Symposium, conducted at the 36th annual meeting of the Association for the Advancement of Behavior Therapy, Reno, NV, November 2002

Frecska E, Arato M: Opiate sensitivity test in patients with stereotypic movement disorder and trichotillomania. Prog Neuropsychopharmacol Biol Psychiatry 26:909–912, 2002

Gluhoski VL: A cognitive approach for treating trichotillomania. J Psychother Pract Res 4:277–285, 1995

Grachev ID: MRI-based morphometric topographic parcellation of human neocortex in trichotillomania. Psychiatry Clin Neurosci 51:315–321, 1997

Hajcak G, Franklin ME, Simons RF, et al: Hair pulling and skin picking in a large college sample: prevalence and relationship to affective distress and obsessive-compulsive symptoms. Manuscript submitted for publication, 2004

Hanna GL: Trichotillomania and related disorders in children and adolescents. Child Psychiatry Hum Dev 27:255–268, 1997

Hayes SC, Strosahl KD, Wilson KG: Acceptance and Commitment Therapy: An Experiential Approach to Behavior Change. New York, Guilford, 1999

Himle JA, Bordnick PS, Thyer BA: A comparison of trichotillomania and obsessive-compulsive disorder. Journal of Psychopathology and Behavioral Assessment 17:251–260, 1995

Iancu I, Weizman A, Kindler S, et al: Serotonergic drugs in trichotillomania: treatment results in 12 patients. J Nerv Ment Dis 184:641–644, 1996

Jenike MA: Obsessive-compulsive and related disorders: a hidden epidemic. N Engl J Med 321:539–541, 1989

Keuthen NJ, O'Sullivan RL, Ricciardi JN, et al: The Massachusetts General Hospital (MGH) Hair Pulling Scale, 1: development and factor analyses. Psychother Psychosom 64:141–145, 1995

Keuthen NJ, Savage CR, O'Sullivan RL, et al: Neuropsychological functioning in trichotillomania. Biol Psychiatry 39:747–749, 1996

Keuthen NJ, Fraim C, Deckersbach TD, et al: Longitudinal follow-up of naturalistic treatment outcome in patients with trichotillomania. J Clin Psychiatry 62:101–107, 2001

Keuthen NJ, Franklin ME, Bohne A, et al: Functional impairment associated with trichotillomania and implications for treatment development. Paper presented at the Trichotillomania: Psychopathology and Treatment Development Symposium, conducted at the 36th annual meeting of the Association for the Advancement of Behavior Therapy, Reno, NV, November 2002

King RA, Scahill L, Vitulano LA, et al: Childhood trichotillomania: clinical phenomenology, comorbidity, and family genetics. J Am Acad Child Adolesc Psychiatry 34:1451–1459, 1995

Koran L, Ringold A, Hewlett W: Fluoxetine for trichotillomania: an open clinical trial. Psychopharmacol Bull 28:145–149, 1992

Koran LM, Thienemann ML, Davenport R: Quality of life for patients with obsessive-compulsive disorder. Am J Psychiatry 153:783–788, 1996

Ladouceur R, Gosselin P, Dugas MJ: Experimental manipulation of intolerance of uncertainty: a study of a theoretical model of worry. Behav Res Ther 38:933–941, 2000

Lenane MC, Swedo SE, Rapoport JL, et al: Rates of obsessive compulsive disorder in first degree relatives of patients with trichotillomania: a research note. J Child Psychol Psychiatry 33:925–933, 1992

Lerner J, Franklin ME, Meadows EA, et al: Effectiveness of a cognitive-behavioral treatment program for trichotillomania: an uncontrolled evaluation. Behav Ther 29:157–171, 1998

Mannino FV, Delgado RA: Trichotillomania in children: a review. Am J Psychiatry 126:505–511, 1969

Mansueto CS: Typography and phenomenology of trichotillomania. Paper presented at the annual convention of the Association for Advancement of Behavior Therapy, San Francisco, CA, November 1990

Mansueto CS, Stemberger RMT, Thomas AM, et al: Trichotillomania: a comprehensive behavioral model. Clin Psychol Rev 17:567–577, 1997

Mouton SG, Stanley MA: Habit reversal training for trichotillomania: a group approach. Cognitive and Behavioral Practice 3:159–182, 1996

Ninan PT, Rothbaum BO, Marsteller FA, et al: A placebo-controlled trial of cognitive-behavioral therapy and clomipramine in trichotillomania. J Clin Psychiatry 61:47–50, 2000

O'Sullivan RL, Keuthen NJ, Hayday CF, et al: The Massachusetts Hospital (MGH) Hair Pulling Scale, 2: reliability and validity. Psychother Psychosom 64:146–148, 1995

O'Sullivan RL, Rauch SL, Breiter HC, et al: Reduced basal ganglia volumes in trichotillomania measured via morphometric magnetic resonance imaging. Biol Psychiatry 42:39–45, 1997

Pollard CA, Ibe IO, Krojanker DN, et al: Clomipramine treatment of trichotillomania: a follow-up report on four cases. J Clin Psychiatry 52:128–130, 1991

Reeve E: Hair pulling in children and adolescents, in Trichotillomania. Edited by Stein DJ, Christenson GA, Hollander E. Washington, DC, American Psychiatric Press, 1999, pp 201–224

Reeve EA, Bernstein GA, Christenson GA: Clinical characteristics and psychiatric comorbidity in children with trichotillomania. J Am Acad Child Adolesc Psychiatry 31:132–138, 1992

Reiss S, Peterson RA, Gursky DM, et al: Anxiety sensitivity, anxiety frequency and the prediction of fearfulness. Behav Res Ther 24:1–8, 1986

Rettew DC, Cheslow DL, Rapoport JL, et al: Neuropsychological test performance in trichotillomania: a further link with obsessive-compulsive disorder. J Anxiety Disord 5:225–235, 1991

Rothbaum BO, Shaw L, Morris R, et al: Prevalence of trichotillomania in a college freshman population (letter to the editor). J Clin Psychiatry 54:72, 1993

Sanderson KV, Hall-Smith P: Tonsure trichotillomania. Br J Dermatol 82:343–350, 1970

Schlosser S, Black DW, Blum N, et al: The demography, phenomenology, and family history of 22 persons with compulsive hair pulling. Ann Clin Psychiatry 6:147–152, 1994

Soriano JL, O'Sullivan RL, Baer L, et al: Trichotillomania and self-esteem: a survey of 62 female hair pullers. J Clin Psychiatry 57:77–82, 1996

Stanley MA, Cohen LJ: Trichotillomania and obsessive-compulsive disorder, in Trichotillomania. Edited by Stein DJ, Christenson GA, Hollander E. Washington, DC, American Psychiatric Press, 1999, pp 225–261

Stanley MA, Swann AC, Bowers TC, et al: A comparison of clinical features in trichotillomania and obsessive-compulsive disorder. Behav Res Ther 30:39–44, 1992

Stanley MA, Borden JW, Mouton SG, et al: Nonclinical hair-pulling: affective correlates and comparison with clinical samples. Behav Res Ther 33:179–186, 1995

Stanley MA, Hannay HJ, Breckenridge JK: The neuropsychology of trichotillomania. J Anxiety Disord 11:473–488, 1997

Stein DJ, Hollander E: Low-dose pimozide augmentation of serotonin reuptake blockers in the treatment of trichotillomania. J Clin Psychiatry 53:123–126, 1992

Stemberger RMT, Thomas AM, Mansueto CS, et al: Personal toll of trichotillomania: behavioral and interpersonal sequelae. J Anxiety Disord 14:97–104, 2000

Stewart RS, Nejtek VA: An open-label, flexible-dose study of olanzapine in the treatment of trichotillomania. J Clin Psychiatry 64:49–52, 2003

Streichenwein SM, Thornby JI: A long-term, double-blind, placebo-controlled crossover trial of the efficacy of fluoxetine for trichotillomania. Am J Psychiatry 152:1192–1196, 1995

Swedo SE: Trichotillomania. Psychiatr Ann 23:402–407, 1993

Swedo SE, Leonard HL: Trichotillomania: an obsessive compulsive spectrum disorder? Psychiatr Clin North Am 15:777–790, 1992

Swedo SE, Leonard HL, Rapoport JL, et al: A double-blind comparison of clomipramine and desipramine in the treatment of trichotillomania hair pulling. N Engl J Med 321:497–501, 1989

Swedo SE, Rapoport JL, Leonard HL, et al: Regional cerebral glucose metabolism of women in trichotillomania. Arch Gen Psychiatry 48:828–833, 1991

Swedo SE, Lenane MC, Leonard HL: Long-term treatment of trichotillomania (hair pulling) (letter to the editor). N Engl J Med 329:141–142, 1993

Tolin DF, Foa EB: Compulsions, in The Corsini Encyclopedia of Psychology and Behavioral Science, 3rd Edition. Edited by Craighead WE, Nemeroff CB. New York, Wiley, 2001, pp 338–339

Tolin D, Franklin ME, Diefenbach G, et al: CBT for pediatric trichotillomania: an open trial. Paper presented at the Trichotillomania: Psychopathology and Treatment Development Symposium, conducted at the 36th annual meeting of the Association for the Advancement of Behavior Therapy, Reno, NV, November 2002

Tolin DF, Abramowitz JS, Brigidi BD, et al: Intolerance of uncertainty in obsessive-compulsive disorder. J Anxiety Disord 17:233–242, 2003

Tukel R, Keser V, Karali NT, et al: Comparison of clinical characteristics in trichotillomania and obsessive-compulsive disorder. J Anxiety Disord 15:433–441, 2001

van Minnen A, Hoogduin KA, Keijsers GP, et al: Treatment of trichotillomania with behavioral therapy or fluoxetine. Arch Gen Psychiatry 60:517–522, 2003

van Nes JJ: Electrophysiological evidence of sensory nerve dysfunction in 10 dogs with acral lick dermatitis. J Am Anim Hosp Assoc 22:157–160, 1986

Ware JE Jr: SF-36 Health Survey Manual and Interpretation Guide. Boston, MA, The Health Institute, New England Medical Center, 1993

8

Kleptomania

Jon E. Grant, J.D., M.D.

History and Classification

One of the first recorded cases of possible kleptomania came from the British legal system at the end of the eighteenth century. This 1799 case involved Mrs. Jane Leigh-Perrot, Jane Austen's aunt and a wealthy woman of Bath, who was arrested for stealing lace. Financially able to purchase the lace, she did in fact buy one piece of lace at the same time she stole another. Given the value of the lace she stole, she faced grand larceny charges punishable by hanging or 14 years in jail. A number of socially and politically prominent people attested to Mrs. Leigh-Perrot's good character in court. Because the defendant was a respectable woman with no apparent reason to steal, the jury found her not guilty (James 1977).

In the early nineteenth century, medical literature began to recognize that a subgroup of shoplifters, like Jane Leigh-Perrot, appeared to steal items they could have obtained by legitimate means. Matthey (1816) described the act of compulsive stealing worthless or unneeded objects "klopemanie" (McElroy et al. 1991a), a term later changed to "kleptomanie" by Marc and Esquirol in 1838 to suggest "stealing madness" (Esquirol 1838). Later in the same century, Lasègue (1880/1881) described the classic kleptomania patient as a "respectable middle-aged housewife shoplifter" (James 1977), a characterization that still persists.

Kleptomania was first officially designated a psychiatric disorder in 1980 in DSM-III (American Psychiatric Association 1980), and in DSM-III-R (American Psychiatric Association 1987) it was grouped under the category "disorders of impulse control not elsewhere classified." As an impulse-control disorder, kleptomania is currently classified in DSM-IV-TR (American Psychiatric Association 2000) with pathological gambling, pyromania, intermittent explosive disorder, and trichotillomania. Although included in DSM-IV-TR, kleptomania is still a poorly understood disorder and has received very little empirical study.

DSM-IV-TR defines *kleptomania* as A) recurrent failure to resist impulses to steal objects that are not needed for personal use or for their monetary value; B) increasing sense of tension immediately before committing the theft; C) pleasure, gratification, or release at the time of committing the theft; D) not committed to express anger or vengeance or in response to a delusion or a hallucination; and E) not better accounted for by conduct disorder, a manic episode, or antisocial personality disorder (American Psychiatric Association 2000, p. 669; see Table 8–1).

Table 8–1.   DSM-IV-TR diagnostic criteria for kleptomania

A. Recurrent failure to resist impulses to steal objects that are not needed for personal use or for their monetary value.

B. Increasing sense of tension immediately before committing the theft.

C. Pleasure, gratification, or relief at the time of committing the theft.

D. The stealing is not committed to express anger or vengeance and is not in response to a delusion or a hallucination.

E. The stealing is not better accounted for by conduct disorder, a manic episode, or antisocial personality disorder.

Criterion A, which focuses on the senselessness of the items stolen, has often been considered the criterion that distinguishes kleptomania patients from ordinary shoplifters (Goldman 1991). Interpretation of this criterion, however, is controversial. The archetype of the middle-aged female kleptomania patient who steals peculiar items may not adequately account for all people with kleptomania (Goldman 1991; McElroy et al. 1991a). Patients with kleptomania may in fact desire the items they steal and be able to use them, but they do not need them. This may be particularly the case with kleptomania patients who hoard items (Goldman 1991). For these patients, multiple versions of the same item are usually not needed, but the item itself may be desired and may be of practical use to the patient.

In addition, patients with kleptomania often report amnesia surrounding the act of shoplifting (Goldman 1991; Grant 2004). These patients deny feelings of tension or arousal prior to shoplifting and deny feelings of pleasure or relief after the thefts. In fact, patients reporting amnesia surrounding thefts often recall entering and leaving a store but have no memory of events in the store, including the theft (Grant 2004). Other patients, who are not amnestic for the thefts, may also deny feelings of tension prior to a theft or pleasure after the act. Instead, these patients describe shoplifting as "automatic" or "a habit." Although they report an inability to control their shoplifting, they deny symptoms that meet criterion B or C of DSM-IV-TR. Do patients who are amnestic for shoplifting or who shoplift "out of habit" represent a subtype of kleptomania? Most clinical samples of kleptomania patients report shoplifting for more than 10 years prior to entering treatment (Goldman 1991; Grant and Kim 2002c; McElroy et al. 1991b). Some patients report that they felt tension and pleasure when they started stealing, but it became a "habit" over time. Do the DSM-IV-TR criteria apply to some kleptomania patients only at a particular time in the course of the illness? Issues of subtyping and the longitudinal course of the illness are only speculative at this time, but ongoing research may assist in better addressing these diagnostic questions.

Epidemiology, Comorbidity, and Relationship to Other Disorders

The prevalence of kleptomania remains unknown. Although preliminary evidence suggests that the lifetime prevalence may be approximately 0.6% (Goldman 1991), this figure possibly underestimates the prevalence of the illness. The shame and embarrassment associated with stealing prevents most people from voluntarily reporting kleptomania symptoms (Grant and Kim 2002c). No national epidemiological study of kleptomania has been performed, but studies of kleptomania in various clinical samples suggest a higher prevalence. A recent study of psychiatric inpatients with multiple disorders revealed that kleptomania may in fact be fairly common. The study of 204 adult psychiatric inpatients in the United States found that 7.8% ($n=16$) endorsed current symptoms consistent with a diagnosis of kleptomania and 9.3% ($n=19$) had a lifetime diagnosis of kleptomania (Grant et al., in press). In addition, kleptomania appeared equally common in patients with mood, anxiety, substance use, or psychotic disorders. These findings are further supported by two French studies. One study examining 107 inpatients with depression found that 4 (3.7%) had kleptomania (Lejoyeux et al. 2002). In a study of 79 inpatients with alcohol dependence, 3 (3.8%) also reported symptoms consistent with kleptomania (Lejoyeux et al. 1999). In two separate studies examining comorbidity in pathological gamblers, rates of comorbid kleptomania were found to range from 2.1% to 5% (Grant and Kim 2003; Specker et al. 1995). A study of bulimia patients found that 24% met DSM-III (American Psychiatric Association 1980) criteria for kleptomania (Hudson et al. 1983).

The literature clearly suggests that the majority of patients with kleptomania are women. Of the four independent studies that have assembled large numbers of patients with kleptomania, 68 of 108 (63.0%) total subjects were female (Grant and Kim 2002b; McElroy et al.1991b; Presta et al. 2002; Sarasalo et al. 1996). Although one explanation for this gender disparity is that kleptomania occurs more frequently in women, another reason may be that women are more likely to present for psychiatric evaluation. The courts may send male shoplifters to prison while sending female shoplifters for psychiatric evaluation (Goldman 1991). Even though the disorder appears to occur more frequently in females, males have also been found to have kleptomania. The severity of kleptomania symptoms and the clinical presentation of symptoms do not appear to differ based on gender (Grant and Kim 2002b).

Although the age at onset of kleptomania appears to be most often late adolescence (Goldman 1991; Grant and Kim 2002b; McElroy et al. 1991b; Presta et al. 2002), there is little information on how kleptomania presents in adolescents. Based on case reports of adolescent kleptomania (Feeney and

Klykylo 1997; Grant and Kim 2002a; Wood and Garralda 1990), there is some evidence that the current DSM-IV-TR criteria apply to adolescents who report being unable to control their shoplifting. More research, however, is needed to understand the presentation of kleptomania among adolescents.

Psychiatric comorbidity is quite common in patients with kleptomania. High rates of other psychiatric disorders have been found in patients with kleptomania. Rates of lifetime comorbid affective disorders range from 59% (Grant and Kim 2002b) to 100% (McElroy et al. 1991b). The rate of lifetime comorbid bipolar disorder has been reported as ranging from 9% (Grant and Kim 2002b) to 27% (Bayle et al. 2003) to 60% (McElroy et al. 1991b). Studies have also found high lifetime rates of comorbid anxiety disorders (60%–80%; McElroy et al. 1991b, 1992), impulse-control disorders (20%–46%; Grant and Kim 2003), substance use disorders (23%–50%; Grant and Kim 2002b; McElroy et al. 1991b), and eating disorders (60%; McElroy et al. 1991b). Personality disorders have been found in 43%–55% of patients with kleptomania, with the most common being paranoid personality disorder and histrionic personality disorder (Bayle et al. 2003; Grant 2004). These high rates of various comorbidities have created much debate over the proper characterization of this disorder.

Substance Use Disorders

Kleptomania and drug addictions appear to share common core qualities: 1) repetitive or compulsive engagement in a behavior despite adverse consequences, 2) diminished control over the problematic behavior, 3) an appetitive urge or craving state prior to engagement in the problematic behavior, and 4) a hedonic quality during the performance of the problematic behavior (Grant and Potenza 2004).

Epidemiological data suggest a relationship between kleptomania and substance use disorders, with high rates of co-occurrence in each direction (Bayle et al. 2003; Lejoyeux et al. 1999; McElroy et al. 1991b). Phenomenological data further support a relationship between kleptomania and drug addictions; for example, the telescoping phenomenon (reflecting the rapid rate of progression from initial to problematic behavioral engagement in women as compared with men) initially described for alcoholism has been applied to kleptomania (Grant and Kim 2002b). Family history data have also suggested a possible common genetic contribution to alcohol use and kleptomania (Grant 2003; McElroy et al. 1991a). In addition, pharmacological data (e.g., the possible effectiveness of the opioid antagonist naltrexone in the treatment of both kleptomania and substance use disorders; Grant and Kim 2002c; Volpicelli et al. 1992) may provide further support for a shared relationship between kleptomania and substance use disorders.

Relationship to Other Disorders

Although much data from diverse sources support a close relationship between kleptomania and substance use disorders, other non–mutually exclusive, proposed models for kleptomania include categorizations as obsessive-compulsive spectrum (Hollander 1993; McElroy et al. 1993, 1994) and affective spectrum (McElroy et al. 1996) disorders. Conceptualization of kleptomania within an obsessive-compulsive spectrum is based on common features of repetitive thoughts and behaviors (Hollander 1993; McElroy et al. 1994) and the high rate (63%) of hoarding found among patients with kleptomania (Grant and Kim 2002b). Although clinical aspects are shared between obsessive-compulsive disorder (OCD) and kleptomania, other aspects seem different, for example, the ego-syntonic nature of shoplifting in kleptomania and the ego-dystonic nature of compulsions in OCD. Although some evidence supports high rates of co-occurring OCD and kleptomania (McElroy et al. 1991b), other studies do not report an association (Bayle et al. 2003; Grant and Kim 2002b). Personality features of individuals with kleptomania (impulsive; reward and sensation seeking) differ from those with OCD (harm avoidant) (Bayle et al. 2003; Grant and Kim 2002d). A family history study also failed to demonstrate an association between kleptomania and OCD (Grant 2003). Thus, there is less evidence linking kleptomania to OCD than to substance use disorders.

The high lifetime comorbidity of kleptomania with mood disorders has led to the possible inclusion of kleptomania within an affective spectrum (McElroy et al. 1996). As mentioned earlier, one study examining 107 French inpatients with depression found that 4 (3.7%) had kleptomania (Lejoyeux et al. 2002). In addition, rates of lifetime comorbid affective disorders range from 59% to 75% (Bayle et al. 2003; Grant and Kim 2002b; Presta et al. 2002) to 100% (McElroy et al. 1991b). Another study found that 32% of a large group of kleptomania patients ($n=37$) had attempted suicide (Sarasalo et al. 1996). Many people with kleptomania report that the pleasurable yet problematic behaviors alleviate negative emotional states (Fishbain 1987; McElroy et al. 1991b), and this may serve as the basis for the close association of kleptomanic behavior and episodes of depression.

Because kleptomanic behavior is risky and self-destructive, the question has been raised whether kleptomania reflects subclinical mania or cyclothymia. Although comorbid mood disorders are common, the rate of comorbid bipolar disorder is unclear. Studies have shown a wide range of lifetime comorbid bipolar types I and II, ranging from 9.1% (Grant and Kim 2002b) to 27% (Bayle et al. 2003) to 60% (McElroy et al. 1991b; Presta et al. 2002). In one study, the onset of the affective disorder preceded the kleptomania symptoms by 1 year in 60% of patients, occurred within the same year in 15%, and occurred after the onset of kleptomania in 25% (McElroy et al. 1991b).

The elevated rates of lifetime comorbid depression and bipolar disorder in patients with kleptomania support kleptomania's possible inclusion within an affective spectrum, as do early reports of treatment response to serotonin reuptake inhibitors, mood stabilizers, and electroconvulsive therapy (McElroy et al. 1991b, 1996). However, depression in kleptomania may be distinct from primary or uncomplicated depression; for example, depression in kleptomania may represent a response to shame and embarrassment (Grant and Kim 2002c). In addition, rates of comorbid kleptomania and bipolar disorder may not be as high as initially thought (Grant and Kim 2002b) and the response to serotonin reuptake inhibitors not as robust as initially anticipated (McElroy et al. 1991b). For these reasons, the relationship between kleptomania and mood disorders requires clarification, particularly because appropriate classification has implications for treatment development.

Functional Impairment, Quality of Life, and Legal Difficulties

Patients with kleptomania experience significant impairment in their ability to function socially and at their occupations. Many patients report intrusive thoughts and urges related to shoplifting that interfere with their ability to concentrate at home and at work (Grant and Kim 2002c). Others report missing work, often in the afternoons, after leaving early to shoplift. The inability to control behavior that an individual does not want to engage in may lead to feelings of shame and guilt, which were reported in 77% of the patients in one study (Grant and Kim 2002b). Shame and guilt also result in secrecy, and less than half (42%) of married patients reported having told their spouses about their behavior (Grant and Kim 2002b; McElroy et al. 1991b).

Further impairment may result from both the elevated rates of stress and the comorbid mood disorders that patients with kleptomania often develop. Patients report levels of perceived stress that worsen as their shoplifting behavior intensifies (Grant et al. 2003). Additionally, many kleptomania patients report the need for psychiatric hospitalization due to the depression they feel was brought on by or exacerbated by the inability to stop their behavior (Grant and Kim 2002b). With the functional impairment that kleptomania patients experience, it is not surprising that they also report poor quality of life. In the only study to systematically evaluate quality of life using a psychometrically sound instrument (Quality of Life Inventory), patients with kleptomania, independent of comorbidity, reported significantly poorer life satisfaction compared with a general, nonclinical adult sample (Grant and Kim 2005). Some patients have even considered suicide as a means by which they could stop themselves from shoplifting (Grant and Kim 2002b).

In addition to the emotional consequences of kleptomania, many patients with kleptomania have faced legal difficulties due to their behavior. Studies have reported that 64%–87% of kleptomania patients have a history of being apprehended (McElroy et al. 1991b; Sarasalo et al. 1996). In fact, one study found that patients reported a mean number of lifetime apprehensions of approximately three per patient (Grant and Kim 2002b). Although most apprehensions do not result in jail time, early evidence suggests that 15%–23% of kleptomania patients have been jailed for shoplifting (Grant and Kim 2002b; McElroy et al. 1991b). In a meta-analysis of 56 subjects, it was determined that although 18% of the patients exhibited antisocial behaviors (lying, fraud, breaking and entering, embezzlement, torturing of animals), none had antisocial personality disorder (McElroy et al. 1991a).

Pathogenesis

Biological Theories

A growing body of literature implicates multiple neurotransmitter systems (e.g., serotonergic, dopaminergic, opioidergic) as well as familial and inherited factors in the pathophysiology of the motivated behaviors associated with impulse-control disorders (Potenza and Hollander 2002). One central aspect of motivated behaviors involves the ventral striatum, a brain region that includes the nucleus accumbens. The ventral striatum receives input from the ventral tegmental area and prefrontal cortex and has direct access to and influence on motor output structures (Kalivas et al. 1999). As such, the ventral striatum is important for controlling motivated behavior that is largely determined through a series of cortical-striatal-thalamic-cortical loops.

Motivated behavior involves integrating a wide array of contextual information, including information regarding a person's internal state (e.g., urges, desires), environmental factors (e.g., presence of danger), and personal experiences (e.g., recollections of rewarding experiences). Specific brain regions are central in providing the primary motivational system with this information. For example, the hypothalamic and septal nuclei provide information about nutrient ingestion, aggression, and reproductive drive; the amygdala provides affective information; and the hippocampus provides contextual memory data (Potenza and Hollander 2002). Although a wide array of neurotransmitters serves to coordinate information processing within this network, the neurotransmitters that are arguably the best characterized that influence motivated behavior are serotonin, dopamine, and the opioid system.

Serotonin and Inhibition

Evidence for serotonergic involvement in impulse-control disorders comes in part from studies of platelet monoamine oxidase B activity, which correlates with cerebrospinal fluid 5-hydroxyindoleacetic acid (CSF 5-HIAA, a metabolite of serotonin) and is considered a peripheral marker of serotonin function (Coccaro et al. 1990; Linnoila et al. 1983). Low CSF 5-HIAA levels have been found to correlate with high levels of impulsivity and sensation seeking (Coccaro et al. 1990). Pharmacological challenge studies that measure hormonal response after the administration of serotonergic drugs also provide evidence for serotonergic dysfunction in impulse-control disorders (DeCaria et al. 1998).

Patients with kleptomania report significant elevations of impulsivity and risk taking compared with control subjects (Bayle et al. 2003; Grant and Kim 2002d), and diminished inhibitory mechanisms may underlie the risk-taking behavior of kleptomania. The most well-studied inhibitory pathways involve serotonin and the prefrontal cortex (Chambers et al. 2003). Decreased measures of serotonin have long been associated with a variety of adult risk-taking behaviors including alcoholism, fire setting, and pathological gambling (Moreno et al. 1991; Virkunnen et al. 1994). Although the precise mechanism has not been fully determined, serotonin projections from the dorsal raphe to motivational circuitry, including the ventral tegmental area, nucleus accumbens, prefrontal cortex, amygdala, and hippocampus, appear to be involved (Chambers et al. 2003). For example, blunted serotonergic responses in the ventromedial prefrontal cortex have been observed in individuals with impulsive aggression (New et al. 2002), and this region has also been implicated in poor decision making (Bechara 2003), as seen in individuals with kleptomania.

Although there have been few biological studies of kleptomania, early evidence may support a theory of serotonergic involvement in the disorder. First, one study examined the platelet serotonin transporter in 20 patients with kleptomania. The number of the platelet serotonin transporter, evaluated by means of binding to [^{3}H]paroxetine, was lower in the kleptomania patients than in the healthy control subjects (Marazziti et al. 2000), thereby suggesting serotonergic dysfunction. Second, pharmacological case studies suggest that serotonin reuptake inhibitors (e.g., clomipramine, selective serotonin reuptake inhibitors [SSRIs]; Lepkifker et al. 1999; McElroy et al. 1991b) may reduce the impulsive behavior associated with kleptomania.

Dopamine and Reward Deficiency

Dopaminergic systems influencing rewarding and reinforcing behaviors have also been implicated in impulse-control disorders and may play a role in the pathogenesis of kleptomania. "Reward deficiency syndrome," a hypothesized hypodopaminergic state involving multiple genes and environmental stimuli that puts an individual at high risk for multiple addictive impulsive and compulsive behaviors, is one proposed mechanism (Blum et al. 2000). Alterations in dopaminergic pathways have been proposed as underlying the seeking of rewards (e.g., shoplifting) that trigger the release of dopamine and produce feelings of pleasure (Blum et al. 2000). Furthermore, dopamine release into the nucleus accumbens has been implicated in the translation of motivated drive into action, serving as a "go" signal (Chambers et al. 2003). Dopamine release into the nucleus accumbens seems maximal when reward probability is most uncertain, suggesting it plays a central role in guiding behavior during risk-taking situations (Fiorillo et al. 2003). The structure and function of dopamine neurons within the nucleus accumbens, in conjunction with glutamatergic afferent and intrinsic GABAergic activities, appear to change in response to experiences that influence the function of the nucleus accumbens. Therefore, future behavior may in part be determined by prior rewarding experiences via neuroplastic changes in the nucleus accumbens. This may explain why, over time, many kleptomania patients report shoplifting "out of habit" even without a pronounced urge or craving.

Opioid System, Cravings, and Pleasure

Preclinical and clinical studies demonstrate that the underlying biological mechanism of urge-based disorders may involve the processing of incoming reward inputs by the ventral tegmental area–nucleus accumbens–orbitofrontal cortex (VTA-NA-OFC) circuit (Hyman 1993; Koob and Bloom 1988; Mogenson et al. 1980). This circuit influences behavior by modulating animal and human motivation (e.g., urges, cravings). Dopamine may also play a major role in the regulation of this region's functioning (Koob 1992; Kuhar et al. 1991).

People with kleptomania report urges to steal (Grant and Kim 2002b); therefore, urges linked to the experiencing of reward and pleasure may represent an important clinical target in treating kleptomania. Most people with kleptomania report fairly frequent urges that result in theft—perhaps two times per week on average (Grant and Kim 2002b). Many indicate that the act of stealing reduces the urges or the tension these urges produce (McElroy et al. 1991b). Although many report the urges as intrusive, the act of stealing is often a "thrill" for some, producing a pleasurable feeling (Goldman 1991; Grant and Kim 2002b). The μ-opioid system is believed to underlie urge regulation through the processing of reward, pleasure, and pain, at least in part via modulation of dopamine neurons in mesolimbic pathway through γ-aminobutyric acid (GABA) interneurons (Potenza and Hollander 2002).

One line of evidence supporting the role of the opioid system in the pathogenesis of kleptomania is found in the treatment literature. Studies of naltrexone in the treatment of kleptomania and other impulse-control disorders have demonstrated its efficacy in reducing urges (Dannon et al. 1999;

Grant and Kim 2002c; Kim et al. 2001). The primary pharmacological action of naltrexone within the central nervous system is the antagonism of the μ-opioid receptor, the site at which β-endorphins, morphine, and heroin act as endogenous and exogenous agonists. The μ-opioid system is involved in the processing of reward, pleasure, and pain. Naltrexone's possible effectiveness in reducing kleptomanic urges may be due to the drug's modulation of dopamine function within the VTA-NA-OFC circuit via the antagonism of opioid receptors in the ventral tegmental area (Broekkamp and Phillips 1979).

In summary, the repeated engagement in kleptomanic behavior may be conceptualized as a result of an imbalance between a pathologically increased urge and a pathologically decreased inhibition. The repeated shoplifting of kleptomania may therefore be due to increased activity of the mesocorticolimbic dopamine circuitry, indirectly enhanced through the opioid system, and decreased activity in the cortical inhibitor processes, which are largely influenced via serotonin.

Psychological Theories

Although biological vulnerabilities may contribute to kleptomanic behavior, the pathogenesis of kleptomania most likely involves multiple factors—psychological, developmental, and biological. Why do kleptomania patients continue to engage in a behavior that results in unneeded items when the possible repercussions are so devastating? In an attempt to address this complex question, many psychological theories of kleptomania have been postulated—for example, gratification of unconscious sexual impulses (Goldman 1991; McElroy et al. 1991a), castration anxiety (Levy 1934), poor self-esteem (Goldman 1991), unresolved dependency (Allen 1965), and masochism (Rado 1933). There are no data, however, to confirm or refute these theories (Goldman 1991).

There are data, however, to support other theories suggesting kleptomania may be related to depression and childhood development. Focusing on the pleasure many patients derive from shoplifting, some have theorized that kleptomania results from an attempt to relieve feelings of depression through stimulation (Goldman 1991; Gudjonsson 1987; McElroy et al. 1991a). Risk-taking behavior may therefore produce an antidepressant effect for some patients (Fishbain 1987; Goldman 1991). It is possible that depressed individuals may engage in shoplifting to distract themselves from life stressors and unpleasant cognitions. Unlike drugs or alcohol, shoplifting leads to neither intoxication nor a directly impaired ability to function at work and as such may be an especially attractive means of escape. Persons who are depressed may also view the objects they steal as a means of significant symptom relief and the possibility of being apprehended as a relatively minor and theoretical setback. Ironically, problems resulting directly from shoplifting (e.g., embarrassment and shame from getting caught) may in turn lead to even more shoplifting as a misguided attempt of symptom management (Goldman 1991).

Evidence for the self-medication hypothesis of shoplifting comes from studies demonstrating that patients with kleptomania report high lifetime rates of depression (45%–100%; Bayle et al. 2003; McElroy et al. 1991b) that usually (60% of cases) precedes the kleptomanic behavior (McElroy et al. 1991b). Furthermore, several case studies report patients who described shoplifting as relief for their depressed moods (Fishbain 1987). Pharmacological case studies also suggest that kleptomania symptoms improved due to treatment with antidepressants (Lepkifker et al. 1999; McElroy et al. 1991b).

Because most people with depression do not shoplift, theories have been offered as to why some depressed people might engage in kleptomanic behavior. One theory has suggested that shoplifting is a symbolic attempt to make up for early deprivations or losses. The shoplifting may therefore be a symbolic compensation for an actual or perceived loss (Cupchick and Atcheson 1983; Goldman 1991). Interestingly, some support for this theory may be found in a recent study of parental bonding that observed that kleptomania patients reported significantly lower maternal and paternal care scores (i.e., parents' expression of affection) than did control subjects (Grant and Kim 2002d). Furthermore, a recent family study found that patients with kleptomania were more likely than control subjects to have a first-degree relative with an alcohol use disorder (Grant 2003). Given the evidence of increased psychiatric stress in the children of alcoholic individuals (Sher 1991), the examination of feelings of deprivation or loss in kleptomania patients merits further attention. Kleptomania patients may have low ego strength, and shoplifting may raise self-esteem by creating feelings of success when a person successfully leaves a store without being apprehended. Early emotional deprivation may therefore play a role in the pathogenesis of kleptomania.

Behavioral models may also provide clues as to the pathogenesis of kleptomania. From an operant standpoint, the positive reinforcer in kleptomania is the acquisition of items for nothing, and the intermittent reinforcement (e.g., not always being able to shoplift because of store security) of kleptomanic behavior may therefore be particularly resistant to extinction. Physiological arousal associated with shoplifting (Goldman 1991) may be yet another reinforcer that initiates and perpetuates the behavior.

Similarly, negative reinforcement (i.e., involving the removal of a punishing stimulus) hypothesizes that initiating but not completing a habitual behavior leads to uncomfortable states of arousal. Applied to kleptomania, this would imply that shoplifting is performed to experience relief from the aversive arousal of urges. Even the self-medication theory of kleptomania may represent a negative reinforcement. This could account for why kleptomanic behavior continues despite the offender's being frequently apprehended.

In addition to a behavioral model, there may also be specific thinking errors that are directly linked to kleptomanic behavior: 1) believing that only shoplifting will reduce the urge or the depressive state, 2) selective memory (e.g., remembering the thrill of shoplifting while ignoring the shame and embarrassment from being apprehended), and 3) erroneous self-assessment (e.g., that one deserves to be caught stealing because one is not intrinsically worth anything). In addition, kleptomania patients score high on indices of impulsivity (Bayle et al. 2003; Grant and Kim 2002d). Impulsive individuals may also be insensitive to internally generated cognitions focusing on restraint (McCown and Chamberlain 2000).

These psychological theories of kleptomania should be understood, however, in the context of the possible biological explanations for kleptomania. For example, although many people shoplift at some time in their lives, it is unclear why all individuals who shoplift more than a few times do not succumb to the disorder-inducing intermittent reinforcement (i.e., positive reinforcement of acquiring items or the negative reinforcement of relief from aversive arousal of urges). One possible explanation is that individual biological differences might regulate individual responses to the positive or negative reinforcement of shoplifting. That is, for some individuals, positive or negative reinforcement may have a more powerful influence on future kleptomanic behavior. Searching for these individual differences may refine both our psychological and our biological understanding of operant processes in the etiology and maintenance of kleptomania.

Integrating cognitive theories of kleptomania with biological processes may also prove useful in understanding the pathogenesis of kleptomania. Does disordered thinking cause individuals to make irrational decisions and, based on this, shoplift? By contrast, perhaps those who are driven to shoplift are prone toward constructing a set of erroneous views that are consistent with their behavior.

Some individuals may possess broad traits or characteristics that leave them vulnerable to kleptomania. For example, extraversion, which we see in people with kleptomania (Grant and Kim 2002d), may be associated with heightened arousal in limbic and cortical areas. If there are common neurobiological processes underlying the urge to engage in a wide range of appetitive behaviors (Kim 1998), then certain traits or dispositions purported to predispose individuals to kleptomania (e.g., impaired impulse control) might reflect an underlying biologically based vulnerability that includes, but is not limited to, kleptomania. Evidence for this position includes 1) neurological data implicating the VTA-NA-OFC circuit as a potential source of an appetitive urge-based brain mechanism; 2) psychopharmacological data indicating that kleptomania, along with a wide range of disorders related to impulse control, responds to the same medication treatments (Grant and Kim 2002c; McElroy et al. 1991b); and 3) epidemiological data demonstrating that having kleptomania substantially increases one's risk of having a number of other impulse-control disorders involving strong appetitive urges (e.g., drug and alcohol use disorders; Bayle et al. 2003; Grant 2003). Therefore, kleptomania vulnerability may be related to one or more broad psychological traits that are themselves manifestations of a specific neurobiological status.

Psychological models provide an important perspective in our attempts to understand the etiology and maintenance of kleptomania. These models are most informative when integrated with what is known about neurobiological processes. A biopsychological perspective will therefore most likely provide the most useful understanding for the treatment and prevention of kleptomania.

Treatment

Pharmacotherapy

No medication is currently approved by the U.S. Food and Drug Administration for treating kleptomania. Therefore, it is important to inform patients of any "off-label" use of medications for this disorder as well as the empirical basis for considering medication treatment.

Only case reports, two small case series, and one open-label study of pharmacotherapy have been conducted for kleptomania. Various medications—tricyclic antidepressants, SSRIs (Lepkifker et al. 1999), mood stabilizers, and opioid antagonists—have been examined for the treatment of kleptomania (Grant and Kim 2002c; McElroy et al. 1989). McElroy et al. (1991b) reported treatment response in 10 of 20 patients with the following single agents: fluoxetine, nortriptyline, trazodone, clonazepam, valproate, and lithium. Other agents used successfully as monotherapy for kleptomania include fluvoxamine (Chong and Low 1996) and paroxetine (Kraus 1999). Combinations of medications have also been effective in case reports: lithium plus fluoxetine (Burstein 1992), fluvoxamine plus buspirone (Durst et al. 1997), fluoxetine plus alprazolam (McElroy et al. 1991b), fluvoxamine plus valproate (Kmetz et al. 1997), and fluoxetine plus imipramine (McElroy et al. 1991b).

The findings from case reports, however, have not been consistent. In fact, seven cases of fluoxetine, three cases of imipramine, two cases of lithium as monotherapy and two cases of lithium augmentation, four cases of tranylcypromine, and carbamazepine in combination with clomipramine all failed to reduce kleptomania symptoms (McElroy et al. 1991b). Additionally, some evidence suggests that SSRIs may actually induce kleptomania symptoms (Kindler et al. 1997).

One case series found that kleptomania symptoms respond to topiramate (Dannon 2003). In a series of three patients treated with a dosage of 100–150 mg/day, all three patients achieved remission of kleptomania symptoms. Two of the patients were also taking an SSRI concomitantly with the topiramate, and two had comorbid diagnoses of attention-deficit/hyperactivity disorder and panic disorder. In another case series examining two subjects treated with naltrexone, both responded to medication (Dannon et al. 1999).

There has been only one open-label trial of medication for kleptomania. In an open-label study of 10 self-referred subjects with kleptomania who were free from other Axis I comorbid disorders, patients were treated with naltrexone (dosage range 50–200 mg/day). All subjects had at least moderate urges to steal at the time of study entry. Patients were assessed weekly for 12 weeks using the Kleptomania Symptom Assessment Scale, a self-report measure of kleptomania symptom severity that has shown good preliminary evidence of reliability and validity in examining kleptomania behavior and urges (Figure 8–1). Naltrexone resulted in a significant decline in the intensity of urges to steal, stealing thoughts, and stealing behavior (Grant and Kim 2002c). The mean dosage of naltrexone for effectiveness was 145 mg/day. A case report of adolescent kleptomania suggests that a lower dosage, possibly 50 mg/day, may be effective in younger people with kleptomania (Grant and Kim 2002a).

Several important findings emerge from these case reports and case series. First, opioid antagonists such as naltrexone may be effective in reducing both the urges to shoplift and the shoplifting behavior seen in kleptomania. In addition, naltrexone often reduces the "thrill" associated with shoplifting and thereby may prevent the positive reinforcement of the behavior. Second, antidepressants, particularly those that influence serotonergic systems (e.g., serotonin reuptake inhibitors), may also be effective in reducing the symptoms of kleptomania. These drugs may operate by targeting serotonergic systems implicated in impaired impulse regulation. Response to antidepressants usually means decreased thoughts about shoplifting, decreased kleptomanic behavior, and improvement in social and occupational functioning. Patients may initially report feeling less preoccupied with shoplifting and less anxious about having thoughts of shoplifting. If kleptomania represents both impaired urge regulation and impaired inhibition of behavior, both opioid antagonists and antidepressants may play a pivotal role in controlling this behavior.

Our understanding of efficacious and well-tolerated pharmacotherapies for kleptomania lags significantly behind that of pharmacotherapies for other major neuropsychiatric disorders. It is hoped that progress in the treatment of kleptomania will continue to be made. More definitive treatment recommendations await the completion of additional, large-scale controlled treatment studies for this disorder and comparative investigations of pharmacological agents. Advances in these areas hold the potential for significantly improving the lives of individuals with kleptomania and those directly or indirectly affected by their conditions.

Psychotherapy

As in the case of medication, many different psychotherapies have been tried in the treatment of kleptomania. The success of these therapies exists only in case reports, with no controlled trials of therapy published.

Kleptomania Symptom Assessment Scale (K-SAS)

The following questions are aimed at evaluating kleptomania symptoms. Please **read** the questions **carefully** before you answer.

1. **If you had urges to steal during the past WEEK, on average, how strong were your urges? Please circle the most appropriate number.**

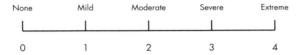

None	Mild	Moderate	Severe	Extreme
0	1	2	3	4

2. **During the past WEEK, how many times did you experience urges to steal? Please circle the most appropriate number.**

   0   None
   1   Once
   2   Two or three times
   3   Several to many times
   4   Constant or near constant

3. **During the past WEEK, how many hours (add up hours) were you preoccupied with your urges to steal? Please circle the most appropriate number.**

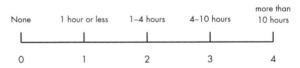

None	1 hour or less	1–4 hours	4–10 hours	more than 10 hours
0	1	2	3	4

4. **During the past WEEK, how much were you able to control your urges? Please circle the most appropriate number.**

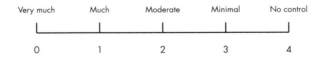

Very much	Much	Moderate	Minimal	No control
0	1	2	3	4

Figure 8–1.   Kleptomania Symptom Assessment Scale (K-SAS).
Source.   Reprinted from Grant JE, Kim SW: "An Open Label Study of Naltrexone in the Treatment of Kleptomania." *Journal of Clinical Psychiatry* 63:349–356, 2002. Copyright 2002, Physicians Postgraduate Press. Used with permission.

5. **During the past WEEK, how often did thoughts about stealing come up? Please circle the most appropriate number.**

   0   None
   1   Once
   2   Two to four times
   3   Several to many times
   4   Constantly or nearly constantly

6. **During the past WEEK, approximately how many hours (add up hours) did you spend thinking about stealing? Please circle the most appropriate number.**

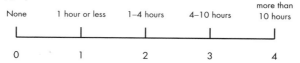

7. **During the past WEEK, how much were you able to control your thoughts of stealing? Please circle the most appropriate number.**

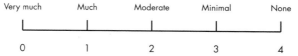

8. **During the past WEEK, on average, how much tension or excitement did you have shortly before you committed a theft? If you did not actually steal anything, please estimate how much anticipatory tension or excitement you believe you would have experienced if you had committed a theft. Please circle the most appropriate number.**

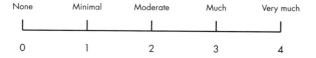

Figure 8–1.   Kleptomania Symptom Assessment Scale (K-SAS) *(continued).*

9. **During the past WEEK, on average, how much excitement and pleasure did you feel when you successfully committed a theft? If you did not actually steal, please estimate how much excitement and pleasure you believe you would have experienced if you had committed a theft. Please circle the most appropriate number.**

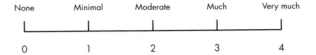

10. **During the past WEEK, how much emotional distress (mental pain or anguish, shame, guilt, embarrassment) has your stealing caused you? Please circle the most appropriate number.**

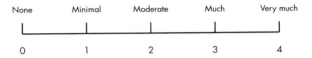

11. **During the past WEEK, how much personal trouble (relationship, financial, legal, job, medical or health) has your stealing caused you? Please circle the most appropriate number.**

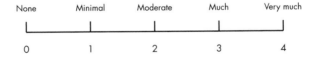

Figure 8–1.   Kleptomania Symptom Assessment Scale (K-SAS) *(continued)*.

Psychoanalysis has resulted in some limited success for kleptomania symptoms, but usually with the addition of medication (Fishbain 1988; Schwartz 1992). Insight-oriented psychotherapy, however, has been unsuccessful in treating this disorder in 11 published cases (McElroy et al. 1991b).

Behavioral therapy appears to have resulted in successfully treated cases of kleptomania. Using covert sensitization combined with exposure and response prevention, Guidry (1969) reported a young man who was able to reduce his stealing frequency. In a total of seven sessions over a 4-month period, the young man imagined stealing as well as the consequences of stealing (being seen, caught, handcuffed, and taken before a judge; feeling embarrassment). In addition, the man went to stores and was asked to imagine that the store manager was observing him. The young man reduced his stealing behavior, although his urges to steal went unchanged.

In another case of covert sensitization, a young woman underwent five weekly sessions wherein she was instructed to practice covert sensitization whenever she had urges to steal. She was able to then go 14 months with only a single lapse in behavior and with no reported urges to steal (Gauthier and Pellerin 1982). Similarly, another woman was instructed to have increasing nausea when tempted to steal, with imagery of vomiting associated with actual stealing (Glover 1985). After four sessions over 8 weeks, the woman was able to go with only a single lapse in behavior over the next 19 months. Finally, aversive breath holding was used whenever a patient reported urges to steal (Keutzer 1972). In combination with keeping a diary of urges to steal and attending six weekly sessions of therapy, the woman was able to significantly reduce her stealing frequency.

Imaginal desensitization uses the idea of imagining the steps of stealing while maintaining a relaxed state. The patient then images the potential scene of stealing but also imagines her ability to not steal in that context. Undergoing fourteen 15-minute sessions over 5 days, two patients reported complete remission of symptoms for a 2-year period (McConaghy and Blaszczynski 1988).

Learning to substitute alternative sources of satisfaction and excitement when the urges to steal occur has been successful in a single case report. The case involved a woman treated weekly for 5 months to assist her in finding alternative sources of excitement, pleasure, and self-fulfillment. She was able to report a 2-year period of remitted symptoms (Gudjonsson 1987).

It should be noted that at present few empirical data are available to guide the selection of one psychotherapy over another in the treatment of kleptomania. This represents an important area of future research. Another important area of study involves the combination of medication and psychotherapy. Clinical experience suggests that this combination may be especially beneficial for treating patients with kleptomania. However, empirical validation of specific well-defined combined pharmacological and psychosocial interventions for the treatment of kleptomania is needed.

Conclusion

This chapter has presented what is currently understood about the phenomenology and treatment of kleptomania. Studies indicate that kleptomania shares features with mood, anxiety, and impulse-control disorders, and this phenomenological overlap may reflect both the limited evidence currently available about kleptomania and the possible heterogeneity of the disorder. Although no uniform pharmacological treatment guidelines are currently available, early evidence supports the possible effectiveness of opioid antagonists, serotonin reuptake inhibitors, and mood stabilizers in the treatment of kleptomania. Furthermore, behavioral therapy also appears to be a promising treatment intervention.

Kleptomania has historically received relatively little attention from clinicians and researchers. As such, our understanding of the basic features of this disorder is relatively primitive. Future research investigating kleptomania, its relationship to other disorders, and its neurobiological underpinnings holds significant promise in advancing treatment strategies for this disabling disorder.

References

Allen A: Stealing as a defense. Psychoanal Q 34:572–583, 1965

American Psychiatric Association: Diagnostic and Statistical Manual of Mental Disorders, 3rd Edition. Washington, DC, American Psychiatric Association, 1980

American Psychiatric Association: Diagnostic and Statistical Manual of Mental Disorders, 3rd Edition Revised. Washington, DC, American Psychiatric Association, 1987

American Psychiatric Association: Diagnostic and Statistical Manual of Mental Disorders, 4th Edition, Text Revision. Washington, DC, American Psychiatric Association, 2000

Bayle FJ, Caci H, Millet B, et al: Psychopathology and comorbidity of psychiatric disorders in patients with kleptomania. Am J Psychiatry 160:1509–1513, 2003

Bechara A: Risky business: emotion, decision-making, and addiction. J Gambling Stud 19:23–51, 2003

Blum K, Braverman ER, Holder JM, et al: Reward deficiency syndrome: a biogenetic model for the diagnosis and treatment of impulsive, addictive, and compulsive behaviors. J Psychoactive Drugs 32 (suppl):1–68, 2000

Broekkamp CL, Phillips AG: Facilitation of self-stimulation behavior following intracerebral microinjections of opioids into the ventral tegmental area. Pharmacol Biochem Behav 11:289–295, 1979

Burstein A: Fluoxetine-lithium treatment for kleptomania. J Clin Psychiatry 53:28–29, 1992

Chambers RA, Taylor JR, Potenza MN: Developmental neurocircuitry of motivation in adolescence: a critical period of addiction vulnerability. Am J Psychiatry 160:1041–1052, 2003

Chong SA, Low BL: Treatment of kleptomania with fluvoxamine. Acta Psychiatr Scand 93:314–315, 1996

Coccaro EF, Siever LJ, Klar HM, et al: Serotonergic studies in patients with affective and personality disorders: correlates with suicidal and impulsive aggressive behavior. Arch Gen Psychiatry 46:587–599, 1990

Cupchick W, Atcheson JD: Shoplifting: an occasional crime of the moral majority. Bull Am Acad Psychiatry Law 11:343–354, 1983

Dannon PN: Topiramate for the treatment of kleptomania: a case series and review of the literature. Clin Neuropharmacol 26:1–4, 2003

Dannon PN, Iancu I, Grunhaus L: Naltrexone treatment in kleptomanic patients. Hum Psychopharmacol 14:583–585, 1999

DeCaria CM, Begaz T, Hollander E: Serotonergic and noradrenergic function in pathological gambling. CNS Spectr 3:38–47, 1998

Durst R. Katz G, Knobler HY: Buspirone augmentation of fluvoxamine in the treatment of kleptomania. J Nerv Ment Dis 185:586–588, 1997

Esquirol E: Des Maladies Mentales. Paris, France, Bailliere, 1838

Feeney DJ, Klykylo WM: Treatment for kleptomania. J Am Acad Child Adolesc Psychiatry 36:723–724, 1997

Fiorillo CD, Tobler PN, Schultz W: Discrete coding of reward probability and uncertainty by dopamine neurons. Science 299:1898–1902, 2003

Fishbain DA: Kleptomania as risk-taking behavior in response to depression. Am J Psychother 41:598–603, 1987

Fishbain DA: Kleptomanic behavior response to perphenazine-amitriptyline HCl combination. Can J Psychiatry 33:241–242, 1988

Gauthier J, Pellerin D: Management of compulsive shoplifting through covert sensitization. J Behav Ther Exp Psychiatry 13:73–75, 1982

Glover JH: A Case of kleptomania treated by covert sensitization. Br J Clin Psychol 24:213–214, 1985

Goldman MJ: Kleptomania: making sense of the nonsensical. Am J Psychiatry 148:986–996, 1991

Grant JE: Family history and psychiatric comorbidity in persons with kleptomania. Compr Psychiatry 44:437–441, 2003

Grant JE: Dissociative symptoms in kleptomania. Psychol Rep 94:77–82, 2004

Grant JE: Co-occurrence of personality disorders in persons with kleptomania: a preliminary investigation. J Am Acad Law Psychiatry 34:395–398, 2004

Grant JE, Kim SW: Adolescent kleptomania treated with naltrexone: a case report. Eur Child Adolesc Psychiatry 11:92–95, 2002a

Grant JE, Kim SW: Clinical characteristics and associated psychopathology of 22 patients with kleptomania. Compr Psychiatry 43:378–384, 2002b

Grant JE, Kim SW: An open label study of naltrexone in the treatment of kleptomania. J Clin Psychiatry 63:349–356, 2002c

Grant JE, Kim SW: Temperament and early environmental influences in kleptomania. Compr Psychiatry 43:223–229, 2002d

Grant JE, Kim SW: Comorbidity of impulse control disorders among pathological gamblers. Acta Psychiatr Scand 108:207–213, 2003

Grant JE, Kim SW: Quality of life in kleptomania and pathological gambling. Compr Psychiatry 46:34–37, 2005

Grant JE, Potenza MN: Impulse control disorders: clinical characteristics and pharmacological management. Ann Clin Psychiatry 16:27–34, 2004

Grant JE, Kim SW, Grosz RL: Perceived stress in kleptomania. Psychiatr Q 74:251–258, 2003

Grant JE, Potenza MN, Levine L, Kim SW: Prevalence of impulse control disorders in adult psychiatric inpatients. Am J Psychiatry (in press)

Gudjonsson GH: The significance of depression in the mechanism of "compulsive" shoplifting. Med Sci Law 27:171–176, 1987

Guidry LS: Use of a covert punishing contingency in compulsive stealing. J Behav Ther Exp Psychiatry 6:169, 1969

Hollander E (ed): Obsessive-Compulsive–Related Disorders. Washington, DC, American Psychiatric Press, 1993

Hudson JI, Pope HG, Jonas JM, et al: Phenomenological relationship of eating disorders to major affective disorder. Psychiatry Res 9:345–354, 1983

Hyman SE: Molecular and cell biology of addiction. Curr Opin Neurol Neurosurg 6:609–613, 1993

James P: A case of shoplifting in the eighteenth century. Med Sci Law 17:200–202, 1977

Kalivas PW, Churchill L, Romanides A: Involvement of the pallidal-thalamocortical circuit in adaptive behavior. Ann N Y Acad Sci 877:64–70, 1999

Keutzer C: Kleptomania: a direct approach to treatment. Br J Med Psychol 45:159–163, 1972

Kim SW: Opioid antagonists in the treatment of impulse-control disorders. J Clin Psychiatry 59:159–164, 1998

Kim SW, Grant JE, Adson DE, et al: Double-blind naltrexone and placebo comparison study in the treatment of pathological gambling. Biol Psychiatry 49:914–921, 2001

Kindler S, Dannon PN, Iancu I, et al: Emergence of kleptomania during treatment for depression with serotonin selective reuptake inhibitors. Clin Neuropharmacol 20:126–129, 1997

Kmetz GF, McElroy SL, Collins DJ: Response of kleptomania and mixed mania to valproate. Am J Psychiatry 154:580–581, 1997

Koob GF: Drugs of abuse: anatomy, pharmacology and function of reward pathways. Trends Pharmacol Sci 13:177–184, 1992

Koob GF, Bloom FE: Cellular and molecular mechanisms of drug dependence. Science 242:715–723, 1988

Kraus JE: Treatment of kleptomania with paroxetine. J Clin Psychiatry 60:793, 1999

Kuhar MJ, Ritz MC, Boja JW: The dopamine hypothesis of the reinforcing properties of cocaine. Trends Neurosci 14:299–302, 1991

Lasègue M: Le vol aux étalages (1880). Abstracted by Motet M. J Ment Sci 26:625–629, 1881

Lejoyeux M, Feuche N, Loi S, et al: Study of impulse-control disorders among alcohol-dependent patients. J Clin Psychiatry 60:302–305, 1999

Lejoyeux M, Arbaretaz M, McLoughlin M, et al: Impulse control disorders and depression. J Nerv Ment Dis 190:310–314, 2002

Lepkifker E, Dannon PN, Ziv R, et al: The treatment of kleptomania with serotonin reuptake inhibitors. Clin Neuropharmacol 22:40–43, 1999

Levy E: Psychoanalytic treatment of a child with a stealing compulsion. Am J Orthopsychiatry 4:1–12, 1934

Linnoila M, Virkunnen M, Scheinen M, et al: Low cerebrospinal fluid 5-hydroxyindoleacetic acid concentration differentiates impulsive from non-impulsive violent behavior. Life Sci 33:2609–2614, 1983

Marazziti D, Presta S, Pfanner C, et al: The biological basis of kleptomania and compulsive buying. Paper presented at the American College of Neuropsychopharmacology 39th Annual Meeting. San Juan, Puerto Rico, December 2000

Matthey A: Nouvelles Recherches sur les Maladies de l'Esprit. Paris, France, JJ Paschoud Libraire, 1816

McConaghy N, Blaszczynski A: Imaginal desensitization: a cost-effective treatment in two shoplifters and a binge-eater resistant to previous therapy. Aust N Z J Psychiatry 22:78–82, 1988

McCown W, Chamberlain L: Best Possible Odds: Contemporary Treatment Strategies for Gambling Disorders. New York, Wiley, 2000

McElroy SL, Keck PE, Pope HG, et al: Pharmacological treatment of kleptomania and bulimia nervosa. J Clin Psychopharmacol 9:358–360, 1989

McElroy SL, Hudson JI, Pope HG, et al: Kleptomania: clinical characteristics and associated psychopathology. Psychol Med 21:93–108, 1991a

McElroy SL, Pope HG, Hudson JI, et al: Kleptomania: a report of 20 cases. Am J Psychiatry 148:652–657, 1991b

McElroy SL, Hudson JI, Pope HG, et al: The DSM-III-R impulse control disorders not elsewhere classified: clinical characteristics and relationship to other psychiatric disorders. Am J Psychiatry 149:318–327, 1992

McElroy SL, Hudson JI, Phillips KA, et al: Clinical and theoretical implications of a possible link between obsessive-compulsive and impulse control disorders. Depression 1:121–132, 1993

McElroy, SL, Phillips KA, Keck PE: Obsessive compulsive spectrum disorder. J Clin Psychiatry 55:33–51, 1994

McElroy SL, Pope HG Jr, Keck PE, et al: Are impulse-control disorders related to bipolar disorder? Compr Psychiatry 37:229–240, 1996

Mogenson GJ, Jones DJ, Yim CY: From motivation to action: functional interface between the limbic system and motor system. Prog Neurobiol 14:69–97, 1980

Moreno I, Saiz-Ruiz J, Lopez-Ibor JJ: Serotonin and gambling dependence. Hum Psychopharmacol 6:9–12, 1991

New AS, Hazlett EA, Buchsbaum MS, et al: Blunted prefrontal cortical 18 fluorodeoxyglucose positron emission tomography response to meta-chlorophenylpiperazine in impulsive aggression. Arch Gen Psychiatry 59:621–629, 2002

Potenza MN, Hollander E: Pathological gambling and impulse control disorders, in Neuropsychopharmacology: The 5th Generation of Progress. Edited by Coyle JT, Nemeroff C, Charney D, et al. Baltimore, MD, Lippincott Williams & Wilkins, 2002, pp 1725–1741

Presta S, Marazziti D, Dell'Osso L, et al: Kleptomania: clinical features and comorbidity in an Italian sample. Compr Psychiatry 43:7–12, 2002

Rado S: Fear of castration in women. Psychoanal Q 2:424–475, 1933

Sarasalo E, Bergman B, Toth J: Personality traits and psychiatric and somatic morbidity among kleptomaniacs. Acta Psychiatr Scand 94:358–364, 1996

Schwartz JH: Psychoanalytic psychotherapy for a woman with diagnoses of kleptomania and bulimia. Hosp Community Psychiatry 43:109–110, 1992

Sher K: Psychological characteristics of children of alcoholics: overview of research methods and findings. Recent Dev Alcohol 9:301–326, 1991

Specker SM, Carlson GA, Christenson GA, et al: Impulse control disorders and attention deficit disorder in pathological gamblers. Ann Clin Psychiatry 7:175–179, 1995

Virkunnen M, Rawlings R, Tokola R, et al: CSF biochemistries, glucose metabolism, and diurnal activity rhythms in alcoholic violent offenders, fire setters, and healthy volunteers. Arch Gen Psychiatry 51:20–27, 1994

Volpicelli JR, Alterman AI, Hayashida M, et al: Naltrexone in the treatment of alcohol dependence. Arch Gen Psychiatry 49:876–880, 1992

Wood A, Garralda ME: Kleptomania in a 13-year-old boy. Br J Psychiatry 157:770–772, 1990

9

Compulsive Shopping

Donald W. Black, M.D.

History

Excessive and uncontrolled buying behavior has been chronicled for centuries, although anecdotal reports mainly involve the wealthy and powerful. Marie Antoinette, Queen of France during the turbulent time prior to the Revolution, was widely observed to spend extravagantly (Erickson 1991). Mary Todd Lincoln, wife of President Abraham Lincoln, was reported to have spending binges that greatly distressed her husband (Baker 1987). During the first half of the twentieth century, publisher William Randolph Hearst was known for his nonstop buying of art and artifacts throughout Europe (Swanberg 1961). His collecting was documented to have occurred over many decades, nearly bankrupting him during the Great Depression of the 1930s. Jacquelyn Kennedy Onassis, known worldwide for her charm and fashion sense, has been described by several biographers as an obsessive shopper, leading both husbands, first President John Kennedy and later Aristotle Onassis, to remark on her uncontrolled shopping behavior (David 1994; Heymann 1989). Even

Princess Diana, before her tragic death in 1997, was considered a clotheshorse by the media, who reported on her intense interest in shopping and spending (Davies 1996).

Most compulsive shopping behavior occurs among ordinary people, and apart from these anecdotal reports of the wealthy and famous, the earliest clinical descriptions date to 1915, when German psychiatrist Emil Kraepelin first used the term *oniomania,* which was later quoted by Swiss psychiatrist Eugen Bleuler in his 1924 *Textbook of Psychiatry:*

> As a last category Kraepelin mentions the buying maniacs (oniomaniacs) in whom even buying is compulsive and leads to senseless contraction of debts with continuous delay of payment until a catastrophe clears the situation a little—a little bit never altogether because they never admit all their debts. According to Kraepelin, here, too, it always involves women. The usual frivolous debt makers, and who in this way wish to get the means for pleasure, naturally do not belong here. The particular element is impulsiveness; they "cannot help it," which sometimes even expresses itself in the fact that not withstanding a good school intelligence the patients are absolutely incapable to think different and to concede to senseless consequences of their act and the possibility of not doing it. They do not even feel the impulse but they act out of their nature like the caterpillar which devours the leaves. (Bleuler 1924, p. 540)

Both Kraepelin and Bleuler considered compulsive buying an example of a *reactive impulse,* or *impulsive insanity,* and grouped it alongside kleptomania and pyromania.

Despite this early work, few psychiatrists held any interest in the disorder until the late twentieth century, when disorders hypothesized to be related to obsessive-compulsive disorder (OCD), including compulsive buying, caught the attention of the psychiatric community (Hollander 1993; Koran 1999). Over the years, interest in compulsive buying has been almost exclusively limited to occasional reports from psychoanalysts (Krueger 1988; Lawrence 1990; Winestine 1985) or from consumer behaviorists (Faber and O'Guinn 1989, 1992; O'Guinn and Faber 1989). By the early 1990s, three independent case series involving a total of 90 persons with compulsive shopping were reported and, along with renewed interest from consumer behaviorists, led to a resurgence of interest in the disorder (Christenson et al. 1994; McElroy et al. 1994; Schlosser et al. 1994).

Definition and Classification

There has been considerable debate in the professional literature about the appropriate classification of compulsive shopping. Some investigators have suggested that compulsive shopping is similar to drug or alcohol addiction (Glatt and Cook 1987; Krych 1989; Scherhorn et al. 1990), whereas other researchers have focused on the disorder's similarity to OCD, placing it within the obsessive-compulsive spectrum (Frost et al. 1998; Hollander 1993). Hollander (1993), for example, described an impulsive-compulsive spectrum of behavior involving many disorders that he related to OCD, including compulsive shopping. Yet other investigators, following in the tradition of Kraepelin and Bleuler, have favored its classification as a disorder of impulse control, similar to such disorders as pathological gambling (Black 2001; Christenson et al. 1994), whereas some have related compulsive buying to the mood and anxiety disorders (Lejoyeux et al. 1996; McElroy et al. 1995). There is currently little evidence to favor its classification as an addiction, an obsessive-compulsive spectrum disorder, or a mood disorder (Black 2000b).

Currently, although DSM-IV-TR (American Psychiatric Association 2000) has no diagnostic category for compulsive buying, individuals with the disorder can be placed in the residual category "disorders of impulse control not otherwise specified." In DSM-IV-TR, impulse-control disorders share an ability to resist an "impulse, drive, or temptation to perform an act that is harmful to the person or to others" (p. 663). One could debate whether compulsive shopping is a harmful act, but as is described later, its secondary consequences frequently are harmful to the individual.

There are several definitions available for compulsive shopping. Consumer behaviorists Faber and O'Guinn (1989) define the disorder as "chronic buying episodes of a somewhat stereotyped fashion in which the consumer feels unable to stop or significantly moderate his behavior" (p. 738). Another consumer behaviorist, Edwards (1993), suggests that compulsive buying is an "abnormal form of shopping and spending in which the afflicted consumer has an overpowering uncontrollable, chronic and repetitive urge to shop and spend [that functions]...as a means of alleviating negative feeling of stress and anxiety" (p. 67). Following the tradition of criteria-based diagnoses, McElroy et al. (1994) developed an operational definition for both clinical and research use (Table 9–1). Their definition recognizes that compulsive buying

Table 9–1.   Diagnostic criteria for compulsive buying

1. Maladaptive preoccupation with buying or shopping, or maladaptive buying or shopping impulses or behavior as indicated by at least one of the following:

    a. Frequent preoccupation with buying or impulses to buy that are experienced as irresistible, intrusive, and/or senseless

    b. Frequent buying of more than can be afforded, frequent buying of items that are not needed, or shopping for longer periods of time than intended

2. The buying preoccupations, impulses, or behaviors cause marked distress, are time consuming, significantly interfere with social or occupational functioning, or result in financial problems (e.g., indebtedness or bankruptcy).

3. The excessive buying or shopping behavior does not occur exclusively during periods of hypomania or mania.

Source.   Reprinted from McElroy S, Keck Jr PE, Pope Jr HG, et al.: "Compulsive Buying: A Report of 20 Cases." *Journal of Clinical Psychiatry* 55:242–248, 1994. Copyright 1994, Physicians Postgraduate Press. Used with permission.

has both cognitive and behavioral components, each potentially causing impairment manifested through personal distress; social, marital, or occupational dysfunction; or financial or legal problems. They exclude from the definition persons whose excessive buying occurs in the context of mania or hypomania. The definition developed by these investigators is now widely used by psychiatric researchers.

Many terms have been used for this condition, including *pathological spending, compulsive consumption, addictive compulsion, addictive shopping, uncontrolled buying, shopaholism,* and even *mall mania.* The most widely used terms are compulsive shopping and compulsive buying, which are used interchangeably in this chapter.

Assessment

As with any clinical disorder, it is important to gather an accurate history through a careful interview (Black 2000a). The goal of evaluation is to define the shopping problem through inquiries regarding the person's attitudes about shopping and spending and then move on to more specific questions about shopping behaviors and patterns. Once acknowledged, the individual can be questioned in detail about the extent of his or her shopping preoccupation and behavior. For general screening purposes, a clinician might ask:

- Do you feel overly preoccupied with shopping and spending?
- Do you ever feel that your shopping behavior is excessive, inappropriate, or uncontrolled?
- Have your shopping desires, urges, fantasies, or behaviors ever been overly time consuming, caused you to feel upset or guilty, or led to serious problems in your life (e.g., financial or legal problems, relationship loss)?

Positive responses should be followed up with more detailed questions, such as how frequently the behavior occurs, what the person prefers to buy, and how much money is spent. Family members and friends can become important informants, able to fill in the gaps in the person's history or to describe behaviors they may have witnessed.

The person's psychiatric history should be carefully explored, because most persons with compulsive shopping have comorbid psychiatric disorders. The presence of specific disorders may suggest particular treatment strategies or approaches as well as provide explanations for the excessive shopping and spending that may be helpful in counseling patients (e.g., treating a patient with comorbid OCD with a serotonin reuptake inhibitor antidepressant).

Clinicians should take note of past psychiatric treatments including medications, hospitalizations, and psychotherapy. A history of physical illness, surgical procedures, drug allergies, or medical treatment is important to note as well, because it may help to rule out medical explanations as a cause of the compulsive buying (e.g., neurological disorders, brain tumors) as well as identify conditions that may contraindicate the use of certain medications prescribed to treat the disorder. Bipolar disorder also needs to be ruled out as a cause of the excessive shopping and spending.

Compulsive shopping and spending need to be distinguished from normal buying behavior, although the distinction is sometimes arbitrary. The clinician should be aware that shopping often occurs within a cultural context, and there are differences between the typical shopping behavior of men and women. In the United States, shopping is often viewed from a woman's perspective, a fact not lost on advertisers. Normal buying behavior can also take on a compulsive quality at times, for example, around special holidays or birthdays. Persons who receive an inheritance or win a lottery may experience one or more spending sprees as well. Finally, it is up to the clinician to exercise appropriate judgment in applying the diagnostic criteria and assessing the evidence for distress or impairment.

Several screening instruments have been developed that appear to reliably separate normal buyers from compulsive shoppers. Perhaps the most widely used is the Compulsive Buying Scale, developed by Faber and O'Guinn (1992). The self-report instrument consists of seven items representing specific behaviors, motivations, and feelings associated with compulsive shopping. This instrument was preceded by the Compulsive Buying Measurement Scale developed in Canada (Valence et al. 1988) and the Addictive Buying Indicator developed by German researchers (Scherhorn et al. 1990). Another useful scale was developed by Edwards (1993); this 13-item scale consists of items selected to measure dimensions of tendency to spend, frequency of shopping and spending, feelings about and experienced while shopping, impulsivity while shopping, unplanned purchasing, postpurchase guilt, and dysfunction surrounding spending (Table 9–2). The scoring can be used to classify consumers according to their level of compulsiveness in buying. Lejoyeux et al. (1997) developed a 19-item questionnaire that is reported to tap the basic features of compulsive buying, but they have not reported on its psychometric properties.

Christenson et al. (1994) developed the Minnesota Impulsive Disorders Interview, a semistructured interview that may be used to assess the presence of compulsive buying, kleptomania, trichotillomania, intermittent explosive disorder, pathological gambling, compulsive sexual behavior, and compulsive exercise. These investigators recommend administering an 82-item expanded module to persons screening positive for compulsive buying.

Monahan et al. (1996) modified the Yale-Brown Obsessive-Compulsive Scale to create the YBOCS–Shopping Version (YBOCS-SV) to assess cognitions and behaviors associated with compulsive shopping. Like the parent instrument, the YBOCS-SV consists of 10 items, 5 rating cognitions and 5 rating behaviors. For both cognitions and behaviors, persons are asked about time involved, interference due to the preoccupations or behaviors, distress associated with preoccupations or the shopping, resistance to the thoughts or behaviors, and the degree of control over the thoughts or behaviors. In the sample described by Monahan and colleagues, the mean YBOCS-SV score for individuals diagnosed with compulsive shopping was 21 (range, 18–25) compared with 4 (range, 1–7) for noncompulsive buyers. The instrument is reported to have adequate interrater reliability and is valid in measuring both severity and change during clinical trials.

Table 9–2.   Edwards 13-item compulsive buying scale

1. I feel driven to shop and spend, even when I don't have the time or energy.
2. (R) I get little or no pleasure from shopping.
3. (R) I hate to go shopping.
4. I go on buying binges.
5. I feel "high" when I go on a buying spree.
6. I buy things even when I don't need anything.
7. I go on a buying binge when I'm upset, disappointed, depressed, or angry.
8. I worry about my spending habits but still go out and shop and spend money.
9. I feel anxious after I go on a buying binge.
10. I buy things even though I cannot afford them.
11. I feel guilty or ashamed after I go on a buying binge.
12. I buy things I don't need or won't use.
13. I sometimes feel compelled to shop.

Note.   R = Point scored when answer is "no."
Source.   Edwards 1993.

Epidemiology

There have been no adequate community studies estimating the prevalence of compulsive buying in the general population, although one small-scale survey has been conducted and suggests a prevalence in the United States between 1.8% and 8.1%. Faber and O'Guinn (1992) developed these figures by administering the Compulsive Buying Scale to 292 individuals responding to a mail survey that was designed to approximate the demographic makeup of the general population of Illinois. The high and low prevalence figures reflect two different thresholds set for the definition of compulsive buying. The high prevalence figure is based on a probability level of 0.70, whereas the lower figure is based on a more conservative probability level of 0.95. Two smaller-scale surveys suggest an even higher prevalence. Magee (1994) reported a figure of 16%, whereas Hassay and Smith (1996) reported a figure of about 12% of respondents classified as compulsive buyers. There are no data to suggest that the prevalence of compulsive shopping is increasing, but Dittmar (2004) pointed out that recent intense media interest and the steady increase in research publications on the topic suggest that the number of people affected is growing.

The disorder shows a female preponderance ranging from 80% to 95% among individuals self-identified as compulsive buyers or who have participated in clinical studies (Table 9–3). Interestingly, Kraepelin (1915) and Bleuler (1924) had observed that compulsive buying mainly involved women. This gender ratio is also found in community samples. Dittmar (2004) reported that in a general population sample drawn in the United Kingdom, 92% of respondents considered compulsive shoppers were women and 8% were men. Using a diagnostic screener, she found that men scored predominantly in the lowest quartile of compulsive buying (69%) and none in the highest quartile. In contrast, more than 70% of women had scores higher than the lowest quartile, with 18% in the highest. Dittmar (2004) concluded that the gender difference is real and not an artifact of men being underrepresented in samples.

Table 9–3.   Case series involving persons with compulsive shopping

Reference	Location	Subjects, N	Mean age, y	Females, %	Mean age at onset, y
O'Guinn and Faber 1989	Los Angeles, CA	386	37	92	—
Scherhorn et al. 1990	Germany	26	40	85	—
McElroy et al. 1994	Cincinnati, OH; Boston, MA	20	39	80	30
Schlosser et al. 1994	Iowa City, IA	46	31	80	19
Christenson et al. 1994	Minneapolis, MN	24	36	92	18
Black et al. 1998	Iowa City, IA	33	40	94	—
Lejoyeux et al. 1999	Paris, France	38	37	95	—
Ninan et al. 2000	Cincinnati, OH; Boston, MA	42	41	81	—
Koran et al. 2002	Stanford, CA	24	44	92	22

The age at onset is uncertain but in clinical studies has ranged from 18 to 30 years (see Table 9–3). The age at the time of interview in the reports cited ranged from 31 to 41 years. These age ranges may differ to some extent because of the way in which the samples were selected. For example, Faber and O'Guinn (1992) recruited compulsive buyers who were in treatment with a psychotherapist, whereas Schlosser et al. (1994) and Christenson et al. (1994) each advertised for study participants in the community.

Compulsive shopping appears to be a worldwide phenomenon. Reports on the disorder have come from Brazil (Bernik et al. 1996), Canada (Valence et al. 1988), England (Elliot 1994), France (Lejoyeux et al. 1997, 1999), Germany (Scherhorn et al. 1990), and the United States (Black et al. 1998; Koran et al. 2002; McElroy et al. 1994).

Psychiatric Comorbidity

Psychiatric comorbidity among compulsive shoppers is the rule, not the exception. Mood, anxiety, substance use, eating, and personality disorders are all reported to be more frequent than would be expected by chance alone. In the only studies in which a comparison group was used, Black et al. (1998) reported that only major depression and "any" mood disorder were excessive, whereas Christenson et al. (1994) reported that the categories of anxiety, substance use, eating, and impulse-control disorders were all excessive. In the six case series summarized in Table 9–4, review of lifetime major mental (Axis I) psychiatric comorbidity confirms high rates across the studies of mood disorders, anxiety disorders, substance use disorders, and eating disorders. The impulse-control disorders have been less commonly assessed, but the rates appear excessive, particularly for pathological gambling and kleptomania. (In some patients, the urge to shop and spend may lead to or be accompanied by stealing behavior.)

The only systematic assessment of personality disorders was conducted by Schlosser et al. (1994), who used both a self-report instrument and a structured interview to assess Axis II disorders. In the sample of Schlosser and colleagues, nearly 60% of subjects met criteria for at least one personality disorder type through a consensus of both instruments, most commonly obsessive-compulsive (22%), borderline (15%), and avoidant (15%). Anecdotally, Krueger (1988) treated four patients with psychoanalysis and observed that each demonstrated aspects of narcissistic character pathology: "They rely on other people for affirmation and esteem regulation and become vulnerably dependent on appearance or possessions to positively influence others" (p. 581).

Table 9–4.   Lifetime psychiatric comorbidity (Axis I) in persons with compulsive shopping

Comorbid disorder	Schlosser et al. 1994 DIS	Christenson et al. 1994 SCID	McElroy et al. 1994 SCID	Lejoyeux et al. 1997[a] MINI	Black et al. 1998[b] SCID	Ninan et al. 2000 SCID	Koran et al. 2002 MINI
Mood disorders, %							
Major depression	28	50	25	100	61	45	8
Dysthymia	—	17	—	—	3	5	13
Mania	—	—	35	10	—	—	—
Any mood disorder	28	54	95	100	64	—	21
Anxiety disorders, %							
Panic	17	13	50	—	15	—	—
Agoraphobia	—	—	—	—	6	—	8
Social phobia	28[c]	21	30	—	9	11	8
Specific phobia	—	17	20	—	24	5	—
Obsessive-compulsive disorder	4	13	35	—	3	10	21
Generalized anxiety disorder	30	21	—	—	12	—	21
Posttraumatic stress disorder	—	—	—	—	—	2	4
Any anxiety disorder	41	50	80	—	42	—	—
Substance use disorders, %							
Alcohol disorder	28	46	35	37	18	14	—
Drug disorder	13	21[d]	20	29	12	14	—
Any substance use disorder	30	46	40	—	21	—	—

Table 9–4. Lifetime psychiatric comorbidity (Axis I) in persons with compulsive shopping *(continued)*

Comorbid disorder	Schlosser et al. 1994 DIS	Christenson et al. 1994 SCID	McElroy et al. 1994 SCID	Lejoyeux et al. 1997[a] MINI	Black et al. 1998[b] SCID	Ninan et al. 2000 SCID	Koran et al. 2002 MINI
Somatoform disorders, %	11	—	10	—	—	—	—
Eating disorders, %	17	21	35	21[c]	15	—	8[e]
Impulse-control disorders, %							
Pathological gambling	20	8	5	10	—	—	—
Kleptomania	37	4	10		—	—	13
Trichotillomania	11	4	10	—	—	—	8
Intermittent explosive disorder	22	4	10	—	—	—	—
Pyromania	2	—	10	—	—	—	—
Paraphilia	13	—	10	—	—	—	—
Any impulse-control disorder	—	21	40	—	—	—	—

Note. DIS = Diagnostic Interview Schedule; MINI = Mini International Neuropsychiatric Interview; SCID = Structured Clinical Interview for DSM-IV.
[a]All subjects were depressed inpatients assessed for buying behavior.
[b]Includes the subjects reported on by Black et al. (1997).
[c]"Phobic disorder."
[d]Cannabis abuse.
[e]Bulimia nervosa.

Course and Outcome

There are no careful longitudinal studies of compulsive shopping, but anecdotal reports suggest that the condition is either chronic or recurrent for most, although it fluctuates in both severity and intensity. In the four studies reported in Table 9–3 in which the mean age at onset at the time of study participation was assessed, subjects reported having had chronic symptoms from 9 to 22 years. In the report by Schlosser et al. (1994), 59% described their course as continuous and 41% as episodic. Similarly, McElroy et al. (1994) reported that 60% of subjects described their course as chronic and 8% as episodic. A recent report (Aboujaoude et al. 2003) suggests that persons who responded to treatment with citalopram were likely to remain in remission during a 1-year follow-up. Thus, it is possible that treatment could alter the natural course of the disorder.

I have observed that subjects will often report that they are able to voluntarily control the behavior for weeks or months at a time, although their shopping urges and preoccupations remain. Reasons given for the improvement in their buying behavior include severe financial or marital problems that force the individual to control their behavior. Onset of the disorder often seems to coincide with an individual's emancipation from the family (e.g., going away to college, moving out on one's own) or obtaining credit cards or a checking account.

Clinical Symptoms

Schlosser et al. (1994) and Christenson et al. (1994) each used the Minnesota Impulsive Disorders Interview to assess buying behaviors and cognitions in their respective samples. These data can be used to paint a broader picture of the individual with compulsive shopping. Christenson et al. (1994) noted that for 47% of the subjects, shopping experiences were associated with irritable urges that prompted the buying. Urges were described as episodic, typically lasting about 1 hour and varying from daily to weekly in occurrence. In a few individuals, urges were reported to occur hourly. Shopping can occur anywhere, but department stores, discount malls, consignment shops, and even television shopping channels are popular with compulsive buyers. Internet shopping has become another way to engage in compulsive shopping behavior (Dittmar 2004).

Shopping was associated with a variety of emotions in the study of Christenson et al. (1994). They reported that many subjects described feeling "happy" (80%), "powerful" (71%), or "elated" (54%). Subsequent to the shopping episode, subjects also reported feeling a "letdown," described as "feeling out of control" (63%), "frustrated" (58%), "irritable" (42%), "depressed" (33%), "hurt" (33%), and "angry" (29%). Interestingly, some subjects (17%) reported that shopping was at times sexually exciting, whereas others described shopping as though in a dissociative state. Nearly all of their sample (96%) reported a release of tension or gratification after buying. However, these initial positive feelings often led to guilt, anger, sadness, or indifference.

Table 9–5 shows the types of merchandise that compulsive shoppers bought during compulsive buying episodes in the studies of Christenson et al. (1994) and Schlosser et al. (1994). Anecdotally, patients often report buying a product based on its attractiveness or because it was a "bargain." In the study by Christenson et al. (1994), compulsive shoppers reported spending an average of $110 during a typical shopping episode, compared with $92 reported in the study by Schlosser et al. (1994).

Inspection of Table 9–5 shows that clothes, shoes, jewelry, makeup, and compact discs/cassettes are the most common items purchased. Individually, the items are not generally large or expensive, and for most persons their purchase would not have led to adverse consequences, yet I have observed that compulsive shoppers often buy in quantity (e.g., five blouses each with a slightly different pattern or color) so that spending gets out of hand. Although neither data set provides gender-specific results, in my experience men are also interested in clothing, shoes, and compact discs/cassettes but tend to have a greater interest than women in electronic, automotive, or hardware goods. In the sample studied by Christenson et al. (1994), 92% of compulsive buyers described attempts to resist urges to buy; those indicating such attempts reported that they tried to resist 43% of the time, although their attempts were often unsuccessful. Subjects indicated that 74% of the time that they experienced an urge to buy, the urge resulted in a purchase. Typically, 1–5 hours passed between initially experiencing the urge to buy and the eventual purchase.

Compulsive buying tends to occur year round; however, Schlosser et al. (1994) found that buying may be even more problematic during the Christmas holidays and the birthdays of family members and friends. Although 96% of subjects said that they use the item that they purchase, subjects described a range of behaviors including returning the item (54%), failing to

Table 9–5.   Merchandise purchased during episode of problem buying

Item	Christenson et al. 1994 (N=24)	Schlosser et al. 1994 (N=46)
Clothing	96%	72%
Shoes	75%	35%
Jewelry	42%	26%
Makeup	33%	22%
Collectibles	25%	20%
Antiques	25%	9%
Compact discs/cassette tapes	21%	35%
Art	17%	4%
Cars/auto parts	17%	–
Electronics	—	15%
Housewares	13%	—
Books	13%	2%
Food	—	11%

remove the item from the packaging (54%), selling the item, or even giving it away. Two individuals described throwing the items out.

Compulsive shoppers tend to rely on credit cards more than do noncompulsive shoppers and tend to have more cards, but they are less likely to pay them off monthly. In one study, individuals who exhibited normal buying behavior reported that 22% of their take-home pay was used to pay off debts (excluding home and car payments). This figure was 46% for compulsive shoppers (O'Guinn and Faber 1989).

Compulsive buying occurs along a spectrum of severity. Black et al. (2001) divided a sample of 44 persons into quartiles from most to least severe depending on their Compulsive Buying Scale score and found that greater severity was associated with lower gross income, less likelihood of having an income above the median, and spending a lower percentage of income on sale items. Subjects with more severe compulsive buying were also more likely to have Axis I or II comorbidity. These results suggest that persons with the most severe buying problems have substantial emotional problems and that their spending is both more impulsive and less well controlled than that of persons with better finances.

Dimensional Traits

Compulsive shoppers often differ from comparison samples when dimensional scales are used. Christenson et al. (1994) reported that compulsive shoppers scored significantly higher on the Beck Depression Inventory (Beck et al. 1961) than did those who exhibited normal buying; their state and trait scores on the Spielberger Trait Anxiety Inventory (Spielberger et al. 1970) were higher, as were their checking/washing, obsessional slowness, and total scores on the Maudsley Obsessive Compulsive Inventory (Hodgson and Rachman 1977). Lejoyeux et al. (1997) reported that compulsive shoppers with depression had significantly higher scores than did individuals with depression who exhibited normal buying on the experience-seeking subscale of the Zuckerman Sensation Seeking Scale (Zuckerman et al. 1978), as well as the cognitive impulsivity, motor impulsivity, nonplanning activity, and total scores for the Barratt Impulsiveness Scale (Barratt 1965). In a study of persons who self-identified as compulsive shoppers, O'Guinn and Faber (1989) identified higher levels of compulsivity, materialism, and fantasy, but lower levels of self-esteem than individuals who engaged in normal buying behavior.

Pathogenesis

The etiology of compulsive shopping is unknown, but investigators have suggested developmental, cultural, neurobiological, and genetic causes. As with any psychiatric disorder, etiology is often multifactorial and involves multiple mechanisms.

Psychoanalysts have suggested that early life events, such as sexual abuse, can lead to compulsive shopping behavior later in life. These same clinicians believe that treatment, described below, necessarily involves uncovering these critical events (Krueger 1988; Lawrence 1990; Winestine 1985). Yet there is little empirical evidence that any consistent pattern of adverse childhood events exists among compulsive buyers.

Cultural influences might help to explain the fact that compulsive shopping is mainly found in developed countries. Essential ingredients for the development of compulsive shopping appear to include a market economy, a diversity of goods, and discretionary income. It seems unlikely that the disorder would occur in poorly developed or undeveloped countries except among the wealthy elite; Imelda Marcos, wife of former Philippine President Ferdinand Marcos, and her penchant for collecting shoes comes to mind (Ellison 1988; Seagrave 1988).

Neurobiological explanations have involved discussion of disturbed serotonin neurotransmission and the role of dopamine in "reward dependence" for perpetuating the behavior. Much of the pharmacological treatment research discussed below has involved the use of selective serotonin reuptake inhibitors (SSRIs). These medications were chosen by investigators who had observed similarities between OCD and compulsive shopping (Hollander 1993). Because initial reports (Black et al. 1997), and at least one recent study (Koran et al. 2003), suggest that SSRIs can help curb a compulsive shopper's urges and preoccupations, serotonin dysregulation is still thought by some to have a role in the etiology of compulsive buying. Although the role of dopamine in other "behavioral addictions" (e.g., pathological gambling) has been discussed (Stahl 2000), there is no evidence that the neurotransmitter plays a role in either initiating or maintaining compulsive shopping behavior.

There is some evidence that compulsive shopping runs in families and that in these same families, mood, anxiety, and substance use disorders are excessive as well. McElroy et al. (1994) reported that of 18 individuals with compulsive shopping, 17 had one or more first-degree relatives with major depression, 11 with alcohol or other substance abuse, and 3 with an anxiety disorder. Three had relatives with compulsive shopping as well. Black et al. (1998) later used the family history method to assess 137 first-degree relatives of 31 individuals with compulsive shopping. In this study, the relatives were significantly more likely than comparators to have depression, alcoholism, a drug use disorder, "any" psychiatric disorder, and "more than one psychiatric disorder." Compulsive buying was identified in 9.5% of the first-degree relatives of subjects with compulsive shopping, although this was not assessed in the comparison group. In the only molecular genetic study of compulsive buying to be reported, Devor et al. (1999) failed to find an association between two serotonin transporter gene polymorphisms and the disorder.

Treatment

Psychotherapy

Psychotherapy has often been described as a mainstay of treatment for compulsive shopping. Krueger (1988), Winestine (1985), and Lawrence (1990), all psychoanalysts, reported that successful treatment of the compulsive shopper requires careful exploration of his or her early life. Krueger (1988) described four cases to show that compulsive shopping was motivated by "a dual attempt to regulate the affect and fragmented sense of self and to restore self-object equilibrium, symbolically or indirectly" (p. 583). Winestine (1985) presented a case of an individual who had a history of sexual abuse and fantasies of being the wife of a famous millionaire who had the power and funds to afford anything she wished. She felt that in identifying with this role, the patient reversed her actual feelings of helplessness and her ability to regulate her shopping and spending behavior. "The purchases offered some momentary fortification against her feelings of humiliation and worthlessness for being out of control" (p. 71). Lawrence (1990) wrote that compulsive shopping stems from an "intrapsychic need for nurturing from the external world" (p. 67). More recently, Krueger (2000) wrote that compulsive shoppers have a fragile sense of self and self-esteem that depend on the responses of others. Goldman (2000) surmised that compulsive buying often follows the disruption of an emotional bond, setting into motion a desperate need to appear attractive and desirable. Benson and Gengler (2004), in considering the different forms of individual therapy, acknowledged that "there are as many different psychodynamic explanations of compulsive buying behavior as there are compulsive buyers" (p. 467).

Cognitive-behavioral therapy (CBT) models have been developed and are now being applied to compulsive shopping, although data regarding their efficacy are limited. Lejoyeux et al. (1996) suggested the use of graded exposure to ever more tempting situations paired with response prevention and instruction and techniques of impulse and condition stimulus control. Bernik et al. (1996) described two patients with comorbid panic disorder and agoraphobia responsive to clomipramine whose compulsive shopping was unaffected by the drug. Each subject responded well to 3 or 4 weeks of daily exposure to shopping stimuli with response prevention, first by an accompanying individual and later by themselves. Follow-up data were not presented.

The use of group therapy for compulsive buying was first described by Damon (1988) in her book *Shopaholics: Serious Help for Addicted Spenders.* Later, Burgard and Mitchell (2000) described a CBT group therapy treatment lasting 8 weeks that focused on factors that maintain the abnormal shopping behavior and on strategies for controlling spending, but not on the individual group member's personal problems. In a preliminary study involving only women, each subject experienced substantial improvement; follow-up data were not presented. In Spain, Villarino et al. (2001) developed a group treatment described in their book *Buying Addiction: Analysis, Evaluation, and Treatment.* These investigators describe the use of in vivo desensitization techniques to control buying impulses; relaxation techniques, visualization exercises, and cognitive restructuring techniques are also embedded in the program. Benson and Gengler (2004) suggested that group therapy may be particularly useful in treating compulsive shoppers, because it may help to "break through the denial of destructive behavior" that they feel are typical of the disorder. They further noted that "the group can grow together in hope and triumph. Individuals can see people at many different stages of recovery and know that others will be there to support them" (p. 467).

Marital counseling can also be helpful, especially when the compulsive spending cannot be dealt with adequately on an individual basis or has disrupted the marriage. To Mellan (1994), the role of the therapist is to aid the couple in restoring financial balance to the relationship through improved communication about money issues and in learning how to relate to money as a tool for managing their lives and not just as an emotionally laden symbol of power, security, and independence.

Because many subjects view compulsive shopping as a financial rather than medical or psychiatric problem, those affected may seek counseling more often from bankers or financial consultants than from mental health professionals (McCall 2000). There are no data on the extent of this form of counseling, but such advice may be helpful. Many compulsive shoppers can also benefit from attending the support group Debtors Anonymous, patterned after Alcoholics Anonymous, which provides an atmosphere of mutual support and encouragement for those who have accumulated substantial debts (Brazer 2000; Levine and Kellen 2000). Simplicity circles have been started in some U.S. cities. These voluntary groups encourage people to adopt a more simple lifestyle and to turn away from their compulsive spending (Andrews 2000).

Self-help books are available, including *Shopaholics: Serious Help for Addicted Spenders* (Damon 1988), *Born to Spend: How to Overcome Compulsive Spending* (Arenson 1991), *Women Who Shop Too Much: Overcoming the Urge to Splurge* (Wesson 1991), *Consuming Passions: Help for Compulsive Shoppers*

(Catalano and Sonenberg 1993), and *Addicted to Shopping...and Other Issues Women Have With Money* (O'Connor 2005). Each of these books provides sensible recommendations that individuals who exhibit compulsive shopping can employ to gain control over their inappropriate shopping and spending behavior.

Psychopharmacology

Interest in drug treatment was spurred by a report by McElroy et al. (1991) of three women who all appeared to demonstrate partial or complete remission of compulsive shopping behavior with fluoxetine, bupropion, or nortriptyline; all had comorbid mood or anxiety disorders. In a later study, McElroy et al. (1994) reported on a series of 20 subjects, 9 of whom had partial or full remission in response to trials of antidepressants, most often SSRIs, often in combination with a mood stabilizer. In most cases, the observation period was limited to a few months. Two of the nine patients who improved had received support or insight-oriented therapy before receiving drug therapy. Black et al. (1997) reported that 9 of 10 individuals with compulsive shopping recruited through a newspaper advertisement improved while receiving fluvoxamine at a mean dosage of 205 mg/day. Three subjects improved in the first week, and all had responded by week 5. Subjects were followed for an additional 4 weeks; by that time, 7 of the 10 patients requested continuation therapy. The authors reported that those who improved were less preoccupied with shopping and spending, spent less time shopping, and reported spending less money. None of the subjects had major depression, refuting the assertion of Lejoyeux et al. (1995) that depressed individuals with compulsive shopping are more likely to improve with antidepressants than those who are not depressed. Koran et al. (2002) reported the results of a 12-week open-label trial of citalopram in 24 compulsive shoppers given a mean dosage of 35 mg/day. They reported that citalopram produced "rapid, marked, and sustained improvements" in 80% of the subjects and that 71% were still considered responders at a 6-month follow-up. Subjects continuing citalopram therapy were less likely to relapse than those discontinuing the medication.

The following is a clinical vignette reported by Black et al. (1997) from their open-label study and illustrates the types of problems typical of compulsive buying.

Heather was an attractive but slightly overweight 35-year-old woman. She had been compulsively shopping and spending since receiving her first credit card in her late teens. Although she knew her behavior was excessive and irrational, her efforts to change always failed. Heather's life revolved around shopping and spending, even though she worked full time and had two young children. She often took them shopping with her, and they, too, expressed keen interest in shopping.

Heather typically bought new clothing for herself or her children, paperback books, cosmetics and hair care products, and numerous small items. Her grocery store purchases included not only the new products ("I just had to sample them") but also nonfood items such as books, greeting cards, and tabloid magazines. Heather's closets and storage spaces were filled with clothing that she did not need and rarely wore, and her kitchen cabinets were packed as well.

Heather loved shopping and was distressed only by its consequences. She admitted that she had sought help mainly because her husband was fed up with her behavior. They were beginning to have financial problems, even though both had adequate incomes. Heather had recurring depression, although she was not clinically depressed at the time of her formal psychiatric assessment. She also had a history of infrequent panic attacks but did not have a panic disorder.

To try to bring her shopping under control, Heather entered an 8-week experimental treatment program. She was started on a low dosage of fluvoxamine (50 mg/day). That dosage was gradually increased, as tolerated, to 150 mg/day. She also met weekly with the researcher to discuss her shopping compulsions and other concerns.

Heather responded well to fluvoxamine. On completing the 8-week treatment period, she reported that she thought less frequently about shopping. She also felt less compelled to shop, and she spent less time actually shopping.

In turn, she began spending more time with her family. She also started to work on hobbies and other special interests. After she was withdrawn from fluvoxamine, however, her symptoms began to recur.

Although the open-label trials have been positive, two double-blind, placebo-controlled trials using fluvoxamine were not; a third double-blind study using citalopram was positive. In a study conducted by Black et al. (2000), 12 subjects were randomly assigned to fluvoxamine and 11 to placebo for a 9-week study. At the conclusion of the trial, 50% of fluvoxamine recipients and 64% of placebo recipients were considered responders. Subjects in both treatment cells showed improvement as early as the second week of the trial and, for most, improvement continued during the 9-week study. There were no significant differences between fluvoxamine- and placebo-treated patients on any of the main outcome measures using an intent-to-treat analysis. Mean YBOCS-SV scores of the fluvoxamine-treated subjects fell from 21 at baseline to 15 at week 9; for the placebo recipients, the scores fell from 24 at baseline to 14 at the end of week 9. Improvement measured from baseline to week 9 was statistically significant for both fluvoxamine and placebo recipients. Ninan et al. (2000) reported results from a double-blind, 12-week trial comparing fluvoxamine with placebo in 37 patients treated at two sites. Intent-to-treat analysis failed to show a significant difference between fluvoxamine and placebo recipients using a version of the YBOCS or the Clinical Global Improvement Scale. Both reports suggest that compulsive shopping has a high placebo response rate, a feature that needs to be considered in planning future studies.

These concerns were partially addressed by Koran et al. (2002) who reported findings from a study in which subjects who improved on citalopram during a 7-week open-label phase (62.5%) were then randomized to drug or placebo. During this phase, 62.5% of those randomized to placebo relapsed versus none of the drug-treated patients, suggesting that citalopram may be effective in treating the symptoms of compulsive shopping.

Finally, in a single case report, Kim (1998) described improvement in a woman with a 5-year history of compulsive buying treated with naltrexone, an opioid antagonist. Kim noted that he had observed three additional cases in which naltrexone produced improvement.

Conclusion

Compulsive shopping is characterized by poorly controlled shopping preoccupations, urges, or behaviors that lead to adverse interpersonal, occupational, legal, or financial consequences. The disorder is estimated to affect from 2% to 8% of the general adult population, and most of those affected are women. Onset occurs in the late teens or early twenties, and the disorder is chronic or intermittent for most. Compulsive shopping behavior has been described by investigators around the globe but appears to occur mainly in developed countries. Comorbid psychiatric disorders are common, especially mood, anxiety, eating, impulse-control, and personality disorders. There is no special "shopping" personality. There are no standard treatments, but recommendations include both individual and group psychotherapy. Results of drug treatment studies are mixed, and most have involved the use of serotonin reuptake inhibitor antidepressants. Financial counseling, 12-Step programs, and self-help books may also be useful to compulsive shoppers.

References

Aboujaoude E, Gamel N, Koran LM: A 1-year naturalistic following of patients with compulsive shopping disorder. J Clin Psychiatry 64:946–950, 2003

American Psychiatric Association: Diagnostic and Statistical Manual of Mental Disorders, 4th Edition, Text Revision. Washington, DC, American Psychiatric Association, 2000

Andrews C: Simplicity circles and the compulsive shopper, in I Shop, Therefore I Am: Compulsive Buying and the Search for Self. Edited by Benson A. New York, Jason Aronson, 2000, pp 484–496

Arenson G: Born to Spend: How to Overcome Compulsive Spending. Blue Ridge Summit, PA, Tab Books, 1991

Baker JH: Mary Todd Lincoln: A Biography. New York, WW Norton, 1987

Barratt ES: Factor analysis of some psychometric measures of impulsiveness and anxiety. Psychol Rep 15:547–554, 1965

Beck AT, Ward CH, Mendelson M, et al: An inventory for measuring depression. Arch Gen Psychiatry 4:561–571, 1961

Benson AL, Gengler M: Treating compulsive buying, in Addictive Disorders: A Practical Handbook. Edited by Coombs R. New York, Wiley, 2004, pp 451–491

Bernik MA, Akerman D, Amaral JAMS, et al: Cue exposure in compulsive buying (letter). J Clin Psychiatry 57:90, 1996

Black DW: Assessment of compulsive buying, in I Shop, Therefore I Am: Compulsive Buying and the Search for Self. Edited by Benson A. New York, Jason Aronson, 2000a, pp 191–216

Black DW: The obsessive-compulsive spectrum: fact or fancy? In Obsessive-Compulsive Disorders. Edited by Maj M, Sartorius N, Okasha A, et al. New York, Wiley, 2000b, pp 233–235

Black DW: Compulsive buying disorder: definition, assessment, epidemiology and clinical management. CNS Drugs 15:17–27, 2001

Black DW, Monahan P, Gabel J: Fluvoxamine in the treatment of compulsive buying. J Clin Psychiatry 58:159–163, 1997

Black DW, Repertinger S, Gaffney GR, et al: Family history and psychiatric comorbidity in persons with compulsive buying: preliminary findings. Am J Psychiatry 155:960–963, 1998

Black DW, Gabel J, Hansen J, et al: A double-blind comparison of fluvoxamine versus placebo in the treatment of compulsive buying disorder. Ann Clin Psychiatry 12:205–211, 2000

Black DW, Monahan P, Schlosser S, et al: Compulsive buying severity: an analysis of Compulsive Buying Scale results in 44 subjects. J Nerv Ment Dis 189:123–127, 2001

Bleuler E: Textbook of Psychiatry. Translated by Brill AA. New York, Macmillan, 1924

Brazer L: Psychoeducation group therapy for money disorders, in I Shop, Therefore I Am: Compulsive Buying and the Search for Self. Edited by Benson A. New York, Jason Aronson, 2000, pp 398–427

Burgard M, Mitchell JE: Group cognitive-behavioral therapy for buying disorders, in I Shop, Therefore I Am: Compulsive Buying and the Search for Self. Edited by Benson A. New York, Jason Aronson, 2000, pp 367–397

Catalano EM, Sonenberg N: Consuming Passions: Help for Compulsive Shoppers. Oakland, CA, New Harbinger, 1993

Christenson GA, Faber JR, de Zwann M: Compulsive buying: descriptive characteristics and psychiatric comorbidity. J Clin Psychiatry 55:5–11, 1994

Damon JE: Shopaholics: Serious Help for Addicted Spenders. Los Angeles, CA, Price Stein Sloan, 1988

David L: Jacqueline Kennedy Onassis: A Portrait of Her Private Years. New York, Birch Lane Press, 1994

Davies N: Diana: The Lonely Princess. New York, Birch Lane Press, 1996

Devor EJ, Magee HJ, Dill-Devor RM, et al: Serotonin transporter gene (5-HTT) polymorphisms and compulsive buying. Am J Med Genet 88:123–125, 1999

Dittmar H: Understanding and diagnosing compulsive buying, in Addictive Disorders: A Practical Handbook. Edited by Coombs R. New York, Wiley, 2004, pp 411–450

Edwards EA: Development of a new scale for measuring compulsive buying behavior. Financial Counseling and Planning 4:67–84, 1993

Elliott R: Addictive consumption: function and fragmentation in post-modernity. Journal of Consumer Policy 17:159–179, 1994

Ellison K: Imelda: Steel Butterfly of the Philippines. New York, McGraw-Hill, 1988

Erickson C: To the Scaffold: The Life of Marie Antoinette. New York, William Morrow, 1991

Faber RJ, O'Guinn TC: Classifying compulsive consumers: advances in the development of a diagnostic tool. Adv Consum Res 16:147–157, 1989

Faber RJ, O'Guinn TC: A clinical screener for compulsive buying. J Consum Res 19:459–469, 1992

Frost RO, Kim HJ, Morris C, et al: Hoarding, compulsive buying and reasons for saving. Behav Res Ther 36:657–664, 1998

Glatt MM, Cook CC: Pathological spending as a form of psychological dependence. Br J Addict 82:1252–1258, 1987

Goldman R: Compulsive buying as an addiction, in I Shop, Therefore I Am: Compulsive Buying and the Search for Self. Edited by Benson A. New York, Jason Aronson, 2000, pp 245–267

Hassay DN, Smith CL: Compulsive buying: an examination of consumption motive. Psychology and Marketing 13:741–752, 1996

Heymann CD: A Woman Named Jackie. New York, Lyle Stuart, 1989

Hodgson RJ, Rachman S: Obsessional-compulsive complaints. Behav Res Ther 15:389–395, 1977

Hollander E (ed): Obsessive-Compulsive Related Disorders. Washington, DC, American Psychiatric Press, 1993

Kim SW: Opioid antagonists in the treatment of impulse-control disorders. J Clin Psychiatry 59:159–164, 1998

Koran L: Obsessive Compulsive and Related Disorders in Adults. New York, Cambridge University Press, 1999

Koran LM, Bullock KD, Hartstan HJ, et al: Citalopram treatment of compulsive shopping: an open-label study. J Clin Psychiatry 63:704–708, 2002

Koran LM, Chuang HW, Bullock KD, et al: Citalopram for compulsive shopping disorder: an open-label study followed by a double-blind discontinuation. J Clin Psychiatry 64:793–798, 2003

Kraepelin E: Psychiatrie, 8th Edition. Leipzig, Germany, Verlag Von Johann Ambrosius Barth, 1915, pp 408–409

Krueger DW: On compulsive shopping and spending: a psychodynamic inquiry. Am J Psychother 42:574–584, 1988

Krych R: Abnormal consumer behavior: a model of addictive behaviors. Adv Consum Res 16:745–748, 1989

Lawrence L: The psychodynamics of the compulsive female shopper. Am J Psychoanal 50:67–70, 1990

Lejoyeux M, Hourtaine M, Andes J: Compulsive buying and depression (letter). J Clin Psychiatry 56:38, 1995

Lejoyeux M, Andes J, Tassian V, et al: Phenomenology and psychopathology of uncontrolled buying. Am J Psychiatry 152:1524–1529, 1996

Lejoyeux M, Tassian V, Solomon J: Study of compulsive buying in depressed patients. J Clin Psychiatry 58:169–173, 1997

Lejoyeux M, Haberman N, Solomon J, et al: Comparison of buying behavior in depressed patients presenting with or without compulsive buying. Compr Psychiatry 40:51–56, 1999

Levine B, Kellen B: Debtors anonymous and psychotherapy, in I Shop, Therefore I Am: Compulsive Buying and the Search for Self. Edited by Benson A. New York, Jason Aronson, 2000, pp 431–454

Magee A: Compulsive buying tendency as a predictor of attitudes and perceptions. Adv Consum Res 21:590–594, 1994

McCall K: Financial recovery counseling, in I Shop, Therefore I Am: Compulsive Buying and the Search for Self. Edited by Benson A. New York, Jason Aronson, 2000, pp 455–483

McElroy S, Satlin A, Pope Jr HG, et al: Treatment of compulsive shopping with antidepressants: a report of three cases. Ann Clin Psychiatry 3:199–204, 1991

McElroy S, Keck Jr PE, Pope Jr HG, et al: Compulsive buying: a report of 20 cases. J Clin Psychiatry 55:242–248, 1994

McElroy SL, Keck PE, Phillips KA: Kleptomania, compulsive buying, and binge-eating disorder. J Clin Psychiatry 56 (suppl):14–26, 1995

Mellan O: Money Harmony: Resolving Money Conflicts in Your Life and Relationships. New York, Walker, 1994

Monahan P, Black DW, Gabel J: Reliability and validity of a scale to measure change in persons with compulsive buying. Psychiatry Res 64:59–67, 1996

Ninan PT, McElroy SL, Kane CP, et al: Placebo-controlled study of fluvoxamine in the treatment of patients with compulsive buying. J Clin Psychopharmacol 20:362–366, 2000

O'Connor K: Addicted to Shopping…and Other Issues Women Have With Money. Eugene, OR, Harvest House, 2005

O'Guinn TC, Faber RJ: Compulsive buying: a phenomenological exploration. J Consum Res 16:147–157, 1989

Scherhorn G, Reisch LA, Raab G: Addictive buying in West Germany: an empirical study. Journal of Consumer Policy 13:355–387, 1990

Schlosser S, Black DW, Repertinger S, et al: Compulsive buying: demography, phenomenology, and comorbidity in 46 subjects. Gen Hosp Psychiatry 16:205–212, 1994

Seagrave S: The Marcos Dynasty. New York, Harper and Row, 1988

Spielberger CD, Gorsuch RL, Luschene RE: Manual for the State-Trait Anxiety Inventory. Palo Alto, CA, Consulting Psychologists Press, 1970

Stahl SM: Essential Psychopharmacology. New York, Cambridge University Press, 2000, pp 503–505

Swanberg WA: Citizen Hearst. New York, Galahad, 1961

Valence G, D'Astous A, Fortier L: Compulsive buying: concept and measurement. Journal of Consumer Policy 11:419–433, 1988

Villarino R, Otero-Lopez JL, Casto R: Adicion a la Compra: Analysis, Evaluaction y Tratamiento [Buying Addiction: Analysis, Evaluation, and Treatment). Madrid, Spain, Ediciones Pirámide, 2001

Wesson C: Women Who Shop Too Much: Overcoming the Urge to Splurge. New York, St. Martin's Press, 1991

Winestine MC: Compulsive shopping as a derivative of childhood seduction. Psychoanal Q 54:70–72, 1985

Zuckerman M, Eysenck S, Eysenck HG: Sensation seeking in England and in America: cross-cultural, age, and sex comparisons. J Consult Clin Psychol 46:139–149, 1978

10

Pyromania

Michel Lejoyeux, M.D., Ph.D.

Mary McLoughlin, Ph.D.

Jean Adès, M.D.

Pyromania is defined as an impulsive behavior leading to motiveless arson. The term *pyromania* was introduced by Marc, a French psychiatrist, in 1833. Marc (cited by West and Walk 1977) described pyromania as a form of "instinctive and impulsive monomania." *Monomania* is an abnormal behavior, "a crime against nature, so monstrous and without reason, as to be explicable only through insanity, yet perpetrated by subjects apparently in full possession of their sanity." Other classic forms of monomania are homicidal monomania, kleptomania, dipsomania, and oniomania (Lejoyeux et al. 1996). The word *pyromania* was transported straight from the French to the English medical vocabulary in the early nineteenth century.

The existence of pyromania as a definite psychiatric disorder was questioned after the first descriptions of monomania (Barker 1994). After Marc, the German physician Griesinger, whose work was published in 1867, stated, "Away with the term *pyromania,* and let there be a careful investigation in every case into the individual psychological peculiarities which lie at the bottom and give rise to this impulse...To include cases of fire setting under the title of 'Pyromania' is the necessary but evil result of a superficial classification" (Griesinger 1867). However, pyromania is still present in DSM-IV-TR (American Psychiatric Association 2000).

Diagnosis and Differential Diagnosis

The essential features of pyromania are deliberate and purposeful (rather than accidental) fire setting on more than one occasion. According to the DSM-IV-TR diagnostic criteria (Table 10–1), the fire setting committed by pyromaniacs is not made for criminal reasons, profit, or sabotage. It is not done for monetary gain or as an expression of sociopolitical ideology (act of terrorism or protest), anger, or vengeance. Another behavior excluded is fire setting directly induced by a psychiatric disorder. The fire setting in response to a delusion of hallucination is not a form of pyromania. DSM-IV-TR criteria also exclude fire setting directly induced by mania, conduct disorders, and antisocial personality disorder. The fire-setting behavior in pyromania is primary, unrelated to another psychiatric state or to ideology, vengeance, or criminality, and does not result from impaired judgment (e.g., in dementia or mental retardation). DSM-IV-TR also excludes "communicative arson," by which some individuals with mental disorders or personality disorders use fire to communicate a desire or need.

The essential feature of pyromania is thus the presence of multiple deliberate and purposeful fire setting. Another important clinical feature of pyromania is the fascination of subjects with fire. People with pyromania like watching fire. They are often recognized as regular "watchers" at fires in their neighborhoods. They may like setting off false fire alarms. Their fascination with fire leads some to seek employment or to volunteer as a firefighter. Patients may be indifferent to the consequences of the fire for life or property, or they may get satisfaction from the resulting destruction. The behavior may lead to property damage, legal consequences, or injury or loss of life to the fire setter or to others.

Table 10–1.   DSM-IV-TR criteria for pyromania

A.   Deliberate and purposeful fire setting on more than one occasion.

B.   Tension or affective arousal before the act.

C.   Fascination with, interest in, curiosity about, or attraction to fire and its situational contexts (e.g., paraphernalia, uses, consequences).

D.   Pleasure, gratification, or relief when setting fires, or when witnessing or participating in their aftermath.

E.   The fire setting is not done for monetary gain, as an expression of sociopolitical ideology, to conceal criminal activity, to express anger or vengeance, to improve one's living circumstances, in response to a delusion or hallucination, or as a result of impaired judgment (e.g., in dementia, mental retardation, substance intoxication).

F.   The fire setting is not better accounted for by conduct disorder, a manic episode, or antisocial personality disorder.

Source.   Reprinted from *Diagnostic and Statistical Manual of Mental Disorders,* 4th Edition, Text Revision. Washington, DC, American Psychiatric Association, 2000. Copyright 2000, American Psychiatric Association. Used with permission.

Recent diagnostic classifications include pyromania among the impulse-control disorders (ICDs). Although the fire setting results from a failure to resist an impulse, there may be important preparation of the fire (Wise and Tierney 1999). The person may leave obvious clues of his fire preparation. Pyromania, however, is considered as an uncontrolled and most often impulsive behavior. Like other ICDs, pyromania is characterized by

- A failure to resist an impulse, drive, or temptation to perform some act harmful to oneself and/or others
- An increasing sense of tension or excitement before acting out
- A sense of pleasure, gratification, or release at the time of committing the act or shortly thereafter (Wise and Tierney 1999)

Older work by Prins et al. (1985) proposed a classification of motives for fire setting. This classification distinguished criminal fire setting and impulsive behaviors more directly related to pyromania (Table 10–2). The most important limitation of this classification is that much of the information concerning causes of fire setting is speculative rather than factual. In some

Table 10–2.   Proposed classification of motives for arson

1. Arson committed for financial reward
2. Arson committed to cover up another crime
3. Arson committed for political purposes (e.g., for specific terrorist or similar activities)
4. Self-immolation as a political gesture
5. Arson committed for mixed motives (e.g., in a state of minor depression [reactive], as a cry for help, or under the influence of alcohol)
6. Arson due to the presence of an actual mental or associated disorder
    a. Severe depression
    b. Schizophrenia
    c. "Organic" disorders (e.g., brain tumor, head injury, temporal lobe epilepsy, dementing processes, disturbed metabolic processes)
    d. Mental subnormality (retardation)
7. Arson due to motive of revenge
    a. Against an individual (specific)
    b. Against society or others (generally)
8. Arson committed as an attention-seeking act (excluding motives set out under #6 above)
9. Arson committed as a means of deriving sexual satisfaction or excitement
10. Arson committed by young adults
11. Arson committed by children

Source.   Adapted from Prins et al. 1985.

cases, no motive at all is apparent. Furthermore, Barker (1994) noted that human motives are rarely pure. In a number of cases, it is very difficult to discern a clearly defined single motive.

Vreeland and Waller (1979) suggested another classification of fire-setting behaviors based on social learning theory (Table 10–3). They took into account four major aspects: antecedents, personal variables, actual behavior, and consequences of fire setting. They provided a unified approach to classification, theory, and therapeutic change.

Table 10–3. Criteria of description of fire-setting behavior

1. Antecedent environmental conditions: referring to the individual's physical and social environment

2. Organismic factors: describing personal variables such as age, sex, genetic factors, physical disabilities, associated behavioral and psychiatric problems, intellectual abilities, and cognitive style

3. Actual fire-setting behavior: may include the degree and sophistication of preparation, the incendiary materials used, the location of the fire, the structures burned, and whether the fire setter flees or remains at the scene of the fire

4. Consequences of fire setting: the actual or potential consequences of the fire-setting act that may serve to reward or otherwise maintain fire-setting behavior, including the warmth and visual stimulation of the fire, the confusion created by the fire, praise from peers for an act of defiance, praise from authority for helping to put out the fire, and economic gains

Source. Adapted from Vreeland and Waller 1979.

Epidemiology

Prevalence

Most epidemiological studies have not directly focused on pyromania. These studies include various populations of arsonists or fire setters. Most reveal a preponderance of males with a history of fire fascination (Barker 1994). They also suggest that true pyromania is rare. Fire setting for profit or revenge or secondary to delusions or hallucinations is more frequent than "authentic" ICD. Fire setting is frequent in children and in adolescents. "True" pyromania in childhood appears to be rare. Juvenile fire setting is most often associated with conduct disorder, attention-deficit/hyperactivity disorder, or adjustment disorder.

The classic study *Pathological Fire-Setting (Pyromania)* by Lewis and Yarnell (1951) is one of the largest epidemiological studies of this topic. The authors included approximately 2,000 records from the National Board of Fire Underwriters. They added cases provided through fire departments, psychiatric clinics and institutions, and police departments near New York City. The authors suggested that the peak incidence of fire setting was between the ages of 16 and 18 years. This observation has not been confirmed by more recent studies. Pyromania is found in adolescents and is also present at any age. Among females, the diversity of ages is particularly apparent (Barker 1994).

Thirty-nine percent of the fire setters from the Lewis and Yarnell (1951) study received the diagnosis of pyromania. Twenty-two percent had borderline to dull normal intelligence, and 13% had between dull and low average intelligence. The authors also described the fire setter as a "pale and yellow, insignificant creature" driven by an irresistible impulse, seeing crime in general as an impulse that has not been resisted.

The high prevalence rates of pyromania have not been confirmed by more recent studies. Robbins and Robbins (1967) identified 23% of a population of 239 convicted arsonists as presenting with pyromania. Koson and Dvoskin (1982) found no cases (0%) of pyromania in a population of 26 arsonists. Ritchie and Huff (1999) identified only three cases of pyromania in 283 cases of arson. According to DSM-IV-TR, pyromania occurs more often in males, especially those with poorer social skills and learning difficulties. This notation confirms the Lewis and Yarnell (1951) data that only 14.8% of those with pyromania are female.

Pyromania and Depression

We (Lejoyeux et al. 2002) assessed the frequency of ICDs in a population of depressed inpatients (Tables 10–4 and 10–5). The study included 107 patients who all met DSM-IV-TR criteria for major depressive episodes. No patient had manic symptoms at the time of the assessment. Mean age of the sample was 41.3. The population consisted of 84 women (78%) and 23 men (22%); 55 (51%) were married or living maritally. ICDs were investigated using the Minnesota Impulsive Disorders Interview. This questionnaire is used to evaluate pyromania and other ICDs. Thirty-one depressed patients met criteria for ICDs: 18 had intermittent explosive disorder, 3 had pathological gambling, 4 had kleptomania, 3 had pyromania, and 3 had trichotillomania.

Patients with co-occurring ICDs were significantly younger (mean ages: 37.7 versus 42.8 years). Patients with pyromania had a higher number of previous depressions (3.3 versus 1.3, $P=0.01$). Bipolar disorders were more frequent in the ICD group than in the group without ICDs (19% versus 1.3%, $P=0.002$). Antisocial personality was not more frequent in the ICD group (3%) versus the control group (1%). Bulimia (42% versus 10.5%, $P=0.005$) and compulsive buying (51% versus 22%, $P=0.006$) were significantly more frequent in the ICD group. Discussion of our results is limited by the small

Table 10–4. Sociological and demographic characteristics of depressed patients with and without impulse-control disorders

	No ICD	Pyromania	Pathological gambling	Intermittent explosive disorder	Kleptomania	Trichotillomania	All ICDs
Patients, N (%)	76 (71.0)	3 (2.8)	3 (2.8)	18 (16.8)	4 (3.7)	3 (2.8)	31 (29.0)
Age, y (mean ± SD)	42.8 (13.9)	49.3 (6.6)	46.6 (13)	35.1 (10)[a]	39.7 (2.5)	30 (5)	37.7 (11)
Gender ratio, men:women	17:59	1:2	2:1	3:15	0:4	0:3	6:25
Married, N (%)	34 (44.7)	3 (100)	3 (100)	9 (50)	3 (75)	3 (100)	21 (67)[b]

Note. ICDs = impulse-control disorders.
[a]Difference statistically significant between the ICD and non-ICD groups, t = 2.19, df = 92, P = 0.03.
[b]Difference statistically significant between the ICD and non-ICD groups, χ^2 = 4.66, df = 1, P = 0.03.
Source. Adapted from Lejoyeux et al. 2002.

Table 10–5. Clinical characteristics of depressed patients with and without impulse-control disorders

	No ICD	Pyromania	Pathological gambling	Intermittent explosive disorder	Kleptomania	Trichotillomania	All ICDs
Patients, N	76	3	3	18	4	3	31
Previous depressive episodes, N (mean ± SD)	1.3 (1.3)	3.3 (1)[a]	1.3 (1.1)	1.3 (1.5)	5.7 (4)[b]	0 (0)	1.9 (2.4)
History of manic episodes (bipolar disorder), N (%)	1 (1.3)	0	0	3 (16)	3 (75)	0	6 (19)[c]
Suicide attempts, N (mean ± SD)	1.1 (2.1)	1 (1)	1 (1.7)	0.5 (0.6)	6 (4.2)[d]	0.6 (0.5)	1.3 (2.3)
Antisocial personality, N (%)	1 (1.3)	0	0	1 (5.5)	0	0	1 (3)
Borderline personality, N (%)	8 (10)	1	1	5	1	0	8 (26)
Bulimia, N (%)	8 (10.5)	0	1 (33)	5 (27)	4 (100)	3 (100)	13 (42)[e]
Compulsive buying, N (%)	17 (22)	0	3 (100)	9 (50)	1 (25)	3 (100)	16 (51)[f]

Note. Student's *t* test was used. ICDs = impulse-control disorders.
[a] Difference between the non-ICD and pyromania groups, $t = 2.46$, $df = 77$, $P = 0.01$.
[b] Difference between the non-ICD and kleptomania groups, $t = 5.33$, $df = 78$, $P < 0.0001$.
[c] Difference between the non-ICD and ICD groups, $\chi^2 = 8.95$, $df = 1$, $P = 0.002$.
[d] Difference between the non-ICD and kleptomania groups, $t = 4.17$, $df = 78$, $P < 0.001$.
[e] Difference between the non-ICD and ICD groups, $\chi^2 = 11.8$, $df = 1$, $P = 0.0005$.
[f] Difference between the non-ICD and ICD groups, $\chi^2 = 7.5$, $df = 1$, $P = 0.006$.
Source. Adapted from Lejoyeux et al. 2002.

number of patients assessed. The selection of subjects entering the hospital for treatment probably reflected the more severe forms of depression.

Thus the findings of the study may suggest higher prevalence rates of ICDs than are found in a less severely ill population. We failed to show a statistically significant gender difference among patients presenting with ICDs because of the size of our population. In all cases, the ICD appeared when patients no longer had mania or hypomania.

Pyromania and Alcohol Dependence

Laubichler et al. (1996) studied the files of 103 fire setters. They compared criminal fire setters and subjects presenting with pyromania. Subjects presenting with pyromania were younger (average age 20 years) than criminal fire setters (average age 30 years). Seventy of the 103 subjects with pyromania had consumed alcohol before setting a fire. Fifty-four presented with alcohol dependence. The authors suggested a correlation between the amount of alcohol consumed and the frequency of fire setting.

Räsänen et al. (1995) found that young arsonists have frequent alcohol problems: 82% had alcoholism. It was also found that 82% of arsonists were intoxicated at the time of committing the crime. The excessive consumption of alcohol had a close connection with the arson committed.

We (Lejoyeux et al. 1998, 1999) also searched for ICDs among consecutive admissions for detoxification of alcohol-dependent patients in a French department of psychiatry. We found 30 alcohol-dependent persons presenting with at least one ICD. The characteristics of these patients were compared with those of 30 alcohol-dependent patients without ICDs matched for gender and age. A control group of subjects without psychiatric disorders matched for gender and age was selected among consultants in general medicine. Diagnoses of ICDs (pyromania, kleptomania, trichotillomania, intermittent explosive disorder, pathological gambling) were based on DSM-IV (American Psychiatric Association 1994) criteria and the Minnesota Impulsive Disorders Interview (Christenson et al. 1994).

ICDs diagnosed in the group included 19 cases of intermittent explosive disorder, 7 cases of pathological gambling, 3 cases of kleptomania, and 1 case of trichotillomania. None of the patients presented with two or more ICDs. No patient presented with pyromania. It cannot be concluded from such a limited population that pyromania is not associated with alcohol dependence. Further studies including a higher number of patients are clearly needed to corroborate or refute this preliminary result.

Fire Setting and Psychiatric Disorders

In most cases, fire-setting behavior is not directly related to pyromania. On the other hand, fire setting in subjects who do not have pyromania appears frequent and often underrecognized. Among psychiatric patients, some research found that 26% of the subjects had a history of fire-setting behavior. Sixteen percent of the same patients had actually set fires (Geller and Bertsch 1985).

In Finland, Räsänen et al. (1995) compared juvenile arsonists with violent juvenile criminals regarding suicide and mental problems. They noted that in recent years the increasing amount of arson committed by juveniles attracted attention worldwide. In 1989, police in Finland registered 748 committed or attempted acts of arson, of which 122 were committed by juveniles ages 15–20 years. In the 1970s, on average, 10% of the persons who had committed arson were young people 15–20 years of age; in the 1980s, the corresponding number was 12%; by 1991, the rate had risen to 21%.

Typical descriptions consider the young arsonist as a juvenile delinquent, typically an unemployed, unmarried male with low social status. Young fire setters are found to have personality disorders, other forms of criminal behavior, early sexual relationships, and impulse-control difficulties. In comparison with other criminals or the general population, arsonists are considered to be more self-destructive.

Räsänen et al. (1995)'s sample consisted of arsonists ages 15–20 years ($n=34$) who had been in the Psychiatric Clinic of the University of Oulu in Finland under forensic psychiatric examination during the period 1983–1993. The control group ($n=33$) consisted of juveniles of the same age who had been under forensic psychiatric examination at the same time because of committing a homicide or a severe act of violence. The data were collected from forensic psychiatric examination pronouncements, case records, and police reports at the time the crime was committed.

Both arsonists and violent offenders were mostly male, poorly educated, unskilled, and unemployed at the time of committing their crimes. Among the arsonists, 79% had used public health services for treatment of their mental symptoms before the impulsive behavior. The most common reason for hospitalization was psychosis, whereas in the outpatient care the juvenile arsonists sought treatment usually because of sleep disorders, excessive use of alcohol, or aggressiveness. Suicide was more common among arsonists; 74% had suicidal thoughts and 44% had tried to commit suicide before setting a fire.

Half of the arsonists had been found guilty of one or several crimes before committing the arson. The difference in the criminal anamnesis compared with the control subjects was statistically nonsignificant. The previous crimes committed by arsonists were larcenies and driving under the influence of alcohol or other traffic offenses. Three fire setters had earlier committed an arson. The arsonists had not earlier committed violent offenses, whereas 27% of the control subjects, who had previous crimes, had committed an aggravated assault before being accused of an assault offense. None of the violent offenders had ever committed an arson. Also, in the control group most previous crimes were larcenies and driving under the influence of alcohol. In the forensic psychiatric examination, personality disorders were the most common diagnoses; 59% of the arsonists had a personality disorder.

Ritchie and Huff (1999) examined psychiatric disorders present in subjects who had set fires. They reviewed mental health records and prison files from 283 arsonists, 90% of whom had a recorded history of mental health problems. Thirty-six percent had schizophrenia or bipolar disorder, and 64% were misusing alcohol or drugs at the time of their fire setting.

Etiology

Psychodynamic Models

Psychodynamic models refer to the symbolism of fire. One of the first descriptions of fire setting refers to Samson, the biblical hero (Barker 1994): "Samson set the torches alight and set the jackal loose in the standing corn of Philistines. And he burnt up standing corn and shocks as well, and vineyards, and olive groves." In nineteenth-century Europe, the typical arsonist was viewed as a female domestic in her teens, uprooted from her home and family and feeling homesick.

The symbolic value of fire is complemented by "normal" human interest in fire. This interest starts between 2 and 3 years of age (Nurcombe 1964).

Kafry's (1980) study of normal schoolboys at ages 6, 8, and 10 years found that fire interest was almost universal. Among children (Kosky and Silburn 1984), the distinction between normal interest in fire and excessive interest leading to pyromania is not always clear. Playing with matches is not a symptom of pyromania. Kolko and Kazdin (1989) showed that "future" pyromaniacs had more curiosity about fire and liked to be in contact with peers of family members involved with fire. According to Geller and Bertsch (1985), children at risk of pyromania were more often involved in fire setting, threatening to set a fire, sounding a false fire alarm, or calling the fire department with a false report of fire than were control subjects. There thus may exist a continuum between excessive interest in fire and "pure" pyromania.

Interest in fire is especially important in populations of firefighters who develop pyromania. Lewis and Yarnell (1951) studied a series of 90 volunteer firemen who deliberately set fires. Fry and Le Couteur (1966) reported the case of a policeman who by hysterical dissociation had set fires and committed crimes and then, being the first on the scene, would set about solving these crimes with great rapidity. Among those with pyromania, working as fire officers or not, there are a notable proportion of fire fetishists. McGuire et al. (1965) showed that a "fire experience" may become a "fire fetish." A fire fantasy—whether imagined or a recollection of a real event—occurring just before orgasm is conditioned by the positive feedback of orgasm to become more and more exciting.

Classical psychodynamic classifications (Lewis and Yarnell 1951) distinguished the most important motivations of fire setting. Lewis and Yarnell (1951) concentrated on fire for psychological reasons and distinguished three main groups of fire setters: the accidental, the occasional, and the habitual. Motivations might be, in cases of pyromania, "a perverted sexual pleasure in the nature of a conversion of a sexual impulse into a special substitutive excitement." Other motivations included accidental or unintentional, delusional, erotic, revenge, or group effect in children and adolescents.

Since the first descriptions by Marc, the symbolic sexual dimension of pyromania has been noted. Marc wrote that "Incendiary acts are chiefly manifested in young persons, in consequence of the abnormal development of the sexual function, corresponding with the period of life between twelve and twenty" (West and Walk 1977)). Later, pyromaniacs were described as fire fetishists. The diverse symbolism of fire is represented in the psychoanalytic interpretations of pyromania. Wilhelm Stekel (1924) discussed 95 cases of patients presenting with pyromania. He noted that "awakening and ungratified sexuality impel the individual to seek a symbolic solution to his conflict between instinct and reality."

Sigmund Freud (1931/1964) considered fire setting, like many other ICDs, to be a masturbatory equivalent. Freud developed his sexual explanation of pyromania and noted that "to gain control over fire, men had to renounce the homosexual desire to put it out with a stream of urine." He also wrote that "the warmth that is radiated by fire calls up the same sensation that accompanies a state of sexual excitation, and the shape and movement of a flame suggest a phallus in activity."

Otto Fenichel (1945) developed the sexual theory of pyromania. He described this behavior as a specific form of urethral–erotic fixation. More recently, Geller and Bertsch (1985) explained fire setting in terms of an attempt at communication by individuals with few social skills.

Noblett and Nelson (2001) studied females presenting with pyromania. Arsonists more frequently had a history of deliberate self-harm and sexual abuse. The researchers' results emphasized the degree of psychosocial traumatisms and difficulties in female arsonists and pyromaniacs. According to the authors, pyromania could be a displacement of aggressivity. This displacement is observed in subjects with a history of sexual trauma. Patients with pyromania could be unable to directly confront people. The channeling of aggression by their fire-setting behavior may be seen as an attempt to influence their environment and improve their self-esteem where other means have failed.

The most frequent motives for arson committed by juveniles (Räsänen et al. 1995) are revenge on parents or other authorities, the search for heroism or excitement, self-destructiveness, and the craving for sensation or an expression of outrage. There is also a great deal of self-destructive behavior by juvenile fire setters before committing arson; 74% of arsonists have suicidal thoughts and 44% have tried to commit suicide before committing their crimes.

Biological Markers

Research has addressed the biological mechanisms of pyromania. Virkkunen and colleagues (Virkkunen 1984; Virkkunen et al. 1987, 1994) first tried to identify biochemical markers of this behavior. They suggested that pyromania could be associated with reactive hypoglycemia and/or lower concentrations of 3-methoxyhydroxyphenylglycol (MHPG) and cerebrospinal fluid 5-hydroxy-indoleacetic acid (CSF 5-HIAA). Their results supported the hypothesis that poor impulse control in criminal offenders is associated with low levels of certain CSF monoamine metabolites and with a hypoglycemic trend. In addition, impulse fire setters who are violent offenders are often dependent on alcohol and have a father who is also alcohol dependent (Linnoila et al. 1989).

Another study (Virkkunen et al. 1996) investigated biochemical and family variables and predictors of recidivism among forensic psychiatric patients who had set fires. One hundred and fourteen male alcoholic patients and fire setters were followed for an average of 4.5 years after their release from prison. Low CSF 5-HIAA and homovanillic acid concentrations were associated with a family history positive for paternal alcoholism with violence.

A low plasma cholesterol concentration was associated with a family history positive for paternal alcoholism without violence. The recidivists, who set fires during the follow-up period, had low CSF 5-HIAA and MHPG concentrations compared with nonrecidivists. Early family environments of the recidivists, compared with those of the nonrecidivists, were characterized by a common paternal absence and the presence of brothers at home. Thus, recidivist violent offenders and fire setters are predicted by low CSF 5-HIAA and MHPG concentrations and a developmental history positive for the early paternal absence from and the presence of brothers in the family of origin.

Impulsivity and Sensation Seeking

We compared (Table 10–6) the level of impulsivity and sensation seeking in depressed inpatients presenting with and without ICDs (Lejoyeux et al. 2002). The Zuckerman Sensation Seeking Scale (Zuckerman et al. 1978) did not reveal statistical differences between subjects with and without ICDs. We did not find a difference in the general factor or in scores of the subscales (thrill and adventure seeking, disinhibition, boredom susceptibility, and experience seeking) of sensation seeking between the groups. We also did not find a difference in terms of sensation seeking between subtypes of ICDs.

Total scores of impulsivity assessed with the Barratt Impulsivity Scale (Barratt and Patton 1983) were not significantly different in the ICD (53.5) and the non-ICD groups (47.8). A significant difference was observed

Table 10–6. Scores of impulsivity (Barratt scale) in depressed patients with and without impulse-control disorders

	No ICD	Pyromania	Pathological gambling	Intermittent explosive disorder	Kleptomania	Trichotillo- mania	All ICDs
Patients, N	76	3	3	18	4	3	31
Total score, N (SD)	47.8 (16.7)	46 (5.1)	82.6 (14.1)[a]	43.7 (17.9)	77 (10)[b]	60 (28.9)	53.5 (22.1)
Nonplanned activity, N (SD)	16.4 (7.4)	9.3 (7)	31 (6)[c]	15 (6.8)	27 (6)[d]	19.3 (14.2)	17.9 (9.5)
Cognitive impulsivity, N (SD)	16.9 (5.6)	15.6 (4.6)	27.6 (2.5)[e]	14.1 (7.3)	26.5 (1)[f]	17 (9.1)	17.4 (5.6)
Motor impulsivity, N (SD)	14.3 (7)	21 (6.9)	24 (7.9)[g]	14.6 (8.1)	23.5 (3)[h]	23.6 (5.7)[i]	18.1 (8.1)[j]

Note. ICDs=impulse-control disorders.
[a]Difference between pathological gambling and non-ICD groups, $t=3.5$, $df=78$, $P<0.0001$.
[b]Difference between kleptomania and non-ICD groups, $t=3.43$, $df=78$, $P=0.0009$.
[c]Difference between pathological gambling and non-ICD groups, $t=3.35$, $df=78$, $P=0.001$.
[d]Difference between kleptomania and non-ICD groups, $t=2.79$, $df=78$, $P=0.006$.
[e]Difference between pathological gambling and non-ICD groups, $t=3.26$, $df=78$, $P=0.001$.
[f]Difference between kleptomania and non-ICD groups, $t=3.36$, $df=78$, $P=0.001$.
[g]Difference between pathological gambling and non-ICD groups, $t=2.34$, $df=78$, $P=0.02$.
[h]Difference between kleptomania and non-ICD groups, $t=2.59$, $df=78$, $P=0.01$.
[i]Difference between trichotillomania and non-ICD groups, $t=2.27$, $df=78$, $P=0.02$.
[j]Difference between ICD and non-ICD groups, $t=6$, $df=105$, $P=0.01$.
Source. Adapted from Lejoyeux et al. 2002.

between the groups for motor impulsivity scores (18.1 in those with ICD versus 14.3 in those without, $P=0.01$).

ICDs in general and pyromania in particular were not associated with antisocial or borderline personalities. These two personalities correspond to a style of behavior that is impulsive and unable to tolerate frustration. In depressed patients, these personalities do not determine impulsive behavior. Pyromania did not appear to be associated with an increased level of sensation seeking.

Depressed patients presenting with pyromania had higher scores of motor impulsivity than those without ICD. Three main impulsiveness subtraits are explored by the Barratt Impulsivity Scale: motor, cognitive, and nonplanned impulsiveness. *Motor impulsiveness* is defined as acting without thinking. *Cognitive impulsiveness* is characterized by quick cognitive decisions, and *nonplanned impulsiveness* by a lack of anticipation. In the ICD group, pathological gambling patients and kleptomania patients scored significantly higher on all three impulsivity subtraits than did patients without ICD. These psychological dimensions of impulsivity were not increased in patients presenting with pyromania.

Surprisingly, patients with ICDs were more often married. Others have suggested that ICDs can induce marital disruption and affective loneliness (McElroy et al. 1992). Comparisons between subcategories of ICDs must be interpreted with caution due to the small number of patients studied.

Independent from studies using scales of impulsivity, clinical pictures of pyromania show that this behavior is not always impulsive. There may be considerable advance preparation for starting the fire, and the person may hesitate for a long time before setting a fire.

Relation to the Obsessive-Compulsive Spectrum

In the past few years, a number of studies have suggested that a range of disorders may belong to the obsessive-compulsive spectrum (Du Toit et al. 2001). In addition to pyromania, disorders hypothesized to belong to this spectrum include eating disorders, tic disorders, somatoform disorders (hypochondriasis, body dysmorphic disorder, pathological "grooming" habits [nail biting or onychophagia, skin picking, trichotillomania]), ICDs, and impulsive personality. Disorders related to the obsessive-compulsive spectrum share characteristics with obsessive-compulsive disorder (OCD). These features include age at onset, clinical course, comorbidity, and response to behavioral and pharmacological therapies (Hollander 1993; Hollander and Benzaquen 1997). Some authors have warned against the risk of being overinclusive in the definition of the obsessive-compulsive spectrum. This spectrum includes quite different disorders in the same diagnostic frame without objective justification of such an association.

Bienvenu et al. (2000) investigated comorbidity and familial relationships between OCD and obsessive-compulsive spectrum conditions including somatoform disorders, eating disorders, pathological grooming conditions, and other ICDs using data from the Johns Hopkins OCD Family Study. They hypothesized that familial spectrum disorders should occur more often in case (OCD) probands and their first-degree relatives compared with control probands and their first-degree relatives.

In the Johns Hopkins OCD Family Study (Bienvenu et al. 2000), the authors recruited adult probands (age 18 years) from five specialty OCD treatment centers in the Baltimore/Washington area. All patients with a diagnosis of OCD who were treated in these centers in the 3 years before the initiation of the study were rostered, and 99 were randomly selected to participate. Case probands were included if they met definite DSM-IV criteria for OCD, scored in excess of 15 on the Yale-Brown Obsessive-Compulsive Scale, and were older than 18 years. Disorders were also grouped together as "either somatoform disorder" (body dysmorphic disorder or hypochondriasis), "any eating disorder" (anorexia nervosa, bulimia nervosa, or eating disorder not otherwise specified), "any grooming disorder" (nail biting, skin picking, trichotillomania, or grooming ICD not otherwise specified), "any other impulse-control disorder" (kleptomania, pathological gambling, pyromania, intermittent explosive disorder, or other ICD not otherwise specified). Bienvenu et al. (2000) did not include a case of pyromania. Their study does not support the possible inclusion of pyromania in the OCD spectrum.

Course and Prognosis

Studies indicate that the recidivism rate for fire setters ranges from 4.5% (Mavromatis and Lion 1977) to 28% (Lewis and Yarnell 1951). In Germany, Barnett et al. (1997, 1999) compared mentally ill and mentally "healthy" fire setters. In that country, trial records are kept by the Federal Central Register.

In this register, all offenses by each delinquent are noted, as well as whether the offender was criminally liable. According to German law, a defendant with a psychiatric disorder can be found to be not responsible, to have diminished responsibility, or to be fully responsible. These categories are mutually exclusive. The files do not contain psychiatric diagnoses. Because the files contain personal data, access to them is restricted to the legal system only. In a complex legal procedure, disclosure of these data was obtained for research purposes.

Barnett's group identified three samples of subjects: 1) all individuals convicted of arson who had been found not guilty by reason of insanity ($n=186$), 2) all individuals convicted of arson who had been found guilty with diminished responsibility ($n=97$), and 3) a random selection of all individuals convicted of arson who had no psychiatric examination in their trial ($n=187$). In Germany, individuals with psychosis, organic brain disease, or severe mental retardation usually obtain exculpation from criminal liability. These disorders were quite common among the arsonists who were found not to be responsible for psychiatric reasons. Subjects with diminished responsibility, however, were not likely to have these disorders.

Previous studies of arsonists remanded for psychiatric examination revealed that personality disorders were the most common diagnoses among arsonists of diminished responsibility and that the diagnosis of psychosis almost always was found among arsonists who were not responsible for psychiatric reasons.

The study by Barnett et al. was not only cross-sectional; follow-up extended for 10 years. Mentally disordered arsonists were more likely than those with no disorder to have a history of arson before their trial. They also were more often convicted of arson again (11% relapse compared with 4%), had fewer registrations of common offenses such as theft as well as traffic violations and alcohol-related offenses, had a higher rate of recurrence, and committed fewer common offenses other than fire setting. Among all arsonists who committed crimes other than arson, those who were found to be partly responsible committed the highest number of offenses followed by those who were deemed not responsible for their actions and those who were fully responsible.

Treatment Possibilities

According to Mavromatis and Lion (1977), treatment for fire setters is problematic because they frequently refuse to take responsibility for their acts, are in denial, have alcoholism, and lack insight. Behavioral treatments have used aversive therapy to help fire setters (McGrath and Marshall 1979). Other methods of treatment rely on positive reinforcement with threats of punishment, stimulus satiation, and operant structured fantasies (Bumpass et al. 1983). Bumpass et al. (1983) treated 29 child fire setters and used a graphing technique that sequentially correlated external stress, behavior, and feelings on graph paper. The authors reported that after treatment (average follow-up, 2.5 years), only 2 of the 29 children continued to set fires.

Franklin et al. (2002) confirmed the positive effect of a prevention program for pyromania. In 1999, they developed the Trauma Burn Outreach Prevention Program. All subjects arrested and convicted after setting a fire received 1 day of information. The program's interactive content focused on the medical, financial, legal, and societal impact of fire-setting behavior. The rate of recidivism was less than 1% in the group who attended the program, compared with 36% in the control group.

Conclusion

Even if studies of pyromania are rare, the recognition of this ICD is important. It has major implications for risk management. The diagnosis of psychiatric disorders and of pathological impulsivity when a subject is arrested after setting a fire allows treatments to be proposed. However, the recognition and management of this disorder is a real challenge for psychiatry. Making a prognosis is difficult, given the lack of clearly established data regarding recidivism and the severity and danger of the disorder.

Repetitive fire setting is in most cases a symptom that can be related to various psychiatric disorders such as ICDs, personality disorders, depression, or anxiety. Recognition and treatment of the psychiatric disorders associated with fire setting are thus crucial to clinical intervention.

In addition, it can be concluded from the literature that little systematic work has been undertaken on the clinical characteristics and treatment of this behavior. Very few individuals who set fires repetitively are caught, and most fire setters with pyromania are minors/juveniles. The clinical concept of pyromania should be more extensively studied as a model of an impulsive and repetitive behavioral disorder.

References

American Psychiatric Association: Diagnostic and Statistical Manual of Mental Disorders, 4th Edition. Washington, DC, American Psychiatric Association, 1994

American Psychiatric Association: Diagnostic and Statistical Manual of Mental Disorders, 4th Edition, Text Revision. Washington, DC, American Psychiatric Association, 2000

Barker AF: Arson: A Review of the Psychiatric Literature. Institute of Psychiatry, Maudsley Monographs No 35. Oxford, England, Oxford University Press, 1994

Barnett W, Richter P, Sigmund D, et al: Recidivism and concomitant criminality in pathological firesetters. J Forensic Sci 42:879–883, 1997

Barnett W, Richter P, Renneberg B: Repeated arson: data from criminal records. Forensic Sci Int 101:49–54, 1999

Barratt ES, Patton JH: Impulsivity: cognitive, behavioral, and psychophysiological correlates, in Biological Bases of Sensation Seeking, Impulsivity, and Anxiety. Edited by Zuckerman M. Hillsdale, NJ, Lawrence Erlbaum, 1983, pp 17–116

Bienvenu OJ, Samuels JF, Riddle MA, et al: The relationship of obsessive-compulsive disorder to possible spectrum disorders: results from a family study. Biol Psychiatry 48:287–293, 2000

Bumpass ER, Fagelman FD, Brix RJ: Intervention with children who set fires. Am J Psychother 37:328–345, 1983

Christenson G, Faber RJ, de Zwaan M, et al: Compulsive buying: descriptive characteristics and psychiatric comorbidity. J Clin Psychiatry 55:5–11, 1994

Du Toit PL, van Kradenburg J, Niehaus D, et al: Comparison of obsessive-compulsive disorder patients with and without comorbid putative obsessive compulsive spectrum disorders using a structured clinical interview. Compr Psychiatry 42:291–300, 2001

Fenichel O: The Psychoanalytical Theory of Neurosis. New York, WW Norton, 1945

Franklin GA, Pucci PS, Arbabi S, et al: Decreased juvenile arson and firesetting recidivism after implementation of a multidisciplinary prevention program. J Trauma 53:260–266, 2002

Freud S: The acquisition and control of fire (1931), in The Complete Psychological Works of Sigmund Freud. Translated and edited by Strachey J. London, Hogarth, 1964, pp 181–193

Fry F, Le Couteur E: Arson. Med Leg J 34:108–121, 1966

Geller J, Bertsch G: Fire-setting behavior in the histories of a state hospital population. Am J Psychiatry 142:464–468, 1985

Griesinger W: Pathologie und Therapie der psychischen Krankheiten, 2nd Edition. Stuttgart, Germany, A. Krabbe, 1867

Hollander E: Introduction, in Obsessive-Compulsive Related Disorders. Edited by Hollander E. Washington, DC, American Psychiatric Press, 1993, pp 1–16

Hollander E, Benzaquen SD: The obsessive-compulsive spectrum disorders. Int Rev Psychiatry 9:99–109, 1997

Kafry D: Playing with matches: children and fire, in Fires and Human Behavior. Edited by Canter D. New York, Wiley, 1980, pp 47–62

Kolko D, Kazdin AE: Assessment of dimensions of childhood fire-setting among patients and nonpatients: the fire-setting risk interview. J Abnorm Child Psychol 17:157–176, 1989

Kosky RJ, Silburn S: Children who light fires: a comparison between fire-setters and non-fire-setters referred to a child psychiatric outpatient service. Aust N Z J Psychiatry 18:251–255, 1984

Koson DF, Dvoskin J: Arson: a diagnostic study. Bull Am Acad Psychiatry Law 10:39–49, 1982

Laubichler W, Kuhberger A, Sedlmeier P: "Pyromania" and arson. A psychiatric and criminological data analysis [in German]. Nervenarzt 67(9):774–780, 1996

Lejoyeux M, Adès J, Tassain V, et al: Phenomenology and psychopathology of uncontrolled buying. Am J Psychiatry 155:1524–1529, 1996

Lejoyeux M, Feuché N, Loi S, et al: Impulse-control disorders in alcoholics are related to sensation seeking and not to impulsivity. Psychiatry Res 81:149–155, 1998

Lejoyeux M, Feuché N, Loi S, et al: Study of impulse control disorders among alcohol-dependent patients. J Clin Psychiatry 40:302–305, 1999

Lejoyeux M, Arbaretaz M, McLoughlin M, et al: Impulse control disorders and depression. J Nerv Ment Dis 190:310–314, 2002

Lewis NDC, Yarnell H: Pathological Firesetting (Pyromania): Nervous and Mental Disease Monograph No 82. New York, Coolidge Foundation, 1951

Linnoila M, De Jong J, Virkkunen M: Family history of alcoholism in violent offenders and impulsive fire setters. Arch Gen Psychiatry 46:613–616, 1989

Mavromatis M, Lion JR: A primer on pyromania. Dis Nerv Syst 38:954–955, 1977

McElroy SL, Hudson JI, Pope HG Jr, et al: The DSM-III-R impulse control disorders not elsewhere classified: clinical characteristics and relationship to other psychiatric disorders. Am J Psychiatry 149:318–327, 1992

McGrath P, Marshall PG: a comprehensive treatment program for a fire-setting child. J Behav Ther Exp Psychiatry 10:69–72, 1979

McGuire RJ, Carlisle JM, Young BG: Sexual deviations as conditioned behaviour: a hypothesis. Behav Res Ther 2:185–190, 1965

Noblett S, Nelson B: A psychosocial approach to arson: a case controlled study of female offenders. Med Sci Law 41:325–330, 2001

Nurcombe B: Children who set fires. Med J Aust 1:579–584, 1964

Prins H, Tennent G, Trick K: Motives for arson (fire-raising). Med Sci Law 25:275–278, 1985

Räsänen P, Hirvenoja R, Hakko H, et al: A portrait of a juvenile arsonist. Forensic Sci Int 73:41–47, 1995

Ritchie EC, Huff TG: Psychiatric aspects of arsonists. J Forensic Sci 44:733–740, 1999

Robbins E, Robbins L: Arson, with special reference to pyromania. N Y State J Med 67:795–798, 1967

Stekel W: Peculiarities of Behaviour: Wandering Mania, Dipsomania, Kleptomania, Pyromania and Allied Impulsive Acts. New York, Liveright, 1924

Virkkunen M: Reactive hypoglycemia tendency among arsonists. Acta Psychiatr Scand 69:445–452, 1984

Virkkunen M, Nuutila A, Goodwin FK: Cerebrospinal fluid monoamine metabolite levels in male arsonists. Arch Gen Psychiatry 44:241–247, 1987

Virkkunen M, Rawlings, Takola R: CSF biochemistries, glucose metabolism, and diurnal activity rhythms in alcoholic, violent offenders, fire setters, and healthy volunteers. Arch Gen Psychiatry 51:20–27, 1994

Virkkunen M, Eggert M, Rawlings R, et al: A prospective follow-up study of alcoholic violent offenders and fire setters. Arch Gen Psychiatry 53:523–529, 1996

Vreeland RG, Waller MB: Personality Theory and Fire-Setting: An Elaboration of a Psychological Model. Washington, DC, U.S. Department of Commerce, National Bureau of Standards, 1979

West DJ, Walk A: Daniel McNaughton: His Trial and the Aftermath. London, Gaskell, 1977

Wise MG, Tierney JG: Impulse control disorders not elsewhere classified, in The American Psychiatric Press Textbook of Psychiatry, 3rd Edition. Edited by Hales RE, Yudofsky SC, Talbott JA. Washington, DC, American Psychiatric Press, 1999, pp 773–794

Zuckerman M, Eysenck S, Eysenck HJ: Sensation seeking in England and in America: cross-cultural, age, and sex comparisons. J Consult Clin Psychol 46:139–149, 1978

11

Pathological Gambling

Stefano Pallanti, M.D., Ph.D.

Nicolò Baldini Rossi, M.D., Ph.D.

Eric Hollander, M.D.

Definition and Clinical Features

Pathological gambling has been considered a distinct diagnostic entity since 1980, when it was first included in DSM-III (American Psychiatric Association 1980) and similarly in ICD-9-CM (World Health Organization 1978). DSM-IV-TR (American Psychiatric Association 2000) currently classifies pathological gambling as an impulse-control disorder (ICD) not elsewhere classified. The essential feature of pathological gambling is recurrent gambling behavior that is maladaptive (i.e., loss of judgment, excessive gambling) and in which personal, family, or vocational endeavors are disrupted, as indicated by five (or more) of the following criteria:

1. Is preoccupied with gambling.
2. Needs to gamble with increasing amounts of money in order to achieve the desired excitement.
3. Has repeated unsuccessful efforts to control, cut back, or stop gambling.
4. Is restless or irritable when attempting to cut down or stop gambling.
5. Gambles as a way of escaping from problems or of relieving a dysphoric mood.
6. After losing money gambling, often returns another day to get even ("chasing" one's losses).
7. Lies to family members, therapist, or others to conceal the extent of involvement with gambling.
8. Has committed illegal acts such as forgery, fraud, theft, or embezzlement to finance gambling.
9. Has jeopardized or lost a significant relationship, job, or educational or career opportunity because of gambling.
10. Relies on others to provide money to relieve a desperate financial situation caused by gambling.

Pathological gambling may be diagnosed only if the maladaptive gambling is not better accounted for by a manic episode in DSM-IV-TR.

Prevalence and Impact of Gambling

Phenomenological and epidemiological studies support the validity and utility of the diagnosis of pathological gambling. Inclusion criteria in the *DSM* and *ICD* systems include specific criteria, thresholds, and durations for pathological gambling patients established by expert consensus via literature review, data analyses, and field trials when available, similar to other DSM-IV-TR psychiatric disorders.

The utility of pathological gambling criteria is underscored by prevalence estimates of 1%–3% of the U.S. population (American Psychiatric Association 1994) and increasing prevalence among females (33% of pathological gambling patients are women; Lesieur 1988a) and high school students (1.7%–5.7%; Ladouceur and Mireault 1988; Lesieur and Klein 1987). Pathological gambling contributes large costs to society and is associated with substantial morbidity; social, family, and job dysfunction; suicide; criminality; and excessive utilization of health care, government, and financial resources.

Lesieur (1998) found in his review of the cost literature that between 69% and 76% of pathological gamblers report having missed work at some time in order to gamble, and they often reveal that they have stolen money or other valuables in order to gamble or pay for gambling debts. Nearly half (46%) of Gamblers Anonymous (GA) participants in Wisconsin reported they had stolen something to gamble, and 39% reported having been arrested (Thompson et al. 1996); a similar GA survey in Illinois found that 56% had stolen to gamble (Lesieur and Anderson 1995). These studies found also that in the GA/treatment populations, 18%–28% of males and 8% of females have declared bankruptcy.

Between 26% and 30% of GA members attribute divorces or separations to their gambling difficulties, and several studies have suggested that pathological and problem gambling are correlated with a decline in health and elevated rates of illness, either physical or mental (Lesieur 1998; Table 11–1).

Table 11–1.   Pathological gambling

Classification
Disorder of impulse control (DSM-IV-TR)
Compulsive disorder
Addictive disorder

Clinical features
Progressive failure to resist impulses to gamble
Gambling disrupts personal, family, and vocational functioning
Gambling increases during stress
Resulting problems intensify gambling

Similarities to Addictive Disorders

Phenomenologically, pathological gambling shares features with substance abuse disorders, because core DSM-IV-TR criteria for substance abuse, including tolerance, dependence, and withdrawal, also apply to pathological gambling (Blume 1987; Dickerson 1984; Dickerson et al. 1987; Greenberg 1980;

Griffiths 1992; Jacobs 1988; Lesieur 1988b; Lesieur and Rosenthal 1991; Martinez-Pina et al. 1991; Wray and Dickerson 1981). In pathological gambling, tolerance develops when the amount or frequency of the wager increases in order to sustain the desired level of arousal. The inability to gamble results in a withdrawal phenomenon in pathological gambling associated with depression, moderate somatic discomfort, restlessness, and irritability. The development of dependence in pathological gambling occurs when 1) larger wagers than intended are made, 2) there are continuous efforts to decrease gambling activity, 3) there is a continuation of gambling in an attempt to reinstate losses rendered, and 4) the gambling activity prevents the individual from participating in otherwise usual social or occupational activities.

The association between pathological gambling and addictive disorders is also evident when one considers the high rates of dually addicted or cross-addicted gamblers (Ciarrochi 1987). Alcohol or drug abuse has been diagnosed in 30%–50% of pathological gambling patients (Lesieur and Rosenthal 1991; Ramirez et al. 1983). One theory of addictions developed by Jacobs (1986, 1988, 1989) relating alcoholism, compulsive eating, and pathological gambling involves detachment and suggests that transient dissociative states occur during the addictive activity. Specifically, dissociative states (e.g., trance-like states, feeling outside of oneself, feeling like one has taken on another identity, hiving memory blackouts while gambling or shortly after) have been found to be experienced more than twice as frequently in pathological gamblers compared with social gamblers.

As a model addiction, pathological gambling is also characterized by similar predisposing factors and symptomatology (Blume 1987; Brown 1987; Greenberg 1980; Jacobs 1988; Lesieur and Rosenthal 1991), and it is often treated in programs modeled on addictive disorders or in the same program as addicts (Blume 1986; Carone et al. 1982; Lesieur and Rosenthal 1991). The development of pathological gambling, as with other addictive disorders, may be associated with both a dysregulated physiological resting state (either aroused or depressed) and childhood feelings of inadequacy (Jacobs 1986). A review of current findings on the genetics of pathological gambling suggests that liability to pathological gambling is in part mediated by genetic factors (Ibanez et al. 2003; Eisen et al. 2001; Walters 2001), and the onset of illness may coincide with the exposure of the predisposed individual to the addictive stimulus.

Gambling dependency may develop over the course of a patient's illness and may be an attempt to guard against stress, anticipated anxiety, or painful realities (Jacobs 1982, 1984). The experience of gambling can be viewed as an addictive psychostimulant substance that reduces tension and anxiety in the afflicted individual (Anderson and Brown 1984), and although money is important, the individual is looking for the "action" or an excited state comparable with a drug-induced "high." Pathological gambling is associated with increased levels of tension prior to the activity followed by a sense of relief after the activity, much like in other addictive disorders. Furthermore, in both pathological gambling and substance abuse, there is a strong sense of pleasure and a release of tension accompanying the completion of the behavior, at least in the initial stages of the disorders (Moran 1970; Peck 1986). Continuation is then promoted by partial reinforcement schedules, craving, and biased cognitions involving changes in the individual's internal state. These include high physiological arousal with sensation-seeking components, euphoria, distraction, perceived control, and magical thinking. Other gambling-relevant cognitive distortions are superstitious beliefs, magnification of one's own gambling skills and minimization of other gamblers' skills, interpretive biases (e.g., internal/external attributions, gambler's fallacy, chasing), predictive skill, selective memory, illusion of control over luck, and illusory correlation.

Identifying Individuals With Pathological Gambling and Measuring Gambling Problems

Numerous terms have been adopted or proposed in the field of gambling research to identify individuals who experience difficulties related to their gambling. The terms *compulsive* (Bergler 1957) and *addictive* (Dickerson 1977) are popular with the public and the media; however, the psychiatric term *pathological gambler* (Moran 1970) is more widely used in the gambling treatment and research communities.

The terms *problem, at risk, potential pathological, subclinical,* and *in transition* have all been proposed by gambling researchers to identify individuals who do not meet the psychiatric criteria for a gambling disorder but who nevertheless appear to experience substantial difficulties related to their gambling. One recent term, *disordered gambling,* was proposed as a way of describing the continuum of problems, from less to more severe levels, noting the similarities and differences among troubled gamblers as observed in a multiplicity of study settings (Shaffer et al. 1999). However, recent findings on biological correlates and pharmacological treatment response have suggested the presence of diagnostic heterogeneity and clinical subtypes.

The only diagnostic tool that has been rigorously developed and tested is the South Oaks Gambling Screen (SOGS; Lesieur and Blume 1987). Based on DSM diagnostic criteria, the SOGS was originally developed to screen for gambling problems in clinical populations, with scores greater than five suggesting pathological gambling. The SOGS is a 20-item scale that includes weighted items to determine whether the subject is hiding evidence of gambling, spending more time or money gambling than intended, arguing with family members over gambling, and borrowing money from a variety of sources to gamble or to pay gambling debts. In developing the SOGS, specific items as well as the entire screen were tested for reliability and validity with a variety of groups, including hospital workers, university students, prison inmates, and inpatients in alcohol and substance abuse treatment programs (Lesieur and Blume 1987).

Although the SOGS diagnostic criteria have demonstrated satisfactory reliability, validity, and classification accuracy, Stinchfield (2003) recently suggested that improvements in classification accuracy could be obtained by lowering the cut-off score to four. False-negative errors may be considered the most serious errors in the diagnosis of pathological gambling because they are likely to have greater consequences than false-positive errors. Clinicians can be fairly confident that the respondent is *not* a pathological gambler if his or her SOGS score is between zero and two, and they can be fairly confident that the respondent *is* a pathological gambler when his or her SOGS score is five or higher.

The National Opinion Research Center Gambling Diagnostic Screen (NODS) is composed of 17 lifetime items and 17 corresponding past-year items, compared with the 20 lifetime items and 20 past-year items that make up the SOGS. Similar to the revised SOGS used in most of the epidemiological research on gambling since 1991, the past-year item is asked for each lifetime NODS item that receives a positive response; the maximum score on the NODS is 10, compared with 20 for the SOGS. Although there are fewer items in the NODS and the maximum score is lower, it is designed to be more demanding and restrictive in assessing problematic behaviors than the SOGS or other screens based on DSM-IV-TR criteria. It examines a number of different impacts of problem and pathological gambling. These include family impact, job impact, financial problems, and criminal or legal problems that are closely related to gambling.

The SOGS is also used to quantify baseline pathological gambling symptom severity and improvement in clinical trials, similar to the pathological gambling modification of the Yale-Brown Obsessive-Compulsive Scale (DeCaria et al. 1998a). This is a 10-item clinician-rated questionnaire that rates on a five-point scale the time spent and the degree of distress, interference, resistance, and control in relation to pathological gambling urges and associated gambling behaviors. A pathological gambling modification of the Clinical Global Impression scale (PG-CGI) has also been adopted (Pallanti et al. 2002b).

In addition, the number of gambling episodes, duration of episode, and percentage of total income lost or gambled are behavioral indicators commonly utilized to assess gambling severity and outcome.

Morbidity and Course of Illness

The course of pathological gambling tends to be chronic, although the pattern of gambling may be regular or episodic. Chronicity is usually associated with increases in the frequency of gambling and the amount gambled. Additionally, gambling may increase during periods of increased stress. The combination of illness chronicity, severe interference with normal life activities, and lack of known expeditious and long-term efficacious treatment frequently lead to severe personal, familial, financial, social, and occupational impairment.

Psychiatric disorders, including major depression and alcohol or substance abuse and dependence, may develop from or be exacerbated by pathological gambling. In addition to such morbidity, there is also a mortality risk associated with pathological gambling such that estimates of suicide attempts in pathological gamblers range from 17% to 24% (Ciarrocchi and Richardson 1989; Custer and Custer 1978; Livingston 1974; Moran 1969). A study by Phillips et al. (1997) indicated that the suicide rate in cities where gambling is legalized is four times higher than in cities without legal gambling. Younger patients are more likely to have suicidal tendencies and major depressive disorders (McCormick et al. 1984).

Gender differences have been described in the course of pathological gambling. In males, the disorder usually begins in adolescence (Custer and Milt 1985; Lesieur and Rosenthal 1991) and may remain undiagnosed for years. When male pathological gamblers are first diagnosed, they often present with a 20–30 year gambling history, with gradual development of dependence. In contrast, onset of pathological gambling in females is more likely to occur later in life. Prior to seeking treatment, the duration of pathological gambling is approximately 3 years. Thus, as a result of the differences in onset and duration, female pathological gamblers generally have a better prognosis than male pathological gamblers (Rosenthal 1992). In addiction, female pathological gamblers tend to be depressed and may use gambling as an anesthetic, accompanied by excitement, to escape from life's problems (i.e., as in a dissociative state; Jacobs 1988; Lesieur 1988b).

Epidemiology

An American national survey suggested that 68% of the general population participated in some form of gambling and that 0.77% of American adults are considered probable pathological gamblers (Commission on the Review of the National Policy Toward Gambling 1976). Prevalence estimates of probable pathological gambling from state surveys range from 1.2% to 3.4%, with increased rates in states that provide greater opportunity for legal gambling (Commission on the Review of the National Policy Toward Gambling 1976; Culleton 1985; Culleton and Lang 1985; Volberg 1990; Volberg and Steadman 1988, 1989). Due to an increase in access to legalized gambling in Italy, for example, our group recently found that approximately 6% of persons who frequented a discotheque in Florence, Italy, had a SOGS score corresponding to a probable diagnosis of pathological gambling (Pallanti et al. 2000).

A meta-analysis by Shaffer et al. (1999) of 120 published studies indicated that the lifetime prevalence of serious gambling (meeting DSM criteria for pathological gambling) among adults is 1.6%. Among persons younger than 18 years, the prevalence is 3.9%, with past-year rates for adults and adolescents being 1.1% and 5.8%, respectively (Shaffer and Hall 1996).

Prevalence estimates of pathological gambling in the general population differ from estimates in a treatment-seeking population. In a statewide epidemiological survey, relative to gamblers identified in treatment programs, there were higher rates of pathological or probable pathological gamblers who were female (36% vs. 7%, respectively), younger (less than 30 years; 38% vs. 18%, respectively), and non-White (43% vs. 9%, respectively) (Volberg and Steadman 1988). Female pathological gamblers clearly represent an understudied and underserved group, because females account for approximately one-third of pathological gamblers (Lesieur 1988a). Prevalence estimates of pathological gambling among high school students range from 1.7% to 3.6% (Ladouceur and Mireault 1988) to 5.7% (Lesieur and Klein 1987). Because most pathological gamblers begin their gambling career during adolescence (Custer 1982; Livingston 1974), early identification and intervention are critical.

Comorbidity

Despite the paucity of clinical samples in which standardized diagnostic instruments have been employed, the literature to date strongly suggests that three Axis I disorders frequently co-occur with pathological gambling: substance abuse or dependence, affective disorders (i.e., bipolar spectrum disorders), and attention-deficit/hyperactivity disorder (ADHD; Figure 11–1).

High rates of comorbid substance abuse and dependency complicate the clinical profile. In one study it was found that 9% of inpatient substance abusers were diagnosed as pathological gamblers (Lesieur et al. 1986) and 17% of alcohol abusers had gambling problems (Haberman 1969). Conversely, 47% of inpatient pathological gamblers (McCormick et al. 1984) and 52% of GA members (Linden et al. 1986) were alcohol or drug abusers. Of note, among a sample of female pathological gamblers, 28% had alcoholic fathers and 5% had alcoholic mothers (Lesieur 1988a). Thus, there appears to be a strong relationship between pathological gambling and substance abuse. Substance abuse should be screened for in routine clinical assessments, because failure to identify and treat comorbid substance use disorders in gamblers may lead to higher relapse rates (Maccallum and Blaszczynski 2002).

Pathological gambling is also highly comorbid with affective disorders. Among inpatient samples of pathological gambling patients, 76% met criteria for a major depressive disorder; 38% were hypomanic; 8% were manic; 2% were diagnosed with schizoaffective disorder, depressed type; and 8% had no comorbid disorder (McCormick et al. 1984). Among outpatient samples,

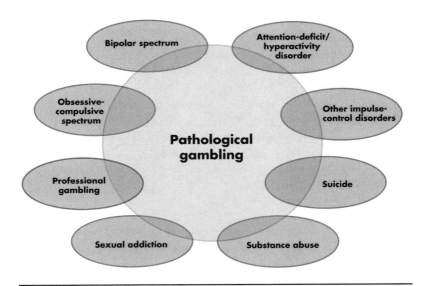

Figure 11–1. Pathological gambling: comorbidity and issues in classification.

28% met criteria for major depressive disorder, 24% had bipolar disorder, and 28% had anxiety disorders (Linden et al. 1986).

Pathological gambling has also been associated with ADHD. Electroencephalographic abnormalities found among pathological gamblers were similar to those found among children with ADHD. Furthermore, results from retrospective questionnaires suggest a greater frequency of ADHD-related behavior during the childhoods of pathological gamblers relative to matched control subjects (Carlton and Goldstein 1987). Interestingly, because an association between alcoholism and childhood ADHD has also been found (Wender et al. 1981; Wood et al. 1983) and a high co-occurrence between pathological gambling and alcohol abuse has been demonstrated (Linden et al. 1986; McCormick et al. 1984), inadequate impulse control may be a key factor that links these three disorders dimensionally (Carlton and Manowitz 1988).

Pathological gambling has also been described as being part of the obsessive-compulsive spectrum and sharing features with both obsessive-compulsive disorder (OCD) and the impulsive cluster of obsessive-compulsive spectrum disorders. ICDs are driven by pleasure, arousal, and gratification, at least initially. However, over time patients may develop unpleasant feelings, physiological activation, and dysphoria, all of which are relieved when the compulsive behavior is performed.

A recent study (Bienvenu et al. 2000) examined the frequency of various obsessive-compulsive spectrum disorders in 80 individuals with OCD and 343 first-degree relatives as well as in 73 control subjects and 300 of their first-degree relatives. Not surprisingly, the lifetime prevalence of any "spectrum" disorder was higher in probands with OCD (57%) than in control subjects (21%). However, only for a few individual disorders—notably hypochondriasis, body dysmorphic disorder, and pathological skin picking but not pathological gambling—did the difference in rates between probands and control subjects reach statistical significance. However, this study did not examine the impact of OCD, ADHD, or bipolar comorbidity and the relationship to pathological gambling.

Compulsive sexual behavior, compulsive buying disorder, and intermittent explosive disorder are relatively frequent, as are personality disorders. Murray (1993) observed that pathological gamblers fit no particular personality profile, but several investigators have reported abnormal personality traits in pathological gamblers based on dimensional assessments such as the Minnesota Multiphasic Personality Inventory or the Eysenck Personality Inventory (Moravec and Munley 1983; Roy et al. 1989). Taber et al. (1987) reported that 20% of 66 inpatients with pathological gambling had personality disorders, but they did not specify which type.

Neurobiology and Genetics

There is evidence of serotonergic, noradrenergic, and dopaminergic dysfunction in pathological gambling, and each of these neurotransmitter systems may play a unique role in the mechanisms that underlie arousal, behavioral initiation, behavioral disinhibition, and reward or reinforcement evident in pathological gambling and other addictive disorders (Table 11–2).

Serotonergic function is linked to behavioral initiation, inhibition, and aggression. Noradrenergic function mediates arousal and detects novel or aversive stimuli. Dopaminergic function is associated with reward and rein-

Table 11–2.   Developmental and neurobiological model of pathological gambling

Vulnerable state

Primed genetically/neurobiologically

Repeated environmental exposure

Gambling cycle: behavioral mechanisms

Stimulation readiness → norepinephrine

Behavioral initiation → serotonin

Reward/reinforcement → dopamine

Behavioral disinhibition → serotonin

forcement mechanisms (Eichelman et al. 1972). Thus, decreased serotonin (Soubrie 1986), increased norepinephrine (Eichelman et al. 1972), and increased dopamine function (Eichelman et al. 1972; Geyer and Segal 1974) facilitate addictive or impulsive behavior (Table 11–3).

Animal and human research suggests that the central serotonin system is involved in the inhibition of impulsive behavior. Evidence of serotonergic dysregulation and a presynaptic deficit of available serotonin has been observed in humans with a variety of impulsive disorders as well as animal models of impulsivity and aggression.

Evidence of serotonergic dysfunction in pathological gamblers comes from neurobiological studies. Pathological gamblers demonstrated dysregulated plasma prolactin response to intravenous clomipramine challenges (Moreno et al. 1991; Vazquez Rodriguez et al. 1991) relative to normal control subjects, indicative of serotonergic dysregulation. Similarly, platelet monoamine oxidase activity, which is a peripheral marker of serotonergic function, was lower in pathological gambling patients compared with control subjects (Carrasco et al. 1994). Our group (DeCaria et al. 1998b) studied serotonin metabolism alteration, examining behavioral ("high") and neuroendocrine (prolactin and cortisol) responses to single-dose (0.5 mg/kg) oral m-chlorophenylpiperazine (m-CPP) and placebo in pathological gamblers and matched control subjects and the relationship with clinical severity. Pathological gamblers had significantly increased prolactin response compared with control subjects at 180 minutes and at 210 minutes after m-CPP administration. Greater pathological gambling severity correlated with increased neuroendocrine responsiveness to

Table 11–3.   Evidence of neurobiological dysfunction in pathological gambling

Norepinephrine dysfunction

Increased urinary norepinephrine levels

Increased cerebrospinal fluid MHPG levels

Enhanced growth hormone response to clonidine

Serotonin dysfunction

Low platelet monoamine oxidase activity

Blunted prolactin response to intravenous clomipramine and increased response to *m*-chlorophenylpiperazine

Response to serotonin reuptake inhibitors

Dopamine dysfunction

Increased prevalence of altered alleles of the genes for dopamine receptors D_1, D_2, D_3, and D_4

Note.   MHPG = methoxyhydroxyphenylglycol.

m-CPP, suggesting greater serotonin dysregulation. Pathological gambling patients had a significantly increased "high" response to m-CPP compared with placebo. Challenge with m-CPP via the hypothalamic-pituitary-adrenal axis provided a dynamic index of central serotonergic function. An enhanced response to direct postsynaptic serotonergic receptor stimulation is consistent with hypersensitive postsynaptic serotonergic function in male pathological gamblers compared with healthy control subjects. This would be consistent with a net deficiency of presynaptic serotonin availability at baseline and a compensatory increase in postsynaptic serotonin receptor sensitivity.

There is evidence of serotonergic dysfunction in depression (Coccaro et al. 1989), impulsivity (Linnoila et al. 1983), suicidality (Gardner et al. 1990; Mann et al. 1992), and alcoholism (Benkelfat et al. 1991; Tollefson 1991). This is of interest because pathological gambling is strongly associated with depression (Roy et al. 1988a, 1988b), impulsivity (Moreno et al. 1991), suicidality (Ciarrochi and Richardson 1989), and alcohol or drug abuse (Linden et al. 1986; McCormick et al. 1984). Thus, pathological gambling may also be associated with serotonergic dysfunction as it relates to these comorbid features.

In addition to being considered an ICD, pathological gambling has also been linked phenomenologically to OCD and obsessive-compulsive related disorders (DeCaria and Hollander 1993; DeCaria et al. 1992; Hollander and Wong 1995a, 1995b; Hollander et al. 1994) in which there is also evidence for serotonergic dysfunction (Hollander et al. 1992a). The phenomenological similarities between pathological gambling and OCD include difficulties controlling and resisting thoughts and urges to perform repetitive behavior, an increased sense of discomfort or tension before engaging in the behavior or when attempting to resist the behavior, and a sense of gratification or tension relief after performing the behavior Clomipramine treatment studies document efficacy in approximately 60% of patients with OCD (Clomipramine Collaborative Study Group 1991). In addition, other obsessive-compulsive spectrum disorders, including Tourette's disorder, body dysmorphic disorder, depersonalization disorder, eating disorders, and trichotillomania, have also shown a possible preferential response to serotonin reuptake blockers such as clomipramine or selective serotonin reuptake inhibitors (SSRIs; Hollander 1993; Hollander et al. 1992b).

The noradrenergic system also seems to play a role in pathological gambling. The greatest concentration of norepinephrine is found in the locus coeruleus. Axons from norepinephrine neurons project to areas of the brain including the limbic system, basal ganglia, and the cortex, mediating physiological functions associated with arousal, mood, and impulse control (Siever et al. 1987). Plasma methoxyhydroxyphenylglycol (MHPG, a norepinephrine metabolite), plasma norepinephrine, and cerebrospinal fluid (CSF) MHPG are highly utilized indices of central norepinephrine function. Studies from the National Institute on Alcohol Abuse and Alcoholism found pathological gambling patients to have significantly higher CSF MHPG levels, a metabolite of norepinephrine, and greater urinary output of norepinephrine than normal control subjects (Roy et al. 1988b). Subsequently, Roy et al. (1989) found significant correlations between measures of extroversion and indices of noradrenergic function, including CSF MHPG, plasma MHPG, and urinary vanillylmandelic acid. Because the noradrenergic system has been associated with arousal (Fuxe et al. 1970; Usdin and Snyder 1973) and pathological gambling has been associated with increased arousal (Anderson and Brown 1984; Boyd 1976; Brown 1986, 1987; Commission on the Review of the National Policy Toward Gambling 1976; Dickerson et al. 1987) as well as increased tonic activity of the central noradrenergic system (Roy et al. 1988b), it is possible that the norepinephrine system also plays a role in the pathophysiology of pathological gambling.

Another index of central norepinephrine function is the neuroendocrine response (e.g., growth hormone) to a norepinephrine agonist (e.g., clonidine) during a pharmacological challenge. Growth hormone response to clonidine challenge reflects the sensitivity of postsynaptic α_2 norepinephrine receptors. Studies in personality disorder patients (Coccaro et al. 1991) with clonidine challenge demonstrate that growth hormone response correlates with risk-taking behavior and the Buss-Durkee Irritability subscale, suggesting that noradrenergic function plays a role in arousal and engagement with the environment. Some preliminary data from our group demonstrate that pathological gambling patients with less control of thoughts or urge to gamble have augmented growth hormone response to clonidine, suggesting increased arousal or response readiness toward gambling. Thus, increased noradrenergic function has been associated with arousal, irritability, and risk-taking behavior. Moreover, noradrenergic mechanisms have been associated with the impulsive and compulsive behavior seen in other related disorders. Hollander et al. (1991) found noradrenergic mechanisms in OCD, because clonidine challenge in OCD patients reduced obsessional thinking, and Glassman et al. (1993) found noradrenergic mechanisms in cigarette craving because there was modest efficacy of clonidine on smoking cessation in nicotine-dependent women.

Serotonergic, noradrenergic, and dopaminergic genes have been investigated because of the putative role of these neurotransmitters in pathological gambling, and a number of molecular genetic studies performed to date have reported findings consistent with the involvement of these neurotransmitter systems in pathological gambling. However, some of the studies performed to date have not been adequately controlled for potential differences in racial and ethnic compositions, factors that could account for differences in allelic variant distributions. As such, findings from the following studies, although promising, should be regarded as preliminary.

Ibanez et al. (2000) found no differences in the frequencies of allelic distribution of a polymorphism in the *MAO-B* gene in a group of pathological gamblers and healthy volunteers. In contrast, they found an association between an allele variant of a polymorphism in the *MAO-A* gene and more severe cases of male pathological gamblers in the sample, suggesting there may be gender differences in the etiology of pathological gambling (Ibanez et al. 2000). Moreover, the low-activity 3-repeat allele of the 30-bp *MAO-A* promoter polymorphism, which is associated with lower transcriptional and enzymatic activity, was found to be significantly increased in male pathological gamblers compared with male control subjects (Ibanez et al. 2000; Perez de Castro et al. 2002). Interestingly, although serotonin is a preferential substrate for monoamine oxidase A, *MAO-A* is expressed in the brain mainly in dopaminergic neurons (Westlund et al. 1993), raising the question of whether those allele variants are more likely to result in changes in serotonergic or dopaminergic transmission.

The same group also found that the less functional short variant of a polymorphism at the serotonin transporter gene (*5-HTTLPR*), a variant associated with decreased promoter activity, was found significantly more frequently in male pathological gamblers than in male control subjects. This finding was not observed in females, further suggesting the existence of gender-related differences in the genetic composition of individuals with pathological gambling (Perez de Castro et al. 1999).

Other studies have investigated the role of genes related to the dopaminergic system in the genesis of pathological gambling. A study by Comings et al. (1996) found a statistically significant association between the *Taq-A1* allele of the *D2* dopamine receptor gene in pathological gamblers compared with control subjects. The *Taq-A1* allele has also been found to be associated with other impulsive-addictive-compulsive behaviors, leading some researchers to propose a reward-deficiency syndrome as an underlying genetic foundation for these disorders (Blum et al. 1995). Ibanez et al. (2001) analyzed another polymorphism within the *D2* dopamine receptor gene and found significant differences in allele distribution in pathological gamblers with—as compared with those without—comorbid psychiatric disorders, a finding supporting the role of this gene as a liability factor for psychiatric disorders. Variants of the dopamine D_1 receptor gene have also been associated with impulsive-addictive-compulsive behaviors, including pathological gambling (Comings et al. 1997). A polymorphism located in exon III of the dopamine D_4 receptor (*DRD4*) gene (encoding a functionally different protein) has been found to be associated with pathological gambling. Specifically, the *DRD4* 7-repeat allele, coding for a "less efficient" version of the *DRD4* receptor, was found significantly more frequently in female pathological gamblers compared with female control subjects. This association was not observed in males. These results suggest that dopaminergic pathways through the involvement of *DRD4* may play a role in the etiology of pathological gambling in females (Perez de Castro et al. 1997).

Family and Twin/Adoption Studies

Initial evidence for the genetic influence on the etiology of pathological gambling came from family studies. Family studies determine the extent to which a disorder clusters in families. Disorders can run in families for many reasons, including common genetic factors, cultural transmission, and shared environments. Studies with clinical samples of pathological gamblers suggest an incidence of about 20% of pathological gambling in first-degree relatives (Ibanez et al. 2003; Lesieur 1988b), and this led to the consideration of the possible role of a genetic component in the development of pathological gambling. Gambino et al. (1993) found that patients at a Veterans Affairs hospital in Boston who perceived that their parents had had gambling problems were three times more likely to score as probable pathological gamblers on the SOGS (Lesieur and Blume 1987). The same study reported that those individuals who also perceived that their grandparents had had gambling problems had a 12-fold increased risk compared with patients who did not perceive gambling problems in their parents and their grandparents.

At present, the main source of evidence for the genetic influence in the etiology of pathological gambling derives from analyses performed on 3,359 male twin pairs of the Vietnam Era Twin Registry cohort (Eisen et al. 1998, 2001; Slutske et al. 2000, 2001). The study was conducted via phone interview and used DSM-III-R (American Psychiatric Association 1987) diagnostic criteria. Results showed that shared factors explained 56% of the report of three or more symptoms of pathological gambling and 62% of the variance in the diagnosis of pathological gambling disorder (Eisen et al. 1998). Analyses of this cohort suggested that gambling problems of increasing severity represent a single continuum of vulnerability rather than distinct entities (Eisen et al. 2001). Initial analysis of the data suggested a genetic susceptibility model in the pathogenesis of pathological gambling (Eisen et al. 1998). Further analysis of this sample supported this interpretation and indicated a common genetic vulnerability for pathological gambling and alcohol dependence in men (Slutske et al. 2000).

In a smaller twin study, Winters and Rich (1999) found a significant heritability explaining "high action" gambling, such as casinos and gambling slot machines, among 92 monozygotic and dizygotic male twin pairs. In contrast, no significant differences in heritability were found among males for "low action" games and among 63 female monozygotic and dizygotic twin pairs for either "high action" or "low action" gambling.

Neuropsychology

Clinical comorbidities, along with observations that pathological gambling involves strong motivations to engage in gambling and subjective feelings of reward, withdrawal, and craving for gambling, supported the categorization of pathological gambling as "a nonpharmacological addiction" (Blanco et al. 2001; Holden 2001). This view is corroborated by neuroimaging findings that gambling-associated cognitive and motivational events, or responses of pathological gamblers to gambling-related stimuli, are associated with metabolic changes in brain regions implicated in studies of substance use disorders (Breiter et al. 2001; Holden 2001; Potenza et al. 2003).

Our group acquired 18-fluorodeoxyglucose (FDG) positron emission tomography scans of seven unmedicated pathological gamblers without comorbid substance use disorders (Hollander et al. 2001). During FDG uptake, patients carried out a computer blackjack task during two different reward conditions presented at least 7 days apart: monetary reward and computer game points only. Monetary-reward blackjack was associated with a significantly higher relative metabolic rate in the primary visual cortex (Brodmann area 17), the cingulate gyrus (Brodmann area 24), the putamen, and prefrontal areas 47 and 10 compared with blackjack playing for points only. No area tested showed a significant decrease. This pattern suggests heightened limbic and sensory activation in the gambling-for-money condition, with increased emotional valence and greater risk and reward, and confirms the salience of monetary reward in the development of pathological gambling.

Data exist to support the notion that individuals with impaired impulse control exhibit abnormalities in risk–benefit decision making in both gambling and nongambling activities and that their cognitive or emotional sense of what distinguishes gambling from other decisions of daily living may be compromised. Individuals with alcoholism, drug dependence, antisocial personality disorder, or pathological gambling have been shown to discount delayed rewards at an excess rate, and such patterns have been thought to represent a functional measure of impulsivity in these groups (Crean et al. 2000;

Madden et al. 1997; Petry 2001b, 2001c; Petry and Casarella 1999). Individuals with substance use disorders and/or pathological gambling have also been shown to perform disadvantageously on gambling tasks used to assess decision-making performance (Bechara 2001; Bechara et al. 2001; Petry 2001a; Potenza 2001; Rogers and Robbins 2001; Rogers et al. 1999). Deficits in emotional or cognitive processes that contribute to neural representations of the possible negative consequences of gambling may impair the capacity to learn from past losses or to assess risks associated with action-oriented decision making (Bechara 2001; Bechara et al. 2000). These deficits could produce an inability to inhibit motivated drives to gamble, leading to persistent gambling. A person may also be attracted to specific features of gambling that distinguish it from usual, nongambling decisions of daily living. A heightened subjective benefit or mental gratification associated with the excitement of participating in a relatively unpredictable risk-decision process may thus also contribute to persistent gambling.

This last scenario represents an increase in the promotion of a motivated drive to gamble. Thus, individuals with impaired impulse control may show persistence in gambling or other addictive behaviors for a variety of reasons, including abnormalities in inhibitory control, decision-making, or motivational proponent processes, or some combination thereof.

Similar characteristics are common in patients with neurological damage to the ventromedial prefrontal cortex; this "myopia for the future" has already been demonstrated in patients with ventromedial prefrontal cortex lesions by Damasio's group (Bechara et al. 1994) using a gambling task that is able to detect and measure, in the laboratory, the decision-making impairment of these subjects, testing the ability to balance immediate rewards against long-term negative consequences. Cavedini et al. (2002) assessed the decision-making function mediated by the ventromedial prefrontal cortex in 20 pathological gambling patients and 40 healthy control subjects using the gambling task, which simulates real-life decision making to test the individual's ability to balance immediate rewards against long-term negative consequence. Significant differences were found in gambling task performance between control subjects and pathological gambling patients, who showed a specific decision-making profile across the sequence of the game.

Attention problems and impulsivity in pathological gamblers could reflect deficits in executive functioning that are often a consequence of minimal brain damage with orbitofrontal cortex impairment (Specker et al. 1995). From a neuropsychological point of view, deficits in executive frontally mediated attention have been observed in these patients, suggesting that attention deficits may be a risk factor for the development of an addictive disorder (Rugle and Melamed 1993).

Treatment

There is a relative lack of effective treatments for pathological gambling reported in the literature. A variety of factors probably account for this circumstance: 1) pathological gambling has only recently received attention from the psychiatric community and been acknowledged as a major mental health problem; 2) the cognitive distortions and denial associated with pathological gambling; 3) the reluctance of patients to reveal their primary and/or comorbid disorders prior to reaching a stage at which pathological gambling becomes obvious to family members, friends, and coworkers; 4) the frequent presentation to self-help groups, which have been known to effectively treat only a small percentage of pathological gamblers; 5) the presentation to mental health clinics for comorbid disorders (i.e., substance abuse and depression) that may mask primary pathological gambling, as well as the patient's denial and mental health professionals' lack of awareness regarding the target signs of pathological gambling; 6) the societal acceptance of gambling as a recreational and financially lucrative and taxable activity; and 7) the consequent lack of exposure of pathological gambling in the literature and at annual conferences.

The uncontrolled and few controlled treatment studies in the literature, although helpful in providing preliminary direction, are frequently methodologically flawed. Imprecise diagnostic criteria, retrospective design, nonstandardized treatment ratings, nonsystematic assessment of comorbid conditions, and small sample sizes confound the conclusions drawn from studies to date, and investigations of long-term efficacy are limited.

Many treatment modalities of pathological gambling are similar to that of other substance abuse disorders and were created based on the addiction model, such as self-help groups, inpatient treatment programs, and rehabilitation programs.

Self-Help, Psychotherapeutic, and Multimodal Interventions

Self-help groups have been available to nearly all gamblers seeking treatment. The most popular intervention for problem gambling is GA, which is similar to Alcoholics Anonymous and Narcotics Anonymous. However, available evidence suggests that GA may not be very effective when used without other treatment modalities (Petry and Armentano 1999). Retrospective studies show a dropout rate of up to 70% within the first year (Stewart and Brown 1988), and overall dropout rates range from 75% to 90% (Moody 1990). Only 8% of GA members report total abstinence at 1-year follow-up and 7% at 2-year follow-up (Brown 1985). Although participation in GA's spousal component, Gam-Anon, may be helpful for some family members, little evidence suggests that it reduces disordered gambling (Johnson and Nora 1992; Petry and Armentano 1999).

Inpatient treatment and rehabilitation programs for pathological gambling were also set up based on similar programs for substance abuse. In fact, pathological gamblers are frequently treated in substance abuse programs for pathological gambling. Programs for pathological gambling have emerged since the early 1970s (Glen 1976; Taber 1981) and have included various combinations of individual and group psychotherapy as well as substance use treatment. Most of them strongly encouraged or required attendance at GA meetings. Substantial numbers of patients improved in all programs, and outcome studies have shown 55% of patients reporting abstinence at 1-year follow-up (Russo et al. 1984; Taber et al. 1987). Although seriously methodologically flawed, these reports suggest that professionally delivered multimodal therapy programs, given alone or in combination with GA, may be more effective than GA alone.

To evaluate other forms of self-help treatment, Dickerson et al. (1990) randomly assigned 29 pathological gamblers to use a self-help manual alone or in conjunction with a single in-depth motivational interview. Both groups had similar reductions in gambling frequency. Although this study was limited by the lack of a control group and failure to assess compliance with the manual, it suggested that self-help manuals may be useful for some problem gamblers. Indeed, other self-help manuals have been published, and studies comparing their effectiveness with professionally delivered cognitive-behavioral therapy are ongoing (Petry and Armentano 1999).

Early reports in the psychoanalytic literature suggested that problem gambling is regressive in nature and representative of various pregenital and genital instincts, unconscious conflicts, or painful affects. Most studies that report good outcome are based on single-case studies (Eissler 1950; Harris 1964; Linder 1950; Simmel 1920), but some authors have commented that purely psychodynamic treatment of pathological gambling is difficult because of patients' denial, refusal to take responsibility for their behavior, lack of desire for treatment, lack of insight, concomitant antisocial behaviors, legal and financial problems, and alcohol and drug abuse. Rosenthal and Rugle (1994) published a contemporary psychodynamic approach to the treatment of pathological gambling in which traditional psychodynamic psychotherapy is integrated with an addiction model. They argued that the goal of treatment is abstinence, which can be achieved by five strategies: 1) breaking through denial, 2) confronting omnipotent defenses, 3) interrupting the chasing cycle, 4) identifying the reasons for gambling, and 5) motivating the patient to become an active participant in treatment. Of note, in contrast to these authors' recommendations, data have shown that controlled gambling can be an acceptable outcome for some pathological gamblers (Blaszczynski et al. 1991).

Behavioral, cognitive, and combined cognitive-behavioral methods have been used in treating pathological gambling. Aversive therapy has been employed (Victor and Cruz 1967) to reach the goal of total abstinence of gambling, as have behavior monitoring, contingency management, contingency contracting, covert sensitization, systematic desensitization, imaginal desensitization, in vivo exposure, imaginal relaxation, psychoeducation, cognitive restructuring, problem-solving skills training, social skills training, and relapse prevention. Use of cognitive restructuring facilitates a decrease in the frequency of gambling and irrational verbalizations associated with gambling (Ladouceur 1990).

Pharmacotherapy

Currently there are only a few controlled pharmacological treatment studies of pathological gambling, although this is a recently developing area of research.

Studies have examined the efficacy of serotonin reuptake inhibitors in patients with pathological gambling. Such studies were initially motivated by the conceptualization of pathological gambling as an obsessive-compulsive spectrum disorder (Hollander 1993). In a single case report, the possible efficacy of the serotonin reuptake blocker clomipramine was demonstrated in a double-blind, placebo-controlled trial, followed by single-blind clomipramine treatment in a 31-year-old woman with a 12-year history of pathological gambling (Hollander et al. 1992b).

Hollander et al. (1998), in a single-blind 8-week trial of the SSRI fluvoxamine, reported that 7 out of 10 pathological gamblers improved, manifesting a significant reduction in gambling urge and gambling behavior. However, fluvoxamine seemed to exacerbate gambling behavior and mood symptoms with dysphoric elation in 2 of the 3 nonresponders who had comorbid cyclothymic disorder. Hollander et al. (2000) reported a superior effect of fluvoxamine (40.6% mean improvement on the PG-CGI) compared with placebo (16.6% mean improvement) in the second phase of a 16-week double-blind, crossover study. In the first phase, a high placebo response rate was noted, such that fluvoxamine did not differ from placebo. In a double-blind study by Blanco et al. (2002) of fluvoxamine treatment in 32 subjects, similar improvement was not observed. Subjects were treated with 200 mg/day of fluvoxamine for 6 months and reduction in money and time spent gambling per week were used as the outcome measures. The authors concluded that, except in the cases of male or young pathological gamblers, treatment with fluvoxamine as compared with placebo did not result in statistically significant improvement. High rates of discontinuation were observed, which were attributed to subjects being "lost to follow-up," further complicating interpretation of the results.

Using fluoxetine in the treatment of pathological gambling, de la Gandara (1999) enrolled 20 patients in a 6-month comparison of fluoxetine (20 mg/day) plus monthly supportive psychotherapy and supportive psychotherapy alone. Efficacy was measured using the PG-CGI, the Ludo-Cage test, and adherence to treatment. At the end of 6 months, the PG-CGI and Ludo-Cage mean scores demonstrated statistically greater improvement in the fluoxetine plus psychotherapy group compared with the psychotherapy group. A greater percentage of the subjects in the combined treatment group maintained better adherence to the treatment compared with those only in psychotherapy, suggesting that combination treatments involving both behavioral and pharmacological therapies may be more effective in the treatment of pathological gambling than either therapy alone. This study exists only as a conference abstract, and details about study design and exclusion criteria are unavailable.

Additionally, the study used a combination of supportive psychotherapy and medication. Because there are no published studies on the effectiveness of supportive psychotherapy in the treatment of pathological gambling, the study design itself is brought into question.

More recently, Zimmerman et al. (2002) studied 15 pathological gambling patients in a 12-week open-label citalopram trial (mean dosage, 34.7 mg/day). They reported a significant improvement on all gambling measures, with 86.7% of the patients rated as responders on the clinician-rated PG-CGI scale. Paroxetine was more effective than placebo (60.8% vs. 22.7%) in an 11-week double-blind trial (Kim et al. 2002). However, a recent multicenter trial comparing paroxetine with placebo did not demonstrate sustained improvement (Grant et al. 2003).

Several important findings emerge from these early studies of SSRIs. First, SSRIs as a group of pharmacological agents may be effective in the short-term reduction of symptoms of pathological gambling. Second, as in the treatment of other disorders, SSRIs are well tolerated, with treatment-emergent adverse events similar in quality and quantity to those documented in prior large-scale investigations of SSRIs (Hollander et al. 2000; Kim and Grant 2001). Third, as in the treatment of OCD, the dosages of serotonin reuptake inhibitors required to treat pathological gambling symptoms appear to be higher than the average dosages generally required to treat depressive disorders. Fourth, SSRIs' treatment effects appear to be independent of underlying depressive symptoms. In studies in which study participants had no or minimal depressive symptoms (Hollander et al. 2000; Kim et al. 2002), SSRIs were still effective in reducing gambling symptoms. Fifth, some placebo-controlled studies (e.g., Hollander et al. 2000) included a significant initial clinical response to placebo, highlighting the importance of monitoring for improvement over an extended period of time and the need for cautious interpretation of open-label studies (Kim and Grant 2001). Sixth, outcome measures that focus on the obsessive gambling preoccupations and urges may be free from external effects, such as bankruptcy, that may limit behavioral manifestations.

Nefazodone, a phenylpiperazine antidepressant that is primarily an antagonist at the serotonin-2 receptors and has mixed noradrenergic/serotonergic reuptake inhibitor effects, has recently been reported to be effective in an 8-week prospective, open-label, controlled clinical trial in 14 pathological gamblers (Pallanti et al. 2002b). Antagonism of serotonin-2 receptors has been associated with a low rate of sexual side effects for nefazodone in comparison with SSRIs (Feiger et al. 1996), which may be of interest in enhancing compliance in this impulsive pathological gambling population.

The core psychopathological features of pathological gambling are mixed: impulsive features (arousal), compulsive features (anxiety reduction), addictive features (symptoms of withdrawal), and features associated with bipolar disorder such as urges, pleasure seeking, and the reduction of judgment capability related to unrealistic appraisal of one's own abilities.

These clinical features suggest the need for studying the efficacy of either mood stabilizers or opiate antagonists in patients with pathological gambling. One report on the use of lithium carbonate demonstrated mild success in three gamblers with an affective mood disorder (Moscowitz 1980). Carbamazepine at a dosage of 600 mg/day was effective in a single-case, double-blind, crossover study with placebo (Haller and Hinterhuber 1994). Lithium carbonate and valproate provided positive results in a 14-week randomized, single-blind study (Pallanti et al. 2002a), with 60.9% responders in the lithium group and 68.4% responders in the valproate group, respectively. Our group also found lithium carbonate superior to placebo in a recent 10-week double-blind trial with bipolar spectrum pathological gamblers (Hollander et al. 2002).

Given naltrexone's ability to modulate the mesolimbic dopamine pathway and this pathway's involvement in rewarding and reinforcing behaviors, one might predict that naltrexone might be efficacious in targeting high urge or craving states. Kim et al. (2001) studied 45 pathological gambling patients in an 11-week double-blind naltrexone versus placebo trial, following a 1-week placebo run-in phase. They reported a significant improvement on PG-CGI scores and a reduction of gambling symptoms in 75% of naltrexone-treated subjects compared with only 24% of placebo-treated subjects. Adverse events included elevated liver enzymes in four patients (20%). In contrast to the greater prevalence of pathological gambling in males in the literature, in this study the sample consisted mainly of female pathological gambling patients.

Emerging data suggest that individuals with schizophrenia treated with atypical as compared with typical antipsychotic drugs show an enhanced ability to diminish or cease addictive behaviors (Albanese et al. 1994; Buckley 2000; George et al. 2000). Consistent with this notion are the findings from a case report demonstrating clinical improvement in psychotic symptoms and cessation of gambling behavior in an individual with comorbid schizophrenia and DSM-IV (American Psychiatric Association 1994) pathological gambling following a change of pharmacotherapy from haloperidol to olanzapine (Potenza and Chambers 2001). Given the ability of atypical antipsychotic drugs to modulate dopamine and serotonin neuronal systems and the role of these neurotransmitter systems in impulse control (Potenza 2001), it seems warranted to investigate the utility of atypical antipsychotics in the treatment of pathological gambling uncomplicated by schizophrenia. In a recent placebo-controlled trial of olanzapine in the treatment of video poker pathological gamblers, initial analyses of the findings did not demonstrate differences in treatment outcome in the placebo- and olanzapine-treated groups. The interpretation of these findings is complicated, however, by differences between the two treatment groups in gambling severity at treatment onset (Rugle 2000).

These pilot data suggest the need for conducting well-designed, controlled clinical trials of various pharmacological agents in the treatment of pathological gambling, according to different clinical presentations and comorbidities.

Treatment Compliance

Compliance with drug treatment in pathological gambling shares similar challenges as in other disorders, including bipolar disorder and substance dependence. Patients with mania may not comply with treatment with mood stabilizers in part because drug treatment may reduce positive or euphoric experiences associated with hypomania or mania. Similarly, with drug use disorders, there exists a hedonic component to drug use that often makes patients ambivalent about their medications to stop using or toward becoming or remaining abstinent. In the treatment of opioid dependence with naltrexone, non–addiction-related rewards have been incorporated into the treatment in a contingency management fashion to substitute for drug-related reward and enhance medication compliance (Carroll et al. 2001). Recruitment of a significant other has also been used to enhance naltrexone treatment compliance in opioid dependence (Carroll et al. 2001). The utility of similar strategies to enhance treatment outcome in pathological gambling remains an important avenue for future investigations.

Duration of Treatment and Medication Dosages

Guidelines for recommended adequate treatment trials have yet to be generated for pathological gambling. In the open-label fluvoxamine study by Hollander et al. (1998), study participants were given placebo for the first 8 weeks followed by 8 weeks of fluvoxamine treatment. During the 8-week placebo phase, the mean baseline score on the pathological gambling version of the Yale-Brown Obsessive-Compulsive Scale dropped from 11.6 to 6.5 at week 2, followed by gradual worsening to 6.9 by week 8. This finding suggests that a sustained drug treatment effect for pathological gambling might require treatment for 4 months or longer. In the subsequent double-blind treatment study, the placebo response was not as pronounced, with an average PG-CGI score of 3.5 at the end of the 7-day placebo lead-in (Hollander et al. 2000). Several studies of SSRI treatment with an 8-week duration have found significant improvement in pathological gambling symptoms by study endpoint. However, the fact that studies have not always documented when symptom improvement began in the course of treatment complicates the extrapolation of guidelines for recommended duration of treatment. An additional difficulty in addressing the question of drug treatment duration is the variability in the magnitude of placebo response observed in various treatment trials. Without a clear understanding of the extent of the placebo response in persons with pathological gambling, clinicians must monitor symptom response over a duration long enough to assess the difference between responses to placebo and active medication.

Questions also exist regarding adequate drug dosing for the treatment of pathological gambling. The placebo-controlled trials performed to date have involved flexible dosing strategies based on clinical response and tolerability. SSRI dosages similar to those typically used for OCD and higher than those typically needed for major depression appear to be necessary for pathological gambling. The authors' clinical experience suggests that an SSRI should not be considered ineffective unless it has been tried for at least 10–12 weeks and the highest dosage tolerated or recommended by the manufacturer has been reached. Because no formal discontinuation studies have been performed to date and only scant data exist on the natural history of gambling behaviors in persons with pathological gambling, the optimal duration of treatment and rates of relapse associated with discontinuation of pharmacological treatment are at present not known.

Conclusion: Subtyping Pathological Gambling

Pathological gambling does not seem to be a homogeneous entity but rather a group consisting of various subtypes (ICD, nonpharmacological addiction, obsessive-compulsive spectrum disorder, mood disorder) that share certain characteristics but differ with regard to choice of gambling setting and activity, motivations to gamble, and the mood state present during gambling or triggered by gambling. Essential features of any therapeutic intervention for pathological gambling include the need to establish both a therapeutic alliance and network, address the underlying pathology, interrupt the behavior and maintain abstinence, problem solve, and improve quality of life.

Pharmacological treatment studies of pathological gambling have demonstrated some promising results with the use of serotonin reuptake inhibitors, serotonin antagonists, opiate antagonists, and mood stabilizers, although some studies have not reported significant findings, primarily due to high placebo response rates. Study design, outcome measure, and subject selection issues are critical in designing and interpreting the large-scale, double-blind, placebo-controlled trials in pathological gambling that are sorely needed in the field. However, findings from psychopharmacological trials that suggest a differential treatment response encourage the evolution of a "tailored" treatment approach according to specific clinical features and comorbid psychiatric conditions. Treatment should ultimately target all symptom domains within the individual pathological gambling patient that contribute to compulsive gambling, including common comorbid conditions such as bipolar spectrum disorder, ADHD, and substance abuse/dependence disorders.

References

Albanese MJ, Khantzian EJ, Murphy SL, et al: Decreased substance use in chronically psychotic patients treated with clozapine. Am J Psychiatry 151:780–781, 1994

American Psychiatric Association: Diagnostic and Statistical Manual of Mental Disorders, 3rd Edition. Washington, DC, American Psychiatric Association, 1980

American Psychiatric Association: Diagnostic and Statistical Manual of Mental Disorders, 3rd Edition, Revised. Washington, DC, American Psychiatric Association, 1987

American Psychiatric Association: Diagnostic and Statistical Manual of Mental Disorders, 4th Edition. Washington, DC, American Psychiatric Association, 1994

American Psychiatric Association: Diagnostic and Statistical Manual of Mental Disorders, 4th Edition, Text Revision. Washington, DC, American Psychiatric Association, 2000

Anderson G, Brown R: Real and laboratory gambling, sensation-seeking and arousal. Br J Psychol 75:401–411, 1984

Bechara A: Neurobiology of decision-making: risk and reward. Semin Clin Neuropsychiatry 6:205–216, 2001

Bechara A, Damasio AR, Damasio H, et al: Insensitivity to future consequences following damage to human prefrontal cortex. Cognition 50:7–15, 1994

Bechara A, Damasio H, Damasio AR: Emotion, decision making and the orbitofrontal cortex. Cereb Cortex 10:295–307, 2000

Bechara A, Dolan S, Denburg N, et al: Decision-making deficits, linked to a dysfunctional ventromedial prefrontal cortex, revealed in alcohol and stimulant abusers. Neuropsychologia 39:376–389, 2001

Benkelfat C, Murphy DL, Hill JL, et al: Ethanol-like properties of the serotonergic partial agonist m-chlorophenylpiperazine in chronic alcoholic patients (letter). Arch Gen Psychiatry 48:383, 1991

Bergler E: The Psychology of Gambling. New York, International Universities Press, 1957

Bienvenu OJ, Samuels JF, Riddle MA, et al: The relationship of obsessive-compulsive disorder to possible spectrum disorders: results from a family study. Biol Psychiatry 48:287–293, 2000

Blanco C, Moreyra P, Nunes EV, et al: Pathological gambling: addiction or compulsion? Semin Clin Neuropsychiatry 6:167–176, 2001

Blanco C, Petkova E, Ibanez A, et al: A pilot placebo-controlled study of fluvoxamine for pathological gambling. Ann Clin Psychiatry 14:9–15, 2002

Blaszczynski A, McConaghy N, Frankova A: Control versus abstinence in the treatment of pathological gambling: a two to nine year follow-up. Br J Addict 86:299–306, 1991

Blum K, Sheridan PJ, Wood RC, et al: Dopamine D2 receptor gene variants: association and linkage studies in impulsive-addictive-compulsive behaviour. Pharmacogenetics 5:121–141, 1995

Blume SB: Treatment for the addictions: alcoholism, drug dependence and compulsive gambling in a psychiatric setting. J Subst Abuse Treat 3:131–133, 1986

Blume SB: Compulsive gambling and the medical model. Journal of Gambling Behavior 3:237–247, 1987

Boyd W: Excitement: the gambler's drug, in Gambling and Society. Edited by Eadington W. Springfield, IL, Charles C Thomas, 1976, pp 371–375

Breiter HC, Aharon I, Kahneman D, et al: Functional imaging of neural responses to expectancy and experience of monetary gains and losses. Neuron 30:619–639, 2001

Brown RI: The effectiveness of Gamblers Anonymous, in The Gambling Studies: Proceedings of the 6th National Conference on Gambling and Risk-Taking. Edited by Eadington WR. Reno, NV, University of Nevada, 1985

Brown RI: Arousal and sensation-seeking components in the general explanation of gambling and gambling addictions. Int J Addict 21:1001–1016, 1986

Brown RI: Classical and operant paradigms in the management of gambling addictions. Behav Psychother 15:111–122, 1987

Buckley PF: Comprehensive disease management for schizophrenia. Drugs Today 36:267–280, 2000

Carlton PL, Goldstein L: Physiological determinants of pathological gambling, in A Handbook of Pathological Gambling. Edited by Glaski T. Springfield, IL, Charles C Thomas, 1987, pp 657–663

Carlton PL, Manowitz P: Physiological factors as determinants of pathological gambling. Journal of Gambling Behavior 3:274–285, 1988

Carone PA, Yolles SF, Kieffer SN, et al (eds): Addictive Disorders Update: Alcoholism, Drug Abuse, and Gambling. New York, Human Sciences Press, 1982

Carrasco J, Saiz-Ruiz J, Moreno I, et al: Low platelet MAO activity in pathological gambling. Acta Psychiatr Scand 90:427–431, 1994

Carroll KM, Ball SA, Nich C, et al: Targeting behavioral therapies to enhance naltrexone treatment of opioid dependence: efficacy of contingency management and significant other involvement. Arch Gen Psychiatry 58:755–761, 2001

Cavedini P, Riboldi G, Keller R, et al: Frontal lobe dysfunction in pathological gambling patients. Biol Psychiatry 51:334–341, 2002

Ciarrochi JW: Severity of impairment in dually addicted gamblers. Journal of Gambling Behavior 3:16–26, 1987

Ciarrochi J, Richardson R: Profile of compulsive gamblers in treatment: update and comparisons. Journal of Gambling Behavior 5:53–65, 1989

Clomipramine Collaborative Study Group: Clomipramine in the treatment of patients with obsessive-compulsive disorder. Arch Gen Psychiatry 48:730–738, 1991

Coccaro EF, Siever LJ, Klar HM, et al: Serotonergic studies in patients with affective and personality disorders: correlates with suicidal and impulsive-aggressive behavior. Arch Gen Psychiatry 46:587–599, 1989

Coccaro EF, Lawrence T, Trestman R, et al: Growth hormone responses to intravenous clonidine challenge correlate with behavioral irritability in psychiatric patients and healthy volunteers. Psychiatry Res 39:129–139, 1991

Comings DE, Rosenthal RJ, Lesieur HR, et al: A study of the dopamine D2 receptor gene in pathological gambling. Pharmacogenetics 6:223–234, 1996

Comings DE, Gade R, Wu S, et al: Studies of the potential role of the dopamine D1 receptor gene in addictive behaviors. Mol Psychiatry 2:44–56, 1997

Commission on the Review of the National Policy Toward Gambling: Gambling in America. Washington, DC, U.S. Government Printing Office, 1976

Crean JP, de Wit H, Richards JB: Reward discounting as a measure of impulsive behavior in a psychiatric outpatient population. Exp Clin Psychopharmacol 8:155–162, 2000

Culleton RP: A survey of pathological gamblers in the state of Ohio. Columbus, OH, Ohio Lottery Commission, 1985

Culleton RP, Lang MH: The Prevalence Rate of Pathological Gambling in the Delaware Valley in 1984. Camden, NJ, Forum for Policy Research and Public Service, Rutgers University, 1985

Custer RL: An overview of compulsive gambling, in Addictive Disorders Update: Alcoholism, Drug Abuse and Gambling. Edited by Carone PA, Yoles SF, Kieffer SN, et al. New York, Human Sciences Press, 1982, pp 107–124

Custer RL, Custer LF: Characteristics of the recovering compulsive gambler: a survey of 150 members of Gamblers Anonymous. Paper presented at the Fourth Annual Conference on Gambling, Reno, NV, December 1978

Custer RL, Milt H: When Luck Runs Out. New York, Facts on File Publications, 1985

DeCaria C, Hollander E: Pathological gambling, in Obsessive-Compulsive Related Disorders. Edited by Hollander E. Washington, DC, American Psychiatric Press, 1993, pp 155–178

DeCaria C, Hollander E, Frenkel M, et al: Pathological gambling: an OCD related disorder? Paper presented at the 145th annual meeting of the American Psychiatric Association, Washington, DC, May 1992

DeCaria CM, Hollander E, Begaz T, et al: Reliability and validity of a pathological gambling modification of the Yale-Brown Obsessive-Compulsive Scale (pathological gambling–YBOCS): preliminary findings. Paper presented at the 12th National Conference on Problem Gambling, Las Vegas, NV, July 1998a

DeCaria CM, Begaz T, Hollander E: Serotonergic and noradrenergic function in pathological gambling. CNS Spectrums 3(6):38-47, 1998b

de la Gandara JJ: Fluoxetine: open-trial in pathological gambling. Paper presented at the 152nd annual meeting of the American Psychiatric Association, Washington, DC, May 1999

Dickerson M: "Compulsive" gambling as an addiction: dilemmas. Scott Med J 22:251–252, 1977

Dickerson MG: Compulsive Gamblers. London, Longmans, 1984

Dickerson M, Hinchy J, Falve J: Chasing, arousal and sensation-seeking in off-course gamblers. Br J Addict 82:673–680, 1987

Dickerson M, Hinchy J, England SL: Minimal treatments and problem gamblers: a preliminary investigation. Journal of Gambling Studies 6:87–102, 1990

Eichelman B, Thoa NB, Ng KY: Facilitated aggression in the rat following 6-hydroxy-dopamine administration. Physiol Behav 8:1–3, 1972

Eisen SA, Lin N, Lyons MJ, et al: Familial influences on gambling behavior: an analysis of 3359 twin pairs. Addiction 93:1375–1384, 1998

Eisen SA, Slutske WS, Lyons MJ, et al: The genetics of pathological gambling. Semin Clin Neuropsychiatry 6:195–204, 2001

Eissler KR: Ego psychological implications of psychoanalytic treatment of delinquents. Psychoanal Study Child 5:97–121, 1950

Feiger A, Kiev A, Shrivastava RK, et al: Nefazodone versus sertraline in outpatients with major depression: focus on efficacy, tolerability, and effects on sexual function and satisfaction. J Clin Psychiatry 57(suppl):53–62, 1996

Fuxe K, Hokfelt T, Ungerstedt U: Morphological and functional aspects of central monoamine neurons, in International Review of Neurobiology, Vol 13. Edited by Pfeiffer CC, Smythies J. New York, Academic Press, 1970, pp 93–126

Gambino B, Fitzgerald R, Shaffer HJ, et al: Perceived family history of problem gambling and scores on SOGS. Journal of Gambling Studies 9:169–184, 1993

Gardner DL, Lucas PB, Cowdry RW: CSF metabolites in borderline personality disorder compared with normal controls. Biol Psychiatry 28:247–254, 1990

George TP, Ziedonis DM, Feingold A, et al: Nicotine transdermal patch and atypical antipsychotic medications for smoking cessation in schizophrenia. Am J Psychiatry 157:1835–1842, 2000

Geyer MA, Segal DS: Shock-induced aggression: opposite effects of intraventricularly infused dopamine and norepinephrine. Behav Biol 10:99–104, 1974

Glassman AH, Covey LS, Dalack GW, et al: Smoking cessation, clonidine, and vulnerability to nicotine among dependent smokers. Clin Pharmacol Ther 54:670–679, 1993

Glen AM: The treatment of compulsive gamblers at the Cleveland VA Hospital, Brecksville Division. Paper presented at the 84th annual convention of the American Psychological Association, Washington, DC, September 1976

Grant JE, Kim SW, Potenza MN, et al: Paroxetine treatment of pathological gambling: a multi-centre randomized controlled trial. Int Clin Psychopharmacol 18:243–249, 2003

Greenberg HR: Psychology of gambling, in Comprehensive Textbook of Psychiatry, 3rd Edition. Edited by Kaplan HI, Freedman AM, Sadock B. Baltimore, MD, Williams & Wilkins, 1980, pp 3274–3283

Griffiths MD: Pinball wizard: the case of a pinball machine addict. Psychol Rep 71:160–161, 1992

Haberman PW: Drinking and other self-indulgences: complements or counter attractions? Int J Addict 4:157–167, 1969

Haller R, Hinterhuber H: Treatment of pathological gambling with carbamazepine. Pharmacopsychiatry 27:129, 1994

Harris HI: Gambling addiction in an adolescent male. Psychoanal Q 33:513–525, 1964

Holden C: "Behavioral" addictions: do they exist? Science 294:980–982, 2001

Hollander E (ed): Obsessive-Compulsive Related Disorders. Washington, DC, American Psychiatric Press, 1993

Hollander E, Wong CM: Introduction: obsessive-compulsive spectrum disorders. J Clin Psychiatry 56(suppl):3–6, 1995a

Hollander E, Wong CM: Body dysmorphic disorder, pathological gambling, and sexual compulsions. J Clin Psychiatry 56(suppl):7–12, 1995b

Hollander E, DeCaria C, Nitescu A, et al: Noradrenergic function in obsessive-compulsive disorder: behavioral and neuroendocrine responses to clonidine and comparison to healthy controls. Psychiatry Res 37:161–177, 1991

Hollander E, DeCaria C, Nitescu A, et al: Serotonergic function in obsessive-compulsive disorder: behavioral and neuroendocrine responses to oral m-CPP and fenfluramine in patients and healthy volunteers. Arch Gen Psychiatry 49:21–28, 1992a

Hollander E, Frenkel M, DeCaria C, et al: Treatment of pathological gambling with clomipramine (letter). Am J Psychiatry 149:710–711, 1992b

Hollander E, Stein DJ, DeCaria CM, et al: Serotonergic sensitivity in borderline personality disorder: preliminary findings. Am J Psychiatry 151:277–280, 1994

Hollander E, DeCaria CM, Mari E, et al: Short-term single-blind fluvoxamine treatment of pathological gambling. Am J Psychiatry 155:1781–1783, 1998

Hollander E, DeCaria CM, Finkell JN, et al: A randomized double-blind fluvoxamine/placebo crossover trial in pathological gambling. Biol Psychiatry 47:813–817, 2000

Hollander E, Pallanti S, Baldini Rossi N, et al: Sustained release lithium/placebo treatment response and FDG-PET imaging of wagering in bipolar spectrum pathological gamblers. Paper presented at the American College of Neuropsychopharmacology Annual Conference, Waikoloa Village, HI, December 2001

Hollander E, Pallanti S, Baldini Rossi N, et al: Sustained release lithium/placebo treatment response in bipolar spectrum pathological gamblers. Paper presented at the New Clinical Drug Evaluation (NCDEU) Annual Meeting, Boca Raton, FL, June 2002

Ibanez A, de Castro IP, Fernandez-Piqueras J, et al: Pathological gambling and DNA polymorphic markers at MAO-A and MAO-B genes. Mol Psychiatry 5:105–109, 2000

Ibanez A, Blanco C, Donahue E, et al: Psychiatric comorbidity in pathological gamblers seeking treatment. Am J Psychiatry 158:1733–1735, 2001

Ibanez A, Blanco C, de Castro IP, et al: Genetics of pathological gambling. Journal of Gambling Studies 19:11–22, 2003

Jacobs DF: Factors alleged as predisposing to compulsive gambling. Paper presented at the 90th annual convention of the American Psychological Association, Washington, DC, August 1982

Jacobs DF: Study of traits leading to compulsive gambling, in Sharing Recovery Through Gamblers Anonymous. Los Angeles, CA, Gamblers Anonymous, 1984, pp 227–233

Jacobs DF: A general theory of addictions: a new theoretical model. Journal of Gambling Behavior 2:15–31, 1986

Jacobs DF: Evidence for a common dissociative-like reaction among addicts. Journal of Gambling Behavior 4:27–37, 1988

Jacobs DF: A general theory of addictions: rationale for and evidence supporting a new approach for understanding and treating addictive behaviors, in Compulsive Gambling: Theory, Research and Practice. Edited by Shaffer H, Stein SA, Gambino B, et al. Lexington, MA, DC Health, 1989, pp 35–61

Johnson EE, Nora RN: Does spousal participation in Gamblers Anonymous benefit compulsive gamblers? Psychol Rep 71:914, 1992

Kim SW, Grant JE: The psychopharmacology of pathological gambling. Semin Clin Neuropsychiatry 6:184–194, 2001

Kim SW, Grant JE, Adson DE, et al: Double-blind naltrexone and placebo comparison study in the treatment of pathological gambling. Biol Psychiatry 49:914–921, 2001

Kim SW, Grant JE, Adson DE, et al: A double-blind placebo-controlled study of the efficacy and safety of paroxetine in the treatment of pathological gambling. J Clin Psychiatry 63:501–507, 2002

Ladouceur R: Cognitive activities among gamblers. Paper presented at the Association for Advancement of Behavior Therapy (AABT) Convention, San Francisco, CA, November 1990

Ladouceur R, Mireault C: Gambling behavior among high school students in the Quebec area. Journal of Gambling Behavior 4:3–12, 1988

Lesieur HR: The female pathological gambler, in Gambling Studies: Proceedings of the 7th International Conference on Gambling and Risk-Taking. Edited by Eadington WR. Reno, NV, University of Nevada, 1988a, pp 230–258

Lesieur HR: Report on pathological gambling in New Jersey, in Report and Recommendations of the Governor's Advisory Commission on Gambling. Trenton, NJ, Governor's Advisory Commission on Gambling, 1988b, pp 103–165

Lesieur HR: Costs and treatment of pathological gambling. Annals of the American Academy of Political and Social Science 556:153–176, 1998

Lesieur HR, Anderson C: Results of a Survey of Gamblers Anonymous Members in Illinois. Park Ridge, IL, Illinois Council on Problem and Compulsive Gambling, 1995

Lesieur H, Blume S: The South Oaks Gambling Screen (SOGS): a new instrument for the identification of pathological gamblers. Am J Psychiatry 144:1184–1188, 1987

Lesieur HR, Klein R: Pathological gambling among high school students. Addict Behav 12:129–135, 1987

Lesieur HR, Rosenthal RJ: Pathological gambling: a review of the literature. Journal of Gambling Studies 7:5–39, 1991

Lesieur H, Blume S, Zoppa R: Alcoholism, drug abuse, and gambling. Alcohol Clin Exp Res 10:33–38, 1986

Linden RD, Pope HG, Jonas JM: Pathological gambling and major affective disorders: preliminary findings. J Clin Psychiatry 47:201–203, 1986

Linder RM: The psychodynamics of gambling. Annals of the American Academy of Political and Social Sciences 269:93–107, 1950

Linnoila M, Virkkunen M, Scheinin M, et al: Low cerebrospinal fluid 5-hydroxyindoleacetic acid concentration differentiates impulsive from nonimpulsive violent behavior. Life Sci 33:2609–2614, 1983

Livingston J: Compulsive Gamblers: Observations on Action and Abstinence. New York, Harper Torchbooks, 1974

Maccallum F, Blaszczynski A: Pathological gambling and comorbid substance use. Aust N Z J Psychiatry 36:411–415, 2002

Madden GJ, Petry NM, Badger GJ, et al: Impulsive and self-control choices in opioid-dependent patients and non-drug-using control participants: drug and monetary rewards. Exp Clin Psychopharmacol 3:256–262, 1997

Mann JJ, McBride PA, Brown RP, et al: Relationship between central and peripheral serotonin indexes in depressed and suicidal psychiatric inpatients. Arch Gen Psychiatry 49:442–446, 1992

Martinez-Pina A, Guirao de Parga JL, Vailverdi RF, et al: The Catalonia Survey: personality and intelligence structure in a sample of pathological gamblers. Journal of Gambling Studies 7:275–299, 1991

McCormick RA, Russo AM, Ramirez LF, et al: Affective disorders among pathological gamblers seeking treatment. Am J Psychiatry 141:215–218, 1984

Moody G: Quit Compulsive Gambling. London, Thorsons, 1990

Moran E: Taking the Final Risk. London, Mental Health, 1969

Moran E: Pathological gambling. Br J Hosp Med 4:59–70, 1970

Moravec JD, Munley PH: Psychological test findings on pathological gamblers in treatment. Int J Addict 18:1003–1009, 1983

Moreno I, Saiz-Ruiz JY, Lopez-Ibor JJ: Serotonin and gambling dependence. Hum Psychopharmacol 6:9–12, 1991

Moscowitz JA: Lithium and lady luck: use of lithium carbonate in compulsive gambling. N Y State J Med 80:785–788, 1980

Murray JB: Review of research on pathological gambling. Psychol Rep 72:791–810, 1993

Pallanti S, Cesarali V, Gotti M, et al: Impulsività, comportamenti a rischio ed epidemiologia del gambling in discoteca. Paper presented at the Italian Group for OCD, Torino, Italy, September 2000

Pallanti S, Quercioli L, Sood E, et al: Lithium and valproate treatment of pathological gambling: a randomized single-blind study. J Clin Psychiatry 63:559–564, 2002a

Pallanti S, Baldini Rossi N, et al: Nefazodone treatment of pathological gambling: a prospective open-label controlled trial. J Clin Psychiatry 63:1034–1039, 2002b

Peck CP: A public mental health issue: risk-taking behavior and compulsive gambling. Am Psychol 41:461–465, 1986

Perez de Castro I, Ibanez A, Torres P, et al: Genetic association study between pathological gambling and a functional DNA polymorphism at the D4 receptor gene. Pharmacogenetics 7:345–348, 1997

Perez de Castro I, Ibanez A, Saiz-Ruiz J, et al: Genetic contribution to pathological gambling: possible association between a functional DNA polymorphism at the serotonin transporter gene (5-HTT) and affected men. Pharmacogenetics 9:397–400, 1999

Perez de Castro I, Ibanez A, Saiz-Ruiz J, et al: Concurrent positive association between pathological gambling and functional DNA polymorphisms at the MAO-A and the 5-HT transporter genes. Mol Psychiatry 7:927–928, 2002

Petry NM: Delay discounting of money and alcohol in actively using alcoholics, currently abstinent alcoholics, and controls. Psychopharmacology (Berl) 154:243–250, 2001a

Petry NM: Pathological gamblers, with and without substance use disorders, discount delayed rewards at high rates. J Abnorm Psychol 110:482–487, 2001b

Petry NM: Substance abuse, pathological gambling, and impulsiveness. Drug Alcohol Depend 63:29–38, 2001c

Petry NM, Armentano C: Prevalence, assessment, and treatment of pathological gambling: a review. Psychiatr Serv 50:1021–1027, 1999

Petry NM, Casarella T: Excessive discounting of delayed rewards in substance abusers with gambling problems. Drug Alcohol Depend 56:25–32, 1999

Phillips DP, Welty WR, Smith MM: Elevated suicide levels associated with legalized gambling. Suicide Life Threat Behav 27:373–378, 1997

Potenza MN: The neurobiology of pathological gambling. Semin Clin Neuropsychiatry 6:217–226, 2001

Potenza MN, Chambers RA: Schizophrenia and pathological gambling. Am J Psychiatry 158:497–498, 2001

Potenza MN, Steinberg MA, Skudlarski P, et al: Gambling urges in pathological gambling: a functional magnetic resonance imaging study. Arch Gen Psychiatry 60:828–836, 2003

Ramirez LF, McCormick RA, Russo AM, et al: Patterns of substance abuse in pathological gamblers undergoing treatment. Addict Behav 8:425–428, 1983

Rogers RD, Robbins TW: Investigating the neurocognitive deficits associated with chronic drug misuse. Curr Opin Neurobiol 11:250–257, 2001

Rogers RD, Everitt BJ, Baldacchino A, et al: Dissociable deficits in the decision-making cognition of chronic amphetamine abusers, opiate abusers, patients with focal damage to prefrontal cortex, and tryptophan-depleted normal volunteers: evidence for monoaminergic mechanisms. Neuropsychopharmacology 20:322–339, 1999

Rosenthal RJ: Pathological gambling. Psychiatr Ann 22:72–78, 1992

Rosenthal R, Rugle L: A psychodynamic approach to the treatment of pathological gambling, part I: achieving abstinence. Journal of Gambling Studies 10:21–42, 1994

Roy A, Custer R, Lorenz V, et al: Depressed pathological gamblers. Acta Psychol Scand 77:163–165, 1988a

Roy A, Adinoff B, Roehrich L, et al: Pathological gambling: a psychobiological study. Arch Gen Psychiatry 45:369–373, 1988b

Roy A, DeJong J, Linnoila M: Extroversion in pathological gamblers: correlates with indexes of noradrenergic function. Arch Gen Psychiatry 46:679–681, 1989

Rugle L: The use of olanzapine in the treatment of video poker pathological gamblers. Paper presented at the 14th National Conference on Problem Gambling, Philadelphia, PA, October 2000

Rugle L, Melamed L: Neuropsychological assessment of attention problems in pathological gamblers. J Nerv Ment Dis 181:107–112, 1993

Russo AM, Taber JI, McCormick RA, et al: An outcome study of an inpatient treatment program for pathological gambling. Hosp Community Psychiatry 35:823–827, 1984

Shaffer HJ, Hall MN: Estimating the prevalence of adolescent gambling disorders: a quantitative synthesis and guide toward standard gambling nomenclature. Journal of Gambling Studies 12:193–214, 1996

Shaffer HJ, Hall MN, Vanderbilt J: Estimating the prevalence of disordered gambling behavior in the United States and Canada: a research synthesis. Am J Public Health 89:1369–1376, 1999

Siever LJ, Coccaro EF, Zemishlany Z, et al: Psychobiology of personality disorders: pharmacological implications. Psychopharmacol Bull 23:333–336, 1987

Simmel E: Psychoanalysis of the gambler. Int J Psychoanal 1:352–353, 1920

Slutske WS, Eisen S, True WR, et al: Common genetic vulnerability for pathological gambling and alcohol dependence in men. Arch Gen Psychiatry 57:666–673, 2000

Slutske WS, Eisen S, Xian H, et al: A twin study of the association between pathological gambling and antisocial personality disorder. J Abnorm Psychol 110:297–308, 2001

Soubrie P: Reconciling the role of central serotonin neurons in human and animal behavior. Behav Brain Sci 9:319–364, 1986

Specker SM, Carlson GA, Christenson GA, et al: Impulse control disorders and attention deficit disorder in pathological gamblers. Ann Clin Psychiatry 7:175–179, 1995

Stewart R, Brown RIF: An outcome study of Gamblers Anonymous. Br J Psychiatry 152:284–288, 1988

Stinchfield R: Reliability, validity, and classification accuracy of a measure of DSM-IV diagnostic criteria for pathological gambling. Am J Psychiatry 160:180–182, 2003

Taber JI: Group psychotherapy with pathological gamblers. Paper presented at the 5th National Conference on Gambling and Risk-Taking. South Lake Tahoe, NV, October 1981

Taber JI, McCormick RA, Russo AM, et al: Follow-up of pathological gamblers after treatment. Am J Psychiatry 144:757–761, 1987

Thompson W, Gazel R, Rickman D: The Social Costs of Gambling in Wisconsin: Report Prepared for the Wisconsin Policy Research Institute (Vol 9, No 6). Thiensville, WI, Wisconsin Policy Research Institute, 1996

Tollefson GD: Anxiety and alcoholism: a serotonin link. Br J Psychiatry 159 (suppl):34–39, 1991

Usdin E, Snyder S (eds): Frontiers in Catecholamine Research. Elmsford, NY, Pergamon, 1973

Vazquez Rodriguez AM, Arranz Pena MI, Lopez Ibor JJ, et al: Clomipramine test: serum level determination in three groups of psychiatric patients. J Pharm Biomed Anal 9:949–952, 1991

Victor R, Cruz C: Paradoxical intension in the treatment of compulsive gambling. Am J Psychother 21:808–814, 1967

Volberg RA: Estimating the prevalence of pathological gambling in the United States. Paper presented at the 8th International Conference on Risk and Gambling, London, August 1990

Volberg RA, Steadman HJ: Refining prevalence estimates of pathological gambling. Am J Psychiatry 145:502–505, 1988

Volberg RA, Steadman HJ: Prevalence estimates of pathological gambling in New Jersey and Maryland. Am J Psychiatry 146:1618–1619, 1989

Walters GD: Behavior genetic research on gambling and problem gambling: a preliminary meta-analysis of available data. Journal of Gambling Studies 17:255–271, 2001

Wender PH, Reimherr F, Wood DR: Attention-deficit disorder (minimum brain dysfunction) in adults. Arch Gen Psychiatry 38:449–456, 1981

Westlund KN, Krakower TJ, Kwan SW, et al: Intracellular distribution of monoamine oxidase A in selected regions of rat and monkey brain and spinal cord. Brain Res 612:221–230, 1993

Winters KC, Rich T: A twin study of adult gambling behavior. Journal of Gambling Studies 14:213–225, 1999

Wood DR, Wender PH, Reimherr FW: The prevalence of attention deficit disorder, residual type, or minimum brain dysfunction in a population of male alcoholic patients. Am J Psychiatry 140:95–98, 1983

World Health Organization: International Classification of Diseases, 9th Revision, Clinical Modification. Ann Arbor, MI, Commission on Professional and Hospital Activities, 1978

Wray I, Dickerson MG: Cessation of high frequency gambling and "withdrawal" symptoms. Br J Addict 76:401–405, 1981

Zimmerman M, Breen RB, Posternak MA: An open-label study of citalopram in the treatment of pathological gambling. J Clin Psychiatry 63:44–48, 2002

12

Problematic Internet Use

Toby D. Goldsmith, M.D.

Nathan A. Shapira, M.D., Ph.D.

Phenomenology

The administration of President William J. Clinton reported in the year 2000 that greater than 50% of all American households possessed a computer and more than 40% of homes in America were connected to the Internet. This report, *Falling Through the Net: Toward Digital Inclusion,* was a collaboration between the Department of Commerce's National Telecommunications and Information Administration and Economics and Statistics Administration (2000). Furthermore, it was reported that between January 1999 and August 2000, the number of users of the Internet increased by nearly one-third to over 116 million. Expansion of the Internet worldwide is also impressive. According to one study, utilization of the Internet has increased worldwide, with over 100 million more individuals accessing the Internet between May 2001 (463 million) and May 2002 (581 million) (Nua Internet Surveys

2002). With the continued rapid expansion and increased availability of the Internet, the number of Internet-associated behavior problems is likely to grow.

The extent of problematic Internet use that actually exists remains in question. There are few studies on problematic Internet use, and most have been conducted online and have lacked control populations (DeAngelis 2000). Given these limitations, it appears that between 6% and 14% of those who use the Internet may be problematic users (DeAngelis 2000). In an attempt to document the scope of "Internet addiction," a study of inappropriate Internet use in the workplace was administered by the Saratoga Institute; 60% of the participating corporations reported employees engaged in various improper Internet use and 30% of the companies reported terminating employees for their behavior (Greenfield 2000). This problem is not limited to the West. In two online studies of Taiwanese college students, including one with more than 753 participants, more than 10% of the students were noted to be potential "Internet addicts" (Chou 2001; Tsai and Lin 2001).

Behavioral problems associated with the Internet have been described utilizing various terms and pseudonyms including computer addiction, Internet addiction (disorder), Internetomania, pathological Internet use, and problematic Internet use (Bai et al. 2001; Beard and Wolf 2001; Belsare et al. 1997; Griffiths 1996, 1997; O'Reilly 1996; Shaffer et al. 2000; Shapira et al. 1998, 2000; Stein 1997a; Young 1996, 1998b; Young and Rogers 1998).

Since the mid-1990s, the media and medical literature have been replete with case reports describing those with problematic Internet use. Problematic Internet use can be typified by the Internet user's inability to limit Internet use, which leads to psychological impairment as well as social, educational, and occupational dysfunction (Shapira et al. 2000). Use of the Internet may be associated with numerous risks to the user. The Internet may be utilized by some to access areas that may be a manifestation of their psychiatric illness, for example, compulsive gambling, paraphilias, and compulsive buying. Small, face-to-face psychiatric studies have demonstrated that many of the evaluated individuals with problematic Internet use have comorbid psychiatric illnesses, especially mood and anxiety disorders (Black et al. 1999; Shapira et al. 2000). These same studies revealed significant distress and daily dysfunction among problematic users.

Whether these aberrant and problematic behaviors are the result of a unique disorder or are simply a manifestation of other psychiatric illnesses remains a pertinent question. In this chapter, we propose to describe the nature of the behavior and to discuss provisional diagnostic criteria for problematic Internet use that fall within the framework of impulse-control disorders. It is imperative that suggested criteria be able to distinguish problematic Internet use from other psychiatric illnesses as well as allow clinicians to consider whether problematic use of the Internet may be a symptom of other psychiatric illnesses.

Background

Initially, the study of technologically related addictions focused on the effects of television and excessive watching (Kubey and Csikszentmihalyi 2002). Renewed interest in this area arose in the early 1990s. "Technological addiction" was coined by Griffiths (1995, 1996) as a term to describe "nonchemical (behavioral) addictions which involve human–machine interaction" (Griffiths 1995, p. 15). In a 1990 case report, Keepers alerted the medical and psychological communities to the potential dangers associated with video and arcade games. A 12-year-old boy was reported to have succumbed to thievery and lying in order to fuel his preoccupation with video games located at a nearby arcade. The adolescent's habit reportedly cost him over $200 per week, and his academic performance was negatively affected. The boy's behavior improved with intense behavioral intervention (Keepers 1990).

Margaret Shotton (1991), well before the Internet was widely available, employed a combination of face-to-face interviews and posted questionnaires in her study of British "computer addiction." Her subjects were noted to have an average age of 29.7 years and had been "dependent" on the computer for more than 5 years. Predominantly they had good academic records. Primarily men answered the surveys, but women who owned computers were noted to be at equivalent risk as men for computer dependency. Shotton described "dependents" as having less satisfying interpersonal relationships and being more likely to characterize their parents as having been insufficiently supportive. Unlike individuals with problematic Internet use, only a few persons with computer dependency described social or occupational difficulties related to their computer use, and very few noted complaints from their spouses regarding their computer usage.

In 1976, William Glasser introduced the notion of "positive addiction"; it has been proposed that this idea may be well suited for Internet addiction (Griffiths 1996). Glasser (1976) described "positive addictions" as behaviors, such as running or knitting, that are beneficial for the individual; these activities may be utilized by those addicted to substances or detrimental behaviors to free them of their negative dependency. Glasser (1976) noted that to be a positive addiction, the behavior had to incorporate the following principles: 1) it did not interfere with everyday activities, 2) it was comparatively facile to perform, 3) it could be performed alone, 4) the individual found it worthwhile, 5) the end result was positive, and 6) the individual could not find fault with his or her involvement with the activity. Although Glasser's criteria may be relevant for some problematic users of the Internet, the notion of positive addiction as addiction has been questioned in view of the fact that positive addictions do not encompass the accepted symptoms of addiction, including tolerance and withdrawal (Griffiths 1996).

Technological addictions, like computer and Internet addiction, may be more similar to drug addiction due to the presence of common components such as euphoria, tolerance, withdrawal, and relapse (Griffiths 1995). In terms of becoming "addicted" to the Internet, several researchers have further described a correlation between the amount of time online and reported negative consequences (Griffiths 2001). "Technological addictions" have been studied primarily using gamblers addicted to slot or "fruit machines" that use operant conditioning to train the gambler to expect a reward for their behavior (Donegan et al. 1983). Not every pull of the lever results in a reward, and thus the gamble ensues (Griffiths 1993). Developers of the fruit machines make every effort to develop machines that are appealing to gamblers, encouraging them to play the game (Griffiths 1993). Griffiths (1995) proposed that two kinds of people become addicted to the Internet—the individual who is intrinsically attracted to the technology and the individual who uses that technology as a diversion from a less-than-pleasing life. As the technology improves (increasing speed, improved graphics), more individuals may be adversely affected by the Internet (Griffiths 1995; Griffiths and Parke 2002).

"Behavioral addiction" has also been proposed as a way of conceptualizing Internet dependence (Bradley 1990; Marks 1990). This variant of the classic addiction model has been used to describe other mental disorders, such as compulsive spending, gambling, compulsive sexual behavior, kleptomania, and overeating, but its utility and reliability have been called into question (Bradley 1990; Holden 2001; Miele et al. 1990). In their survey of 129 college students, Greenberg et al. (1999) noted a trend toward multiple addictions, with students with behavioral addictions (Internet, exercise, gambling) also being addicted to substances, including nicotine and alcohol. Psychological dependence is present in both substance and behavioral addictions; symptoms may occur even in the absence of substance use (Bradley 1990; Marks 1990). Individuals use various Web sites and forums on the Internet. For a given person, only a particular activity (or activities) may promote the development of an Internet addiction or compulsion (Griffiths 1995, 1996, 1997; Turkle 1995). Individuals with problematic Internet use have been noted to prefer computer activities that entail large amounts of interpersonal interaction, such as e-mail, chat rooms, and interactive gaming (Black et al. 1999; Chou 2001; Shapira et al. 2000; Young 1998a, 1998b). Studies demonstrate that Internet usage is gender and age dependent, with females and mature "addicts" preferring chat rooms that contain sexual material, and males and younger "addicts" more tempted by pornographic and gaming sites (P. Mitchell 2000).

Online pornography, "cybersex," and "cyberrelationships" are integral elements of the Internet (Cooper 1998; Cooper and Sportolari 1997). Sexually related Web sites are a major constituent element of the Internet, and it is believed that more than 50% of revenues earned on the Internet are related to these sites (Griffiths 2001). Although sexually related material and activities are prevalent, their importance in problematic Internet use is controversial (P. Mitchell 2000), and some of these activities may be more symptomatic of hypersexual disorder (Stein et al. 2001). There are also those who have suggested that "Internet sex addiction" be considered a unique subset of "Internet addiction" (Griffiths 2001).

Current Conceptual Approaches

There have been several attempts to formulate a diagnostic structure for problematic Internet use. One of the first conceptualizations was by Young (1996), who described an individual with "Internet addiction" using DSM-IV (American Psychiatric Association 1994) criteria for substance dependence. The individual was diagnosed with "Internet addiction" if he or she had three of seven of the modified criteria. Young went on to say that those with problematic Internet use may have symptoms similar to those addicted to drugs, alcohol, or gambling. Brenner (1997) developed an exploratory scale for "Internet addiction," the Internet-Related Addictive Behavior Inventory, which included adapting DSM-IV criteria for substance abuse. He noted that the scale had a good internal consistency ($\alpha = 0.87$) and that all of the 32 questions from the 563 online survey results correlated moderately with the total score (average 0.44; Brenner 1997). Brenner (1997) concluded that there was a subgroup of Internet users who endorsed various problems related to their Internet use, including domains often seen in addictions. Armstrong et al. (2000) also created their 20-question scale (Internet Related Problem Scale) in part from DSM-IV criteria for substance abuse/dependence and administered it to 50 subjects recruited through the Internet, who demonstrated internal consistency ($\alpha = 0.877$) and correlations ($r = 0.759$, $P < 0.001$) between high scores and hours spent online as well as correlations with a scale previously established for addiction, the Minnesota Multiphasic Personality Inventory–2 Addiction Potential Scale ($r = 0.297$, $P < 0.05$). The authors concluded that the Internet Related Problem Scale demonstrated construct validity and supported the concept of Internet addiction. However, it has also been argued by Satel (1993) that to expand addictions to include all "compulsive self-destructive behaviors" is problematic because such an expansion would weaken the concept of addiction as an actual illness and would risk treating all such behaviors with 12-Step programs without determining whether other treatment modalities might be more beneficial.

Since 1998, Young has reconceptualized problematic Internet use as an impulse-control disorder not unlike pathological gambling (Young 1998a, 1998b; Young and Rogers 1998) and subsequently has developed new criteria based on pathological gambling (Young 1998b). Using DSM-IV gambling criteria, Young developed an eight-item questionnaire; two criteria from the pathological gambling diagnosis were not considered to be applicable to problematic Internet users (Young 1998b). A survey was given to 396 "dependents" and 100 "nondependents" via telephone or electronic means. The dependency state was determined based on the individual's usage of the Internet, his or her online activities, and the negative impact the usage had on his or her life. The survey found that dependents were more likely to experiencing negative consequences in their lives (Young 1998b).

In an attempt to improve these criteria, Beard and Wolf (2001) reformulated Young's DSM-IV pathological gambling–based Internet addiction criteria. Their concern was based on the observation that several of the behaviors included by Young could be behaviors other than addiction. Subsequently, they modified the number of criteria required for a diagnosis of Internet addiction. Furthermore, utilizing a factor analysis investigation of 47 computer usage variables given via a survey to college students, Charlton (2002) concluded that adapting DSM criteria for pathological gambling likely overestimates the number of people addicted because there is no distinction made between the milder "engagement-related" criteria and the stronger criteria of the DSM checklist. In 1999, Praterelli et al. (1999) administered a 94-item survey to college students. This factor analysis supported a psychiatric component to "computer/Internet addiction" in that affected individuals were noted to have obsessive traits associated with their Internet and computer usage, prefer virtual relationships to vital ones, and use the computer to self-soothe or increase sexual feelings (Praterelli et al. 1999).

The umbrella of impulse-control disorders has also been used by others to characterize problematic Internet use (Shapira et al. 2000; Treuer et al. 2001). Shapira et al. (2000) evaluated Internet users whose problematic Internet use was broadly predefined as "1) uncontrollable, 2) markedly distressing, time-consuming or resulting in social, occupational or financial difficulties and 3) not solely present during hypomanic or manic symptoms" (p. 268). In their face-to-face interviews with 20 individuals with problematic Internet use, Shapira et al. (2000) found that all 20 of these subjects' Internet use would meet DSM-IV criteria for an impulse-control disorder not otherwise specified, whereas only 3 of the subjects would meet criteria for obsessive-compulsive disorder. Treuer et al. (2001) further described a high prevalence of features of impulse-control disorders among 86 Internet users who completed questionnaires after visiting the authors' Internet home page. Results from an online survey of these 86 Internet users included an increase in impulse-control disorder symptoms (Treuer et al. 2001).

Recently, Shapira et al. (2003) expressed the importance of provisionally developing specific problematic Internet use criteria that reflected their and others' observations; such criteria would ease the diagnosis of problematic Internet use in the clinic as well as foster further research in the area. As in other impulse-control disorders, problematic Internet users would experience a subjective feeling of tension before engaging in the specific behavior, followed by the experience of contentment or gratification upon the completion of the act. Although the category of impulse-control disorders already contains a variety of different diagnoses, these diagnoses (such as compulsive gambling, kleptomania, and intermittent explosive disorder) have been found to be beneficial in terms of patient education and treatment planning (Shapira et al. 2003). The criteria proposed by Shapira et al. (2003) were formatted in the style of the DSM-IV-TR (American Psychiatric Association 2000) criteria and those developed by McElroy et al. (1994) for compulsive shopping, because the authors thought that the criteria needed be inclusive enough to recognize problematic Internet users but not so inclusive that they included individuals whose symptoms were due to another psychiatric disorder. Shapira et al. (2003) did not feel that criteria for problematic Internet use based on compulsive gambling or substance addiction allowed appropriate examination of other potentially treatable psychiatric illnesses and thus put forth the diagnostic criteria for problematic Internet use described in Table 12–1.

Table 12–1. Proposed diagnostic criteria for problematic Internet use

A. Maladaptive preoccupation with Internet use, as indicated by at least one of the following:
Preoccupations with use of the Internet that are experienced as irresistible
Excessive use of the Internet for periods of time longer than planned

B. The use of the Internet or the preoccupation with its use causes clinically significant distress or impairment in social, occupational, or other important areas of functioning.

C. The excessive Internet use does not occur exclusively during periods of hypomania or mania and is not better accounted for by other Axis I disorders.

Source. Reprinted from Shapira NA, Lessig MC, Goldsmith TD, et al.: "Problematic Internet Use: Proposed Classification and Diagnostic Criteria." *Depression and Anxiety* 17:207–216, 2003. Copyright 2003, John Wiley & Sons. Used with permission.

Distinctness and Comorbidity

Several studies have looked at the comorbidity between problematic Internet use and other psychiatric disorders and symptoms. In one study of the comorbidity of addictions, Greenberg et al. (1999) found that those "addicted" to the Internet were more likely to abuse alcohol and other substances. Both Black et al. (1999) and Shapira et al. (2000) systematically evaluated smaller numbers of problematic Internet users and noted high rates of mood, substance use, anxiety, impulse-control, and personality disorders among them. Although Black et al. (1999) revealed numerous psychiatric diagnoses among the 21 individuals who presented requesting treatment for computer addiction, they were fewer in number than those found by Shapira et al. (2000) in their group of 20 individuals. All 20 were noted to have at least one major psychiatric diagnosis that predated their use of the Internet (Shapira, unpublished data, 2000). Also separating the two studies was the percentage of patients meeting criteria for a bipolar disorder, with 70% of Shapira et al.'s group meeting lifetime criteria for bipolar I or II versus 10% for Black et al.'s group. The demographics of the individuals were similar in both studies, with the average subjects being in their 30s and with problematic use occurring for approximately 3 years. The estimated time online was 27–28 hours per week that was not work or school related. Many of the individuals in both studies described problems in work, home, or school related to their use of the Internet (Black et al. 1999; Shapira et al. 2000). Fifteen of the 20 studied by Shapira et al. (2000) reported receiving psychopharmacological treatment at some time prior to their evaluation, and overall subjects retrospectively rated improved control over their Internet use when the medications were appropriate for comorbid psychiatric illnesses. To be effective, the treatment of problematic Internet use may need to be comprehensive, including use of biological and psychological remedies such as cognitive-behavioral therapy (Orzack 1999; Orzack and Orzack 1999; Orzack and Ross 2000).

There are also those who take issue with existence of problematic Internet use as a unique entity. P. Mitchell (2000) called into question the "chicken or the egg" issue of Internet addiction—is the problematic Internet use a disorder unique in itself or is it a symptom of another psychiatric illness? Griffiths (1999, 2000) noted that in most cases, excessive use of the Internet appears to be an expression of rewarding behaviors in which the Internet is mostly used solely to perform these behaviors. Furthermore, Shaffer et al. (2000) indicated that it is premature to define problematic Internet use as a unique psychiatric disorder before there has been systematic research to comprehensively and rigorously evaluate the construct. Recently, Pratarelli and Browne (2002), utilizing a factor analysis approach, reported that their survey data (when evaluated for sexual and other functional uses of the Internet) support the belief that the "Internet addict" has an "addictive" predisposition or susceptibility that leads to excessive Internet use.

Pathogenesis

Although it is fundamentally accepted that there are individuals who display patterns of problematic Internet use, how that problematic behavior develops is not understood (P. Mitchell 2000), and until longitudinal studies are performed, an adequate answer to this query may not be found.

Various researchers have commented on the use of the Internet as an alternative to socialization and interpersonal relationships. An individual with "pathological computer use disorder" may view the computer as either a vehicle for thrill seeking or a source of comfort (Orzack 1999). The addicted individual risks substituting vital relationships with virtual ones (Stein 1997a). Griffiths (1997) added that the Internet permits an individual to hide him- or herself within computer games, further avoiding real human relationships. This concern was demonstrated by Kraut et al. (1998) in a prospective study of 169 individuals (73 homes) over 2 years; higher use of the Internet was correlated with reduced engagement in family events, a decrease in the size of the individuals' social network, and an increase in depression and loneliness. Armstrong et al. (2000) found that subjects who had poorer self-esteem but not impulsivity had higher scores on their Internet-Related Problem Scale and predicted heavier personal/voluntary Internet use. In some vulnerable individuals, there is the risk that the isolation incurred by the use of the Internet may encourage further time online, exacerbating the individual's feelings of estrangement (Pratarelli et al. 1999). Morahan-Martin and Schumacher (2003) found that "lonely" undergraduate individuals used the Internet and e-mail more than did "nonlonely" individuals and also used the Internet more for emotional support. They found that socialization was enhanced in these individuals reportedly due to the Internet and that lonely subjects reported increased rates of meeting friends online and a heightened satisfaction with these relationships. However, these subjects were also more likely to report disturbances in their daily functioning due to the Internet.

Beyond the risks to the individual brought on by Internet use, there are the risks to society. As many as 5% of all Internet users have accessed Internet gambling sites (Pew Internet and American Life 2000). In a commentary in the *Journal of the American Medical Association,* Mitka (2001) wrote of the need to monitor online gambling given its accessibility to susceptible adolescents as well as the problems associated with greater availability of gambling in general. Many of the virtual gaming sites specifically target adolescents and children, enticing them with prizes and financial incentives (Levy and Strombeck 2002). Problems specific to online gambling among adolescents include the inability to prevent their access to gambling Web sites, the possibility of gambling while under the influence of a substance, and the 24-hour/day accessibility to the Web sites. Also, the use of credit cards rather than cash to finance the gaming may further impair an adolescent's judgment (Griffiths and Wood 2000).

Promiscuity and dangerous sexual behaviors may also be cultivated by Internet relationships (Benotsch et al. 2002; Elford et al. 2001; Kim et al. 2001; McFarlane et al. 2000; Toomey and Rothenberg 2000). For example, in a study of men who reported accessing gay-oriented Web sites, over one-third admitted having sexual relations with an individual they initially met through the Internet (Benotsch et al. 2002). In 1999, San Francisco health officials noted an increase in syphilis among gay men; this upsurge in the sexually transmitted disease was traced back to participants in a chat room (Klausner et al. 2000). Adolescents are also vulnerable to receiving unsolicited sexual invitations (K.J. Mitchell et al. 2001). There is also considerable concern regarding the availability of pornography to youngsters (Griffiths 2001).

The Internet has become a major resource for those seeking medical information as well as those seeking support as they struggle with their own illnesses. There have been numerous studies evaluating the accuracy of information on the Internet (Chen et al. 2000; Jejurikar et al. 2002; Karp and Monroe 2002; Kunst et al. 2002; Latthe et al. 2000; Lee et al. 2003; Lissman and Boehnlein 2001; Madan et al. 2003; Martin-Facklam et al. 2002; Roberts and Copeland 2001; Stapleton 2001; Tatsioni et al. 2003). Although there have been some recent signs of improvement in the completeness and accuracy of information (Karp and Monroe 2002), most studies indicate that the Internet is not a dependable source of patient information. Additionally, there are those who in their quest for attention have abused the sympathy and empathy of others. In one case series, several accounts of "virtual" factitious disorder and Munchausen syndrome by proxy were presented (Feldman 2000). Users of particular chat rooms reported spurious accounts of their own personal illnesses or troubles. Feldman (2000) recognized that the Internet can be a genuine tool for many, but may be abused by others, thus requiring all Internet consumers to be wary. An additional health-related problem associated with the Internet is the availability of prescription medications. Certain pharmacy Web sites allow easy access to pharmaceuticals without proper medical guidance or monitoring, putting the buyer at risk of complications (Levy and Strombeck 2002).

The Internet is having both positive and negative effects on mental health and mental health care. The Internet as a venue for psychotherapy and self-help has been discussed (Stein 1997b), and the Internet as a site for a mental health clinic for those with problematic Internet use has been considered (Bai et al. 2001).

Although the Internet can be beneficial as a tool, it can also negatively influence the psychiatric patient. The Internet can be incorporated into an individual's psychiatric symptoms. Two individuals whose delusions involved the control of their thoughts and bodies by computers, the Internet, and the World Wide Web have been reported; interestingly, neither had ready access to a computer (Catalano et al. 1999). A case of erotic transference that evolved through e-mail has also been documented (Gabbard 2001). A case patient (a composite of two individuals) with hypersexual disorder whose behaviors revolved around numerous Internet relationships has been described (Stein et al. 2001). A woman with posttraumatic stress disorder and multiple personality disorder was described by Podoll et al. (2002); two of the woman's 48 alters often frequented chat rooms. The patient's Internet use was viewed as symptom of her dissociative disorder rather than as a separate illness (Podoll et al. 2002).

Treatment

Pharmacotherapy

There have been no published systematic studies evaluating the effect of pharmacotherapy for problematic Internet use. Shapira et al. (2000) reported that when retrospectively evaluating medication effects in 15 of the 20 problematic Internet use subjects who had taken psychotropic medications, mood stabilizing medication was associated with a higher rate of moderate or marked reduction in problematic Internet use. However, these findings are limited by several factors, including the study's small size, retrospective nature, lack of a control group, and self-reported interviews (Shapira et al. 2000).

Psychotherapy

There have been no published systematic studies evaluating psychotherapy for problematic Internet use. Currently, cognitive-behavioral therapy has been the primary proposed treatment to interrupt problematic computer use and replace these routines with other activities (Orzack 1999; Young 1999). Also, support groups and family therapy are often recommended to help repair relationship discord and engage friends and family in the treatment.

Conclusion

As a result of the expanding technology, problematic Internet use is a new phenomenon, and much about it remains unknown. At the crux of the issue is whether problematic Internet use is a distinct entity or simply a symptom of other psychiatric illnesses. It is currently unknown whether problematic Internet use, commonly and probably erroneously called "Internet addiction," represents symptoms of preexisting psychiatric illnesses. Yet there is some evidence that problematic Internet use cannot always be explained by other conditions and that like other impulsive disorders, it can be distressing, disabling, and quite prevalent. It is also unclear what are the most effective treatment or treatment strategies for this proposed entity. Because of the Internet's rapidly expanding availability, more systematic research is needed to characterize problematic Internet use and to understand the interactions between the Internet and psychiatric illness.

References

American Psychiatric Association: Diagnostic and Statistical Manual of Mental Disorders, 4th Edition. Washington, DC, American Psychiatric Association, 1994

American Psychiatric Association: Diagnostic and Statistical Manual of Mental Disorders, 4th Edition, Text Revision. Washington, DC, American Psychiatric Association, 2000

Armstrong L, Phillips JG, Saling LL: Potential determinants of heavier Internet usage. Int J Hum Comput Stud 53:537–550, 2000

Bai YM, Lin CC, Chen JY: Internet addiction disorder among clients of a virtual clinic. Psychiatr Serv 52:1397, 2001

Beard KW, Wolf EM: Modification in the proposed diagnostic criteria for Internet addiction. Cyberpsychol Behav 4:377–383, 2001

Belsare TJ, Gaffney GR, Black DW: Compulsive computer use (letter). Am J Psychiatry 154:289, 1997

Benotsch EG, Kalichman S, Cage M: Men who have met sex partners via the Internet: prevalence, predictors, and implications for HIV prevention. Arch Sex Behav 31:177–183, 2002

Black DW, Belsare G, Schlosser S: Clinical features, psychiatric comorbidity, and health-related quality of life in persons reporting compulsive computer use behavior. J Clin Psychiatry 60:839–844, 1999

Bradley BP: Behavioural addictions: common features and treatment implications. Br J Addict 85:1417–1419, 1990

Brenner V: Psychology of computer use, XLVII: parameters of Internet use, abuse and addiction. The first 90 days of the Internet Usage Survey. Psychol Rep 80:879–882, 1997

Catalano G, Catalano MC, Embi CS, et al: Delusions about the Internet. South Med J 92:609–610, 1999

Charlton JP: A factor-analytic investigation of computer "addiction" and engagement. Br J Psychol 93:329–344, 2002

Chen LE, Minkes RK, Langer JC: Pediatric surgery on the Internet: is the truth out there? J Pediatr Surg 35:1179–1182, 2000

Chou C: Internet heavy use and addiction among Taiwanese college students: an online interview study. Cyberpsychol Behav 4:573–585, 2001

Cooper A: Sexuality and the Internet: surfing into the new millennium. Cyberpsychol Behav 1:181–187, 1998

Cooper A, Sportolari L: Romance in cyberspace: understanding online attraction. J Sex Educ Ther 6:79–104, 1997

DeAngelis T: Is Internet addiction real? Monitor on Psychology (American Psychological Association Publication—serial online) 31(4), 2000. Available at: http://www.apa.org/monitor/apr00/. Accessed September 7, 2004

Donegan NH, Rodin J, O'Brien CP, et al: A learning-theory approach to commonalities, in Commonalities in Substance Abuse and Habitual Behavior. Edited by Levison PK, Gerstein DR, Maloff DR. Lexington, MA, DC Heath, 1983, pp 111–156

Elford J, Bolding G, Sherr L: Seeking sex on the Internet and sexual risk behaviour among gay men using London gyms. AIDS 15:1490–1415, 2001

Feldman MD: Munchausen by Internet: detecting factitious illness and crisis on the Internet. South Med J 93:669–672, 2000

Gabbard GO: Cyberpassion: e-rotic transference on the Internet. Psychoanal Q 70:719–737, 2001

Glasser W: Positive Addiction. New York, Harper & Row, 1976

Greenberg JL, Lewis SE, Dodd DK: Overlapping addictions and self-esteem among college men and women. Addict Behav 24:565–571, 1999

Greenfield D: Lost in cyberspace: the web @ work, 2000. Available at: http://www.virtual-addiction.com/pdf/lostincyberspace.pdf. Accessed on September 7, 2004

Griffiths MD: Fruit machine gambling: the importance of structural characteristics. Journal of Gambling Studies 9:101–119, 1993

Griffiths MD: Technological addictions. Clin Psychol Forum 95:14–19, 1995

Griffiths MD: Internet addiction: an issue for clinical psychology? Clinical Psychology Forum 97:32–36, 1996

Griffiths MD: Psychology of computer use, XLIII: some comments on "Addictive Use of the Internet" by Young (comment). Psychol Rep 80:81–82, 1997

Griffiths MD: Internet addiction: fact or fiction? Psychologist 12:246–250, 1999

Griffiths MD: Does Internet and computer "addiction" exist? Some case study evidence. Cyberpsychol Behav 3:211–218, 2000

Griffiths MD: Sex on the Internet: observations and implications for Internet sex addiction. J Sex Res 38:331–351, 2001

Griffiths MD, Parke J: The social impact of Internet gambling. Social Science and Computer Review 20:312–320, 2002

Griffiths M, Wood RTA: Risk factors in adolescence: the case of gambling, videogame playing, and the Internet. Journal of Gambling Studies 16:199–225, 2000

Holden C: "Behavioral" addictions: do they exist? Science 294:980–982, 2001

Jejurikar SS, Rovak JM, Kuzon WM, et al: Evaluation of plastic surgery information on the Internet. Ann Plast Surg 49:460–465, 2002

Karp S, Monroe AF: Quality of health care information on the Internet: caveat emptor still rules. Manag Care Q 10:3–8, 2002

Keepers GA: Pathological preoccupation with video games. J Am Acad Child Adolesc Psychiatry 29:49–50, 1990

Kim AA, Kent C, McFarland W, et al: Cruising on the Internet highway. J Acquir Immun Defic Syndr 28:89–93, 2001

Klausner JC, Wolf W, Fischer-Ponce L, et al: Tracing a syphilis outbreak through cyberspace. JAMA 284:447–449, 2000

Kraut R, Lundmark V, Patterson M, et al: Internet paradox: a social technology that reduces social involvement and psychological well-being? Am Psychol 53:1017–1031, 1998

Kubey R, Csikszentmihalyi M: Television addiction is no mere metaphor. Sci Am 286:74–80, 2002

Kunst H, Groot D, Latthe PM, et al: Accuracy of information on apparently credible websites: survey of five common health topics. BMJ 324:581–582, 2002

Latthe PM, Latthe M, Khan KS: Quality of medical information about menorrhagia on the World Wide Web. BJOG 107:39–43, 2000

Lee CT, Smith CA, Hall JM, et al: Bladder cancer facts: accuracy of information on the Internet. J Urol 170:1756–1760, 2003

Levy JA, Strombeck R: Health benefits and risks of the Internet. J Med Syst 26:495–510, 2002

Lissman TL, Boehnlein JK: A critical review of Internet information about depression. Psychiatr Serv 53:1046–1050, 2001

Madan AK, Frantzides CT, Pesce CE: The quality of information about laparoscopic bariatric surgery on the Internet. Surg Endosc 17:685–687, 2003

Marks I: Behavioural (nonchemical) addictions. Br J Addict 85:1389–1394, 1990

Martin-Facklam M, Kostrzewa M, Schubert F, et al: Quality markers of drug information on the Internet: an evaluation of sites about St. John's wort. Am J Med 15:740–745, 2002

McElroy SL, Keck PE Jr, Harrison PG, et al: Compulsive buying: a report of 20 cases. J Clin Psychiatry 55:242–248, 1994

McFarlane M, Bull SS, Rietmeijer CA: The Internet as a newly emerging risk environment for sexually transmitted diseases. JAMA 284:443–446, 2000

Miele GM, Tilly SM, First M, et al: The definition of dependence and behavioural addictions. Br J Addict 85:1421–1423, 1990

Mitchell KJ, Finkelhor D, Wolak J: Risk factors for and impact of online sexual solicitation of youth. JAMA 285:3011–3014, 2001

Mitchell P: Internet addiction: genuine diagnosis or not? Lancet 355:632, 2000

Mitka M: Win or lose, Internet gambling stakes are high. JAMA 285:1005, 2001

Morahan-Martin J, Schumacher P: Loneliness and social uses of the Internet. Comput Human Behav 19:659–671, 2003

National Telecommunications and Information Administration and Economics and Statistics Administration: Falling through the Net: toward digital inclusion (executive summary) [Online NTIA Release], 2000. Available at: http://www.ntia.doc.gov/ntiahome/digitaldivide/execsumfttn00.htm. Accessed September 7, 2004

Nua Internet Surveys. 2002. Available at: http://www.nua.ie/surveys/how_many_online/world.html. Accessed September 7, 2004

O'Reilly M: Internet addiction: a new disorder enters the medical lexicon. Can Med Assoc J 154:1882–1883, 1996

Orzack MH: How to recognize and treat computer.com addictions. Directions in Mental Health Counseling 9:13–20, 1999

Orzack MH, Orzack DS: Treatment of computer addicts with complex comorbid psychiatric disorders. Cyberpsychol Behav 2:465–473, 1999

Orzack MH, Ross CR: Should virtual sex be treated like other sex addictions? Sexual Addictions and Compulsivity 7:113–125, 2000

Pew Internet and American Life: New Internet users: what they do online, what they don't, and implications for the Net's future, 2000. Available at: http://www.pewInternet.org/reports/toc.asp?Report=22. Accessed September 7, 2004

Podoll K, Morth D, Sass H, et al: Self-help via the Internet: chances and risks of communication in electronic networks [in German]. Nervenarzt 73:85–89, 2002

Pratarelli ME, Browne BL: Confirmatory factor analysis of Internet use and addiction. Cyberpsychol Behav 5:53–64, 2002

Pratarelli ME, Browne BL, Johnson K: The bits and bytes of computer/Internet addiction: a factor analytic approach. Behav Res Methods Instrum Comput 31:305–314, 1999

Roberts JM, Copeland KL: Clinical websites are currently dangerous to health. Int J Med Inform 62:181–187, 2001

Satel SL: The diagnostic limits of "addiction" (letter; comment). J Clin Psychiatry 54:237–238, 1993

Shaffer HJ, Hall MN, Bilt JV: Computer addiction: a critical consideration. Am J Orthopsychiatry 70:162–168, 2000

Shapira NA, Goldsmith TD, Keck PE, et al: Psychiatric evaluation of individuals with problematic use of the Internet. Poster presented at the 151st annual meeting of the American Psychiatric Association, Toronto, Ontario, Canada, June 1998

Shapira NA, Goldsmith TG, Keck PE, et al: Psychiatric features of individuals with problematic Internet use. J Affect Disord 57:267–272, 2000

Shapira NA, Lessig MC, Goldsmith TD, et al: Problematic Internet use: proposed classification and diagnostic criteria. Depress Anxiety 17:207–216, 2003

Shotton MA: The costs and benefits of "computer addiction." Behav Inf Technol 10:219–230, 1991

Stapleton JL: A comprehensive review of selected cancer websites. Can Oncol Nurs J 11:146–148, 2001

Stein DJ: Internet addiction, Internet psychotherapy (letter; comment). Am J Psychiatry 154:890, 1997a

Stein DJ: Psychiatry on the Internet: survey of an OCD mailing list. Psychiatr Bull 21:95–98, 1997b

Stein DJ, Black DW, Shapira NA, et al: Hypersexual disorder and preoccupation with Internet pornography. Am J Psychiatry 158:1590–1594, 2001

Tatsioni A, Gerasi E, Charitidou E, et al: Important drug safety information on the Internet: assessing its accuracy and reliability. Drug Saf 26:519–527, 2003

Toomey KE, Rothenberg RB: Sex and cyberspace: virtual networks leading to high-risk sex. JAMA 284:485–487, 2000

Treuer T, Fábián Z, Füredi J: Internet addiction associated with features of impulse control disorder: is it a real psychiatric disorder? J Affect Disord 66:283, 2001

Tsai CC, Lin SS: Analysis of attitudes toward computer networks and Internet addiction of Taiwanese adolescents. Cyberpsychol Behav 4:373–376, 2001

Turkle S: Life Behind the Screen: Identity in the Age of the Internet. New York, Simon & Schuster, 1995

Young KS: Psychology of computer use, XL: addictive use of the Internet: a case that breaks the stereotype. Psychol Rep 79:899–902, 1996

Young KS: Caught in the Net: How to Recognize the Signs of Internet Addiction and a Winning Strategy for Recovery. New York, Wiley, 1998a

Young KS: Internet addiction: the emergence of a new clinical disorder. Cyberpsychol Behav 1:237–244, 1998b

Young KS: Internet addiction: symptoms, evaluation and treatment. Innovations in Clinical Practice 17:19–31, 1999

Young KS, Rogers RC: The relationship between depression and Internet addiction. Cyberpsychol Behav 1:25–28, 1998

13

Treatment of Impulse-Control Disorders

Dan J. Stein, M.D., Ph.D.

Brian Harvey, Ph.D.

Soraya Seedat, M.B., Ch.B., F.R.C.Psych.

Eric Hollander, M.D.

This chapter focuses on the treatment of impulse-control disorders (ICDs). On the one hand, ICDs are complex conditions for which there is no magic bullet. Unfortunately there is no U.S. Food and Drug Administration (FDA)–approved medication and no standardized cognitive-behavioral manual for impulsivity in general. Furthermore, relatively few controlled clinical trials have been undertaken on individual ICDs. Nevertheless, significant progress has been made in delineating, diagnosing, and assessing these conditions. Fluoxetine is FDA approved for the treatment of bulimia, and the selective serotonin reuptake inhibitors (SSRIs) and a number of mood stabilizers/anticonvulsants have been studied in several ICDs. Cognitive-behavioral therapy (CBT) provides treatment principles for the management of a number of these conditions, and psychodynamically informed psychotherapy also has a useful role. The field is therefore able to outline the basis of a rational approach to treatment. Rather than focusing on any one ICD, this chapter focuses on general principles for the management of adult patients with ICDs. More specific details of the pharmacotherapy and psychotherapy approaches to each of the individual ICDs are covered in prior chapters.

Diagnosis

The development of specific diagnostic criteria for ICDs in DSM-III (American Psychiatric Association 1980) provided an important step forward for research on these conditions. The DSM system provides criteria not only for the diagnosis of several Axis I ICDs but also for a number of Axis II disorders characterized by impulsivity. Nevertheless, a number of other ICDs are not included as independent diagnoses and fall into the residual category of ICD not otherwise specified. Similarly, widely used screening questionnaires, such as the Primary Care Evaluation of Mental Disorders, and structured diagnostic clinical interviews, such as the Mini International Neuropsychiatric Inventory, focus primarily on mood and anxiety disorders, giving rather short shrift to impulsive and aggressive symptoms.

This relative neglect may reflect concerns about the validity of ICDs. Throughout this volume, contributors have raised questions about whether ICDs are best conceptualized as specific psychiatric conditions or simply entail symptoms that should be understood as manifestations of other disorders. The heterogeneity of impulsive symptoms and conditions, their frequent culture boundedness (e.g., problematic Internet use), and their high comorbidity with mood and anxiety disorders raise skepticism about whether these are specific entities. On the other hand, there are consistent features that characterize the ICDs and are important in their diagnosis and treatment. Given the large burden of illness caused by the ICDs, there is a clear need to screen for their presence.

In our view, it is therefore important to include questions about impulsivity and aggression in the standard psychiatric history. Screening questions can include, "Do you have a temper?" "Do you hurt yourself in any way (e.g., hair pulling, skin picking)?" "Are there repetitive behaviors you feel driven to perform, but later regret (e.g., gambling, sexual behavior)?" In more specialized clinics, structured diagnostic clinical interviews, such as the Minnesota Impulsivity Interview or the Structured Clinical Interview for Diagnosis of Obsessive-Compulsive Spectrum Disorders are useful because they cover many of the ICDs, thus allowing diagnosis of the range of comorbid ICDs often present in patients presenting with any one ICD (du Toit et al. 2001).

Given the heterogeneity of the ICDs, diagnostic interviews must, however, be supplemented by more detailed kinds of individualized assessment. Impulsivity is not a unitary construct, with multiple definitions in both the animal and clinical literature (Evenden 1999). Key dimensions within the ICDs that may be targeted in treatment include cognitive impulsivity (to what extent is there a lack of planning?), emotional impulsivity (to what extent is there an inability to delay gratification?), attentional impulsivity (to what extent is there distractibility?), and moral processing (to what extent is there empathy and a conscience?). We discuss the assessment of patients with ICDs in more detail in the next section. The management of the acutely agitated or aggressive patient can overlap with the treatment of ICDs but also involves somewhat different principles (DosReis et al. 2003; Swann 2003) and is not discussed further here.

Assessment

Individual assessment of the patient with an ICD must cover a range of issues. A first question is the severity of the primary symptoms and the consequent distress and disability. Several standardized rating scales are available for the assessment of symptom severity and quality of life. Scales are also available for the measurement of externalizing symptoms in children and adolescents (Collett et al. 2003). Nevertheless, impulsive patients may overestimate or underestimate the extent of both their symptoms and their impairment, and where feasible, additional sources of history should be considered. Interviewing family members or others involved in the patient's life (e.g., teachers) may be an important first step in developing a treatment plan.

A second important issue is that of comorbidity. Given the high comorbidity between the ICDs and mood, anxiety, and substance use disorders, it is crucial to assess any patient with an ICD with a comprehensive psychiatric history and examination. A careful assessment of suicidal and homicidal ideation must be included. Structured clinical interviews such as the Mini International Neuropsychiatric Interview may be useful in addressing a range of common psychiatric disorders other than ICDs (Sheehan et al. 1998). In addition, the importance of excluding general medical disorders should not be underestimated. Physical history and examination, with special attention to neurological issues, should be a routine consideration.

Some comorbid conditions, such as mood and anxiety disorders, may respond to similar interventions as are usually employed in the treatment of ICDs. Comorbidity of other conditions may, however, demand considerable changes in the approach toward evaluation and management. Comorbidity of impulsivity with antisocial personality disorder, for example, is not uncommon and presents a particular challenge for treatment. Basic cognitive-affective neuroscience suggests a division between impulsive-affective and controlled-predatory subtypes of aggression (Miczek et al. 2002), and indeed, interventions for impulsive patients who also have psychopathy may require significant modification. Similarly, comorbidity of impulsivity with substance use disorders, eating disorders, and attention-deficit/hyperactivity disorder (ADHD) is frequently seen and demands that clinicians focus their interventions to address these conditions (Lavine 1997).

A number of contributors to this volume have emphasized an association between childhood trauma and adult impulsivity. Our view is that assessment of childhood trauma should be a routine part of the evaluation of patients with ICDs. Although the suggestibility of some patients with ICDs is a valid concern, it is also important not to ignore the reality of this association; questions about childhood adversity should be straightforward and direct. If there is any evidence of childhood abuse, additional corroboration is valuable, and a scale such as the Childhood Trauma Questionnaire (Bernstein et al. 1994) may be useful in assessing the nature and severity of such traumas.

Current stress may also be a key precipitant of impulsive symptoms; this phenomenon is consistent with basic work demonstrating the exacerbation of impulsive and aggressive behavior after particular stressors (Miczek et al. 2002) and deserves particular clinical consideration. The role of past and current stressors in the pathogenesis of impulsivity should be understood within an integrated psychobiological framework; genetic vulnerabilities may confer risk to pathological responses to stress (Caspi et al. 2003), and stressors also have specific chronic neurobiological sequelae (Heim and Nemeroff 2001).

It is also important to determine the meaning of ICD symptoms within the person's life as a whole. Early authors emphasized that such symptoms often represented particular kinds of emotional conflict and could therefore be understood in the context of the patient's current circumstances and life history. Understanding the person as a whole, including his or her intrapsychic life, family system and social supports, and any pertinent cultural factors remains a key goal of the clinical assessment of ICD symptoms. Furthermore, it is important to determine patients' own explanatory model—how do they understand their symptomatology, and what is their belief about its etiology? Impulsive symptoms are often experienced as shameful, and it is also important to address this issue.

There is an increasing appreciation of the underlying neurocircuitry that mediates the different dimensions of impulsivity. The dorsolateral frontal cortex plays a crucial role in cognitive operations such as planning; the orbitofrontal cortex and amygdala play a key role in emotional regulation and behavioral control; the nucleus accumbens is a neural substrate for motivational processes and may also be involved in processing delay of gratification; and parietal structures are key in attention. Complex phenomena such as empathy integrate both cognitive and affective processes and are distributed across different neuronal circuits. Serotonin is a particularly crucial neurotransmitter in the mediation of behavioral control and impulsive aggression, and the dopamine system may be particularly relevant to the reinforcement of impulsive behaviors, but a range of other monoamine systems and other neurochemical and neurohormonal systems are also important. Neurobiological substrates of impulsivity change throughout life, and there is growing information, including animal data, about the basis for periods of increased impulsivity, such as adolescence (Laviola et al. 2003). Although much work on the neural substrate of impulsivity remains in the realm of research, neuropsychological and neuropsychiatric evaluation, including determination of soft neurological signs, electroencephalography, and, in specialized settings, positron emission tomography or single photon emission computed tomography, may provide useful information.

In the absence of comprehensive integrated psychobiological models of ICD symptoms, it may be useful to draw eclectically on a range of different models during the assessment and evaluation process. In addition to considering different proximal factors that may contribute to ICD symptoms (e.g., neurobiological, general medical, psychological), it may be useful to bear in mind more distal evolutionary mechanisms that could be relevant. Although such models are currently speculative, they remind the clinician that within particular evolutionary contexts, impulsive and aggressive symptoms can be adaptive and thus may help to emphasize resilience and counter stigmatization (Gerald and Higley 2002; Scott 1958).

Pharmacotherapy

A range of different medication classes have been investigated in the treatment of ICDs and borderline personality disorder. In this section, we briefly summarize the evidence for the use of antidepressants such as the SSRIs; mood stabilizers/anticonvulsants such as lithium, valproate, and topiramate; and antipsychotic agents. Agents from each of these classes may be useful in particular patients with ICDs; it is therefore important to individualize treatment decisions based on the limited evidence base, the patient's presenting problems, and history. There is some evidence that different symptom dimensions within the ICDs are particularly responsive to different medication classes. Some symptom dimensions (e.g., antisocial traits) may be less responsive to medication, and some classes of medication, including the benzodiazepines, do not appear particularly effective for the treatment of ICDs and should therefore generally be avoided.

Antidepressants

There are multiple case reports of tricyclic antidepressants (TCAs) and monoamine oxidase inhibitors (MAOIs) being useful in different ICDs, including binge eating disorder, kleptomania, and trichotillomania. The efficacy of MAOIs is consistent with genetic work showing that variants in the MAO-A gene are associated with impulsivity and aggression. Nevertheless, apart from some trials in borderline personality disorder, there is a paucity of controlled trials with these older agents for impulsive symptoms; in addition, these agents have a relatively poor tolerability profile and significant potential for serious adverse events (e.g., in overdose or when dietary precautions are not followed). For this reason, MAOIs are not generally considered as first-line medications in the treatment of ICDs. However, in individual patients who have failed trials of other agents, they may have a role. In particular, they can be considered in patients with comorbid depression that is refractory to new-generation antidepressants. TCAs should, however, generally be avoided in patients with evidence of bipolarity and may exacerbate impulsivity in patients with borderline or schizotypal personality disorder (Soloff et al. 1987).

Controlled trials of SSRIs have been undertaken in a range of ICDs and in borderline personality disorder. Part of the impetus for this work are the data that serotonergic hypofunction can be a key factor in mediating impulsivity. Trials of SSRIs have been positive in binge eating disorder, borderline personality disorder, compulsive shopping, intermittent explosive disorder, and pathological gambling. Methodological problems associated with such trials include a high placebo rate, and effect sizes do not always indicate a robust response. In a minority of individuals, it is possible that SSRIs increase impulsivity (Walsh and Dinan 2001). This may be especially true in patients with comorbid bipolar spectrum disorders.

The heterogeneity of the data reflects in part the heterogeneity of these disorders. Once again, an individualized approach is required. The SSRIs can be given particular consideration in the treatment of ICD patients with comorbid depression or anxiety disorders. Optimal dosage and duration of the SSRIs in treating ICDs have not been fully characterized; our approach is to begin with a low dosage and gradually increase to those that are maximally tolerated. Although responses may be seen relatively quickly, we typically use any one SSRI for 10–12 weeks before making a final determination about its value for a particular patient.

Selective norepinephrine reuptake inhibitors (SNRIs) such as venlafaxine are better tolerated than the older TCAs and may therefore also be useful in the treatment of some patients with ICDs. The use of such agents is given theoretical support by evidence that the noradrenergic system contributes to impulsivity, perhaps by modulating irritability and mood. They can perhaps be considered in patients with comorbid ADHD. β-Blockers have been studied in a broad range of populations and have a role in the treatment of aggression across various diagnoses including head injury and mental retardation (Haspel 1995). In addition, α_2-adrenergic autoreceptor agonists such as clonidine are widely used to reduce symptoms of ADHD including impulsivity. Nevertheless, the database of studies using SNRIs and adrenergic medications in ICDs is at present rather limited, and some caution is warranted given previous findings that TCAs can exacerbate impulsivity in some patients (Soloff et al. 1987).

Agents that act at specific serotonin receptors, such as 5-HT_{1A}, are currently not often used in the treatment of impulsivity. Nevertheless, basic work suggests that certain serotonin receptors are particularly important in mediating impulsivity and aggression. There are open-label data supporting the value of buspirone, a 5-HT_{1A} partial agonist, for aggression, but little controlled work. A class of so-called serenic drugs with a primary site of action at 5-HT_{1B} receptors did not come to market. New generation antipsychotic agents that have a robust action on 5-HT_2 receptors may, however, act to decrease impulsivity and aggression in part via their actions on the serotonergic system.

Anticonvulsants/Mood Stabilizers

A second class of medication often used in the pharmacotherapy of ICDs are the mood stabilizers or anticonvulsants. Early work suggested that lithium was useful in decreasing aggression in a broad range of populations (Sheard et al. 2003), and more recent controlled studies in younger patients have supported this contention (Malone et al. 2000). In view of its adverse event profile, lithium is generally no longer used as a first-line medication for the ICDs unless there is comorbid bipolarity. For example, lithium was effective in a recent controlled trial in subjects with pathological gambling and bipolar conditions (Hollander et al. 2002).

Phenytoin and carbamazepine have also been used for many years to treat patients with impulsive symptoms secondary to neurological lesions, and there is some controlled evidence that they are able to reduce impulsive aggression, although there is little work on these agents in patients with ICDs (Barratt et al. 1997; Cueva et al. 1996; Stanford et al. 2001). Their use is supported in part by basic evidence that alterations in the balance of excitatory glutamatergic and inhibitory GABAergic tone contributes to the regulation of impulsivity and that anticonvulsants modify this balance. More recent work has established the value of several new generation anticonvulsants in patients with bipolar disorder and has led to several controlled trials of these agents in patients with ICDs.

New-generation anticonvulsants can be given particular consideration when patients with ICDs have comorbid cyclothymia or bipolar disorder (including bipolar type II), when there is a suspicion of underlying temporal lobe involvement (e.g., on the basis of electroencephalography), or when outwardly directed irritable aggression is a key target symptom (Donovan et al. 2000). In particular, a number of controlled trials of valproate for impulsive aggression now exist, supporting the use of this agent for such symptoms (Hollander et al. 2003; Lindenmeyer and Kotsaftis 2000). There are also persuasive data from controlled trials of topiramate in binge eating disorder (McElroy et al. 2003) and in alcohol dependence (Johnson et al. 2003) that suggest the efficacy of this medication for these indications. In the absence of published trials on specific indications, the choice of a particular anticonvulsant for a patient with an ICD may be made on the basis of more subtle considerations such as side-effect profile and family history of response to medication. Optimal dosage and duration have not been fully determined, and in general it may be useful to assume that dosages in the antiseizure range and relatively long treatment trials (10–12 weeks) will be required.

Antipsychotics

New-generation antipsychotics are another consideration in the pharmacotherapy of ICDs. The dopamine system plays a key role in motivation and in reward processing, and changes in this system may theoretically help reduce the reinforcement associated with impulsive symptoms. Early controlled trials demonstrated the efficacy of first-generation antipsychotics in borderline personality disorder, and more recent trials have indicated the value of new-generation agents in borderline personality disorder, conduct disorder, and trichotillomania. These agents also reduce aggressive symptoms in a range of different psychiatric diagnoses, including primary psychotic illness, pervasive developmental disorders, and dementia (Aleman and Kahn 2001).

Despite the improved adverse effect profile of the new-generation antipsychotics, caution is still warranted before using these agents, and in most cases of ICD they will not be a first-line choice. They may be more strongly considered when there are micropsychotic episodes (in borderline personality disorder) or when there is comorbid schizotypal or paranoid personality disorder. They may also have a role in augmenting SSRIs in patients with particularly severe and refractory symptoms and those with Cluster B personality disorders. There is also a growing database of studies of antipsychotics in aggressive youth (Schur et al. 2003). In general, when prescribed for ICDs, relatively low dosages of antipsychotics are used in order to minimize adverse effects. Interestingly, in this population, there is also evidence that psychostimulants have an antiaggressive role independent of their effect on ADHD symptoms (Connor et al. 2002; Pine and Cohen 1999).

Benzodiazepines

Benzodiazepines are generally not recommended for the treatment of ICDs and likely should be restricted to the acute administration to treat acute agitation and aggression under emergency circumstances. In laboratory settings, benzodiazepines produce bitonic effects on aggressive behavior, with lower dosages causing increasing aggression. In the clinic, there is concern about possible behavioral disinhibition after benzodiazepine administration, about difficulties in ultimately withdrawing patients from medication, and about the fact that these agents are not useful for comorbid mood disorders. There is evidence that behavioral disinhibition with benzodiazepines is particularly likely in individuals with a history of impulsive disorders (Bond 1998).

Miscellaneous Agents

Opioid antagonists, in particular naltrexone, may decrease impulsive symptoms in alcohol dependence, bulimia nervosa, kleptomania, pathological gambling, and repetitive self-injury by inhibiting dopaminergic neurons in reward neurocircuitry. Nevertheless, few controlled and dose-ranging studies exist, so further work is needed to consolidate such findings (Kim et al. 2001; Srisurapanont and Jarusuraisin 2005). Recent work has suggested that particular dietary interventions may be useful in decreasing impulsive aggression (Gesch et al. 2002). There is growing evidence that dietary supplementation, for example with omega-3 and omega-6 fatty acids, can have behavioral effects, but in the context of the treatment of ICDs, this research remains preliminary. Hormonal interventions have been used in treatment of paraphilias and severe aggression, but here again there is no evidence base to suggest the value of extending such interventions to patients with ICDs. Further work is needed to provide a complete understanding of the mechanisms that might be relevant to the efficacy of a range of agents used in preliminary studies of ICD and to replicate and clarify this early work.

Psychotherapy

The development of a working alliance is a first crucial step in the treatment of patients with ICDs. Although this is relatively easy in some conditions (e.g., trichotillomania), in other ICDs (e.g., impulsive personality disorders) development of such an alliance can be a significant challenge. An initial period of negotiating therapist and patient responsibilities and determining the structure and limits of the relationship may be required. In many cases, it is necessary to ensure external structure, whether this occurs in the form of a period of hospitalization, by means of family and social supports, or by using 12-Step programs. In patients with antisocial personality traits, limit setting is particularly key. Impulsive symptoms are often subject to positive reinforcement, and limit setting can therefore also be understood in more cognitive-behavioral terms.

A second issue that can be briefly mentioned in this context is the importance of the countertransference. Treatment of patients with ICDs can bring a range of intense reactions to the fore. Clinicians may overidentify with the excitement or pleasure of the patient's impulses and underestimate their dangers. Alternatively, clinicians may find the patient's impulses scary and avoid the treatment. The psychodynamic principle of identifying and attempting to understand one's feelings during the encounter with the impulsive patient remains key. Cognitive-behavioral constructs, such as schemas, can also be used to conceptualize these phenomena. Appropriate structure, boundaries, and limit setting play a key role in allowing feelings in the transference and countertransference to be contained and prevent their being acting out.

Past traumas may play an important role in the psychodynamics of many patients with ICDs. The effects of early adverse environments can be conceptualized in terms of their effects on maladaptive schemas (Young 1994) or their long-term neurobiological sequelae (Heim and Nemeroff 2001). In psychotherapy, it is important to provide an environment where the patient is able to experience a more nurturing relationship and where the patient's negative transference or maladaptive schemas can be articulated and addressed. In some patients, high levels of negative affect are at the fore; in other patients, affect may need to be mobilized in order for maladaptive schemas to be identified and worked with. Current stressors may be particularly likely to precipitate impulsivity in patients with a history of early trauma, and stress management techniques are therefore also relevant.

Psychotherapeutic intervention may also play a key role during pharmacotherapy. The high placebo response of ICDs to pharmacotherapy and the high rates of relapse during medication maintenance suggest that factors such as the therapeutic relationship play a critical role in determining response to medication treatment. Patients who experience strong negative transference may also be particularly prone to experiencing adverse effects of medication. Psychotherapeutic work to prevent overidealization and demonization of pharmacotherapy can be a crucial component of work with ICD patients, and a close understanding of how symptoms respond to changes in the environment over time are needed in order to help determine the efficacy of an particular trial of medication.

Manualized psychotherapies for the treatment of ICDs are now available and provide a standardized method for tackling issues such as these. Dialectical behavioral therapy (DBT), for example, has been studied in different populations of impulsive patients and appears effective in both individual and group formats. As discussed in previous chapters, specific and systematic CBT approaches have also been developed for several individual ICDs such as pathological gambling and trichotillomania as well for impulsive symptoms such as anger, and there is growing evidence of the efficacy of such treatments, again in both individual and group formats (Tavares et al. 2003). Cognitive-behavioral programs for the treatment of impulsivity in children have also been developed (Kendall and Wilcox 1980).

Cognitive-behavioral psychotherapies for ICDs incorporate the general principles of CBT as well as additional techniques to address the specific symptoms of ICDs. CBT treatments are typically multimodal and may vary in the extent to which they focus on cognitive versus behavioral change techniques. Strategies relevant to particular ICDs include assertiveness training for intermittent explosive disorder, financial counseling for pathological gambling, and parent management training for aggressive youth. Although the research database demonstrating the efficacy of such interventions is growing, at this stage there is often insufficient information available to determine which are the most active ingredients of multimodal interventions. As in the case of pharmacotherapy, psychotherapy of impulsive disorders therefore relies on individualization of interventions for each particular patient.

Cognitive interventions include education, promoting awareness of cognitive errors, raising doubt about the validity of irrational cognitions, and cognitive restructuring. Both socratic questioning by the therapist and self-monitoring of cognitions by the patient (e.g., using the standard thought record) are used to uncover and to combat cognitive errors and irrational cognitions. More behavioral approaches emphasize the value of a functional analysis to determine triggers of impulsive behaviors and to assess their positive and negative consequences using behavioral techniques (including behavioral aversion, imaginal and in vivo desensitization, and relaxation training) to manage triggers, decrease the positive reinforcement associated with impulsive symptoms, and increase reinforcement from nonimpulsive activities.

In our view, given the relatively early stage of our understanding of precisely how psychotherapy effects changes in the ICDs and the relatively underdeveloped clinical trials database, maintaining a flexible and eclectic approach seems reasonable. It is also reasonable for even experienced clinicians to obtain professional supervision or guidance during the treatment of difficult cases of impulsive patients. Additional research is required on determining the efficacy of individual components of psychotherapy, on addressing abstinence versus control as treatment goals, on comparing individual versus group approaches, and on developing effective interventions for patients with comorbidity and for prevention of emergence of ICDs (e.g., school-based curriculums on aggression or gambling).

Conclusion

The management of patients with impulsive disorders is one of psychiatry's perennial challenges. Nevertheless, there has been progress in this field, and we are now able to offer our patients a broader array of rational and evidence-based interventions. There are reliable diagnostic criteria for the ICDs and standardized rating scales for their assessment. The development of cognitive-affective neuroscience models of impulsivity has provided a basis for the development of specific pharmacotherapeutic and psychotherapeutic interventions. This chapter reviewed some of the key principles of pharmacotherapy and psychotherapy of patients with ICDs, and previous chapters have provided detailed reviews of the efficacy of particular medications and psychotherapies in the management of specific ICDs. We can look forward to further progress in our models of impulsivity and aggression in the years to come and to concomitant progress in our therapeutic armamentarium. Ultimately, early assessment of dimensions such as behavioral disinhibition or school-based preventive programs may be successful in preventing later psychopathology (Hirshfeld-Becker et al. 2003).

References

Aleman A, Kahn RS: Effects of the atypical antipsychotic risperidone on hostility and aggression in schizophrenia: a meta-analysis of controlled trials. Eur Neuropsychopharmacol 11:289–293, 2001

American Psychiatric Association: Diagnostic and Statistical Manual of Mental Disorders, 3rd Edition. Washington, DC, American Psychiatric Association, 1980

Barratt ES, Stanford MS, Felthous AR, et al: The effects of phenytoin on impulsive and premeditated aggression: a controlled study. J Clin Psychopharmacol 17:341–349, 1997

Bernstein DP, Fink L, Handelsman L, et al: Initial reliability and validity of a new retrospective measure of child abuse and neglect. Am J Psychiatry 151:1132–1136, 1994

Bond AJ: Drug-induced behavioural disinhibition: incidence, mechanisms and therapeutic implications. CNS Drugs 9:41–57, 1998

Caspi A, Sugden K, Moffitt TE, et al: Influence of life stress on depression: moderation by a polymorphism in the 5-HTT gene. Science 301:291–293, 2003

Collett BR, Ohan JL, Myers KM: Ten-year review of rating scales, VI: scales assessing externalizing behaviors. J Am Acad Child Adolesc Psychiatry 42:1143–1170, 2003

Connor DF, Glatt SJ, Lopez ID, et al: Psychopharmacology and aggression, I: a meta-analysis of stimulant effects on overt/covert aggression-related behaviors in ADHD. J Am Acad Child Adolesc Psychiatry 41:253–261, 2002

Cueva JE, Overall JE, Small AM, et al: Carbamazepine in aggressive children with conduct disorder: a double-blind and placebo-controlled study. J Am Acad Child Adolesc Psychiatry 35:480–490, 1996

Donovan SJ, Stewart JW, Nunes EV, et al: Divalproex treatment for youth with explosive temper and mood lability: a double-blind, placebo-controlled crossover design. Am J Psychiatry 157:818–820, 2000

DosReis S, Barnett S, Love RC, et al: A guide for managing acute aggressive behavior of youths in residential and inpatient treatment facilities. Psychiatr Serv 54:1357–1363, 2003

du Toit PL, van Kradenburg J, Niehaus DJH, et al: Comparison of obsessive-compulsive disorder patients with and without comorbid putative obsessive-compulsive spectrum disorders using a structured clinical interview. Compr Psychiatry 42:291–300, 2001

Evenden JL: Varieties of impulsivity. Psychopharmacol 146:348–361, 1999

Gerald MS, Higley JD: Evolutionary underpinnings of excessive alcohol consumption. Addiction 97:415–425, 2002

Gesch CB, Hammond SM, Hampson SE, et al: Influence of supplementary vitamins, minerals and essential fatty acids on the antisocial behaviour of young adult prisoners: randomised, placebo-controlled trial. Br J Psychiatry 181:22–28, 2002

Haspel T: Beta-blockers and the treatment of aggression. Harv Rev Psychiatry 2:274–281, 1995

Heim C, Nemeroff CB: The role of childhood trauma in the neurobiology of mood and anxiety disorders: preclinical and clinical studies. Biol Psychiatry 49:1023–1029, 2001

Hirshfeld-Becker DR, Biederman J, Calltharp S, et al: Behavioral inhibition and disinhibition as hypothesized precursors to psychopathology: implications for pediatric bipolar disorder. Biol Psychiatry 53:985–999, 2003

Hollander E, Pallanti S, Baldini-Rossi N, et al: Sustained release lithium/placebo treatment response in bipolar spectrum pathological gamblers. Poster presented at the 42nd Annual New Clinical Drug Evaluation Unit Meeting, Boca Raton, FL, June 2002

Hollander E, Tracy KA, Swann AC, et al: Divalproex in the treatment of impulsive aggression: efficacy in Cluster B personality disorders. Neuropsychopharmacology 28:1186–1197, 2003

Johnson BA, Ait-Daoud N, Bowden CL, et al: Oral topiramate for treatment of alcohol dependence: a randomised controlled trial. Lancet 361:1677–1685, 2003

Kendall PC, Wilcox LE: Cognitive-behavioral treatment for impulsivity: concrete versus conceptual training in non-self-controlled problem children. J Consult Clin Psychol 48:80–91, 1980

Kim SW, Grant JE, Adson DE, et al: Double-blind naltrexone and placebo comparison study in the treatment of pathological gambling. Biol Psychiatry 49:914–921, 2001

Lavine R: Psychopharmacological treatment of aggression and violence in the substance abusing population. J Psychoactive Drugs 29:321–329, 1997

Laviola G, Macri S, Morley-Fletcher S, et al: Risk-taking behavior in adolescent mice: psychobiological determinants and early epigenetic influence. Neurosci Biobehav Rev 27:19–31, 2003

Lindenmeyer JP, Kotsaftis A: Use of sodium valproate in violent and aggressive behaviors: a critical review. J Clin Psychiatry 61:123–128, 2000

Malone RP, Delaney MA, Luebbert JF, et al: A double-blind placebo-controlled study of lithium in hospitalized aggressive children and adolescents with conduct disorder. Arch Gen Psychiatry 57:649–654, 2000

McElroy SL, Arnold LM, Shapira NA, et al: Topiramate in the treatment of binge eating disorder associated with obesity: a randomized, placebo-controlled trial. Am J Psychiatry 160:255–261, 2003

Miczek KA, Fish EW, de Bold JF, et al: Social and neural determinants of aggressive behavior: pharmacotherapeutic targets at serotonin, dopamine and g-aminobutyric acid systems. Psychopharmacology 163:434–458, 2002

Pine DS, Cohen E: Therapeutics of aggression in children. Paediatr Drugs 1:183–196, 1999

Schur SB, Sikich L, Findling RL, et al: Treatment recommendations for the use of antipsychotics for aggressive youth (TRAAY), part I: a review. J Am Acad Child Adolesc Psychiatry 42:132–144, 2003

Scott JP: Aggression. Chicago, IL, Chicago University Press, 1958

Sheard MH, Marini JL, Bridges CI, et al: The effect of lithium on impulsive aggressive behavior in man. Am J Psychiatry 133:1409–1413, 2003

Sheehan DV, Lecrubier Y, Sheehan KH, et al: The Mini-International Neuropsychiatric Interview (MINI): the development and validation of a structured diagnostic psychiatric interview for DSM-IV and ICD-10. J Clin Psychiatry 59:22–33, 1998

Soloff PH, George A, Nathan RS, et al: Behavioral dyscontrol in borderline patients treated with amitriptyline. Psychopharmacol Bull 23:177–181, 1987

Srisurapanont M, Jarusuraisin N: Opioid antagonists for alcohol dependence. Cochrane Database Syst Rev. CD001867, 2005

Stanford MS, Houston RJ, Mathias CW, et al: A double-blind placebo-controlled crossover study of phenytoin in individuals with impulsive aggression. Psychiatry Res 103:193–203, 2001

Swann AC: Neuroreceptor mechanisms of aggression and its treatment. J Clin Psychiatry 64:26–35, 2003

Tavares H, Zilberman ML, el-Guebaly N: Are there cognitive and behavioral approaches specific to the treatment of pathological gambling? Can J Psychiatry 48:22–27, 2003

Walsh MT, Dinan TG: Selective serotonin reuptake inhibitors and violence: a review of the available evidence. Acta Psychiatr Scand 104:84–91, 2001

Young EJ: Cognitive Therapy for Personality Disorders: A Schema-Focused Approach. Sarasota, FL, Professional Resources Press, 1994

Index

*Page numbers printed in **boldface** type refer to tables or figures.*